STOP, THAT and One Hundred Other Sleep Scales

Azmeh Shahid • Kate Wilkinson
Shai Marcu • Colin M. Shapiro
(Editors)

STOP, THAT and One Hundred Other Sleep Scales

Springer

Editors
Azmeh Shahid, M.D
University of Toronto
The Youthdale Child and Adolescent
Sleep Centre
227 Victoria Street
M5B 1T8 Toronto, Canada
azmehs@hotmail.com

Kate Wilkinson, Ph.D
University of Toronto
The Youthdale Child and Adolescent
Sleep Centre
227 Victoria Street
M5B 1T8 Toronto, Canada

Shai Marcu, M.D
University of Toronto
The Youthdale Child and Adolescent
Sleep Centre
227 Victoria Street
Toronto, Canada

Colin M. Shapiro, MBChB., Ph.D.,
MRCPsych, FRCP(C)
Department of Psychiatry
University of Toronto
The Youthdale Child and Adolescent
Sleep Centre
227 Victoria Street
M5B 1T8 Toronto, Canada

ISBN 978-1-4419-9892-7 e-ISBN 978-1-4419-9893-4
DOI 10.1007/978-1-4419-9893-4
Springer New York Dordrecht Heidelberg London

Library of Congress Control Number: 2011944754

Printed on acid-free paper

Springer is part of Springer Science+Business Media (www.springer.com)

We dedicate this book to our immediate and extended families and to Ian Oswald, a pioneer in sleep research.

Introduction

There are at least four reasons why a sleep clinician should be familiar with rating scales that evaluate different facets of sleep.

Firstly, the use of scales facilitates a quick and accurate assessment of a complex clinical problem. In 3 or 4 minutes (the time to review ten standard scales), a clinician can come to a broad understanding of the patient in question. For example, a selection of scales might indicate that an individual is sleepy but not fatigued; lacking alertness with no insomnia; presenting with no symptoms of narcolepsy or restless legs but showing clear features of apnea; exhibiting depression and a history of significant alcohol problems. This information can be used to direct the consultation to those issues perceived as most relevant, and can even provide a springboard for explaining the benefits of certain treatment approaches or the potential corollaries of allowing the status quo to continue.

Secondly, rating scales can provide a clinician with an enhanced vocabulary or language, improving his or her understanding of each patient. For example, a medical student or resident in psychiatry may erroneously think that she has performed a comprehensive assessment of Obsessive Compulsive Disorder (OCD) by asking whether the patient repeatedly checks that the door is locked or the stove is switched off. By reading a scale on OCD, the student may develop a deeper appreciation of the condition and its sequelae in a way that is distinctly different – and perhaps more practical – than simply reading a chapter in a textbook. In the case of the sleep specialist, a scale can help him or her to distinguish fatigue from sleepiness in a patient, or elucidate the differences between sleepiness and alertness (the latter is not merely the inverse of the former). Sleep scales are developed by researchers and clinicians who have spent years in their field, carefully honing their preferred methods for assessing certain brain states or characteristic features of a condition. Thus, scales provide clinicians with a repertoire of questions, allowing them to draw upon the extensive experience of their colleagues when attempting to tease apart nuanced problems.

Thirdly, some scales are helpful for tracking a patient's progress. A particular patient may not remember how alert he felt on a series of different stimulant medications. Scale assessments administered periodically over the course of treatment provide an objective record of the intervention, allowing the clinician to examine and possibly reassess her or his approach to the patient. Furthermore, evaluation with the same rating scale on a longitudinal basis may facilitate compliance with treatment, particularly if it provides objective evidence that the treatment has made positive change in a patient's problem or illness. For this reason, an assessment at the "baseline period" (prior to the first contact with the sleep specialist) is highly desirable.

Finally, for individuals conducting a double-blind crossover trial scales are imperative. However even those doing a straightforward clinical practice audit, and who are interested in research will find that their own clinics become a source of great discovery. Scales provide standardized measures that allow colleagues across cities and countries to coordinate their practices. They enable the replication of previous studies and facilitate the organization and dissemination of new research in a way that is accessible and rapid. As the emphasis placed on evidence-based care grows, a clinician's ability to assess his or her own practice and its relation to the wider medical community becomes invaluable. Scales make this kind of standardization possible, just as they enable the research efforts that help to formulate those standards.

Though the potential for these instruments is great, the key to unlocking that potential lies in the selection of the appropriate scales. A clinician will want to cover those issues that are most applicable to his or her practice, while also querying additional problems or symptoms that could be relevant to a patient's care. For example, a sleep specialist is likely to focus her attention on scales designed to assess both specific sleep disorders and sleep problems in general. However, if a patient is well treated for sleep apnea but has many complaints about low energy and sleepiness, it may be very useful to know that the person scores 25 on the Center for Epidemiological Studies of Depression Scale (where a score of above 16 is suggestive of depression). Information garnered through objective questionnaires can help clinicians to recognize manifestations of problems and disorders that fall outside of their specific disciplines. In the case of the patient with apnea, the identification and treatment of depression could mean the difference between CPAP noncompliance and successful sleep therapy.

While the impulse may be to administer as many scales as possible in the hope that at least one will prove illuminating, the patient's tolerance vis-a-vis lengthy questionnaires must also be considered. When selecting a group of scales for routine use, balance is necessary: the physician requires enough information to make the endeavor useful, but it is vital that he does not overload the patient with too much "homework." In general, we have found that most patients appreciate being asked to complete scales. They view the process as an indicator of the physician's thoroughness (which it is), and are willing to endure more than most clinicians are likely to request. Our anecdotal observation is that only two groups of patients tend to have difficulty with the task: those who are not fluent in the language in which the questionnaires are written and medical professionals who tend to view themselves as exempt from the process. In general, however, it is not difficult to convince patients to participate in their care, and most will not refuse to complete a few well-chosen questionnaires.

Thus, all that remains is to choose the questionnaires that are most pertinent for your clinic or research project. With such a wide range of scales available, a clinician may find the selection process daunting. What are the most important issues to query? How many scales should be used? Ultimately, the clinician's particular practice and focus will dictate the kind of measures that are needed. A researcher in the field of insomnia, for example, will have different needs than a clinician interested in improving quality of life in patients with sleep apnea, and these two individuals will select scales accordingly. At the end of this book we have included several scales along with a simple scoring guide to help those who are new to such instruments. These materials can be either distributed to patients in the form of a booklet or used to guide the assembly of a similar instrument tailored to one's specific clinical needs. Similarly, the scoring guide can be employed by medical students, residents, fellows, sleep technologists, or other members of the medical team, allowing physicians themselves to focus on the clinical interview.

Clinicians may find the task of selecting questionnaires for use in pediatric populations particularly complex. These scales are often designed for very specific age ranges. While this ensures that appropriate issues and developmental milestones are taken into account, it makes it more difficult to create a consolidated set of scales for routine use in pediatric clinics. Similarly, deciding who to solicit responses from when assessing children is important. For younger patients, questions are usually answered by a parent or guardian and they tend to refer to behaviors rather than emotional states. In the case of adolescent clients, the clinician may desire a response from both the patient and the guardian, requiring multiple separate measures.

For adults, a broad set of standard questionnaires may include the following:

General

The Epworth Sleepiness Scale (ESS), a widely used measure of sleepiness
The Fatigue Severity Scale (FSS), a widely used measure of fatigue
The Toronto Hospital Alertness scale (THAT), an easy-to-use measure of alertness
Owl Lark Self-Test, which helps assess body clock rhythm

Specific

Athens Insomnia Scale, to quickly assess features of insomnia
STOP Bang, easy-to-use inquiry regarding sleep apnea
The Restless legs questionnaire is for trying to detect Restless Legs syndrome and the PLMS

Related Subjects

CAGE, a quick screening measure for alcohol dependence
CES-D, screen for mood-related problems which are common in patients with sleep disorders
Zung Anxiety scale
Illness intrusiveness scale

This set of 11 scales (see Appendix) is short, and would take someone with a little experience only three minutes to assess. While no substitute for a clinical interview, these scales provide a vast amount of information and take only a modest amount of time to complete and review. Provided that they have been scored, a physician familiar with these scales would require less than a minute to glean a reasonably comprehensive sketch of an individual patient. For convenience, the set could be mailed out and completed at home prior to a clinical appointment, or a patient could be asked to complete these scales while waiting in the doctor's office.

The large part of this book is devoted to briefly discussing individual scales. When possible (for copyright reasons), an example of the scale is provided so that readers may gain a sense of the instrument's content. The individual using the scales needs to ensure that they have appropriate copyright permission where necessary.

As we acquire new scales (and add omissions from the list we have created in this book and which should have been included), we will add information about these scales on a section of our website (www.sleepontario.com). We hope that these scales may appear in a future edition of the book. We will also endeavour to keep this as a repository of translations of scales and we would welcome submissions of translations and recommendations of scales to be added to suzanne.alves@uhn.ca. The scale STOP-Bang has eleven translations in this book (see Chap. 92).

Note on the Text

We would like to thank all the authors and publishers who allowed us to reprint their scales and questionnaires. We acknowledge that the copyrights belong to their respective owners and the scales are reprinted with their permission.

If a reader would like to obtain a copy of any of the scales, he or she must contact the copyright owner. Reproduction, duplication, or modification of any of these scales is strictly prohibited without the copyright owner's consent.

Contents

Contributors

Shai Marcu, M.D The Youthdale Child and Adolescent Sleep Centre, University of Toronto, Toronto, Canada

Azmeh Shahid, M.D The Youthdale Child and Adolescent Sleep Centre, University of Toronto, Toronto, Canada

Colin M. Shapiro, MBChB., Ph.D., MRCPsych, FRCP(C) The Youthdale Child and Adolescent Sleep Centre, University of Toronto, Toronto, Canada

Kate Wilkinson, Ph.D., M.Sc The Youthdale Child and Adolescent Sleep Centre, University of Toronto, Toronto, Canada

1 Adolescent Sleep Habits Survey

Purpose A structured survey featuring both open-ended and multiple-choice questions. Intended as a clinical tool, the instrument allows for the collection of demographic details, familial and medical histories, and information regarding sleep habits, schedules, and behaviors [1]. Three versions of the survey have been created: two designed for self-report (differing only in their mention of either male- or female-related developmental milestones), and one for the adolescent's parent or guardian to complete.

Population for Testing Age range is less of an issue for this survey since it is not intended to be a standardized measure – any youth considered an "adolescent" may be surveyed, though the questionnaire itself specifically refers to grades 4 through 12.

Administration All three versions are pencil-and-paper instruments, consisting of between 61 and 65 questions – each version should require between 20 and 30 min for completion. When choosing whether to administer the self-report or parent version, consider the different foci of the two tests: Parents/guardians may be able to provide more detailed developmental histories and important third-party observations of behaviors (e.g., snoring), while self-reports allow the patients themselves to clarify personal sleep preferences and habits.

Reliability and Validity Designed simply as a tool for collecting qualitative information, the psychometric properties of the scale have not been analyzed.

Obtaining a Copy All three versions can be found at http://www.kidzzzsleep.org

Reprint requests should be directed to:
Dr. Judith Owens
Rhode Island Hospital, Division of Pediatric Ambulatory Medicine
593 Eddy Street, Potter Building, Suite 200
Providence, RI 02903, USA
Telephone: (401) 444-8280
Email: owensleep@aol.com

Scoring The survey was developed predominantly as an instrument for screening, and is not often used in research as its open-ended format precludes attempts at standardization. Since interpretation of the survey's answers requires at least some training in sleep medicine, the questionnaire is largely used by sleep specialists to gain an overall understanding of the familial, medical, and behavioral history of patients presenting at specialized clinics.

A. Shahid et al. (eds.), *STOP, THAT and One Hundred Other Sleep Scales*,
DOI 10.1007/978-1-4419-9893-4_1, © Springer Science+Business Media, LLC 2012

TODAY'S DATE: ____/____/____

PARENT QUESTIONNAIRE

SCHOOL-AGED CHILDREN (4-12 years old)

PEDIATRIC SLEEP CLINIC QUESTIONNAIRE (4-12 YEAR OLDS)

1. Name of Patient: ______________________ 2. Date of Birth:___/___/___
3. Name of person completing questionnaire ______________________
   Relationship to child ______________________
   Referred by ______________________
   Pediatrician ______________________
4. A copy of the sleep clinic evaluation will be sent to you, your pediatrician, and any referring physician. Please indicate anyone else who should receive a copy:

Name: ______________________ Address: ______________________

____

5. What are your major concerns about your child's sleep? ______________________

____

____

6. What do you think is causing your child's sleep problem? ______________________

____

7. When did your child's sleep problems start? ______________________

____

FAMILY INFORMATION

8. Please list all members of the households in which your child lives full or part-time:

Name/Relationship to Child	Age	Child lives with (please indicate full-time or part-time)

9. Mother's Marital Status: Married Divorced Separated Widowed Single
   If divorced, child custody with: ______________________
10. Mother's education: ______________________
11. Mother's occupation: ______________________
    Does mother work outside of home? ☐ yes ☐ no
    If yes, mark each label that best describes her work:

☐ day shift	☐ full time
☐ evening shift	☐ part time
☐ night shift (graveyard)	☐ one job
☐ changing shifts	☐ more than one job

12. Fathers's Marital Status: Married Divorced Separated Widowed Single
If divorced, child custody with: ________________________
13. What is father's education: ____________________________
14. Father's occupation: ______________________________
Does father work outside of home? ☐ Yes ☐ No

If yes, mark each label that best describes his work:

☐ day shift	☐ full time
☐ evening shift	☐ part time
☐ night shift (graveyard)	☐ one job
☐ changing shifts	☐ more than one job

15. What best describes your child's racial/ethnic background?

White/Caucasian_____________	Asian/Asian American _____________
Black/African American __________	Native American ___________________
Hispanic/Latino _________________	Multiracial (Please specify)___________

Other (Please specify)____

16. Please list family members (parents, grandparents, siblings, aunts/uncles) with a history of any SLEEP PROBLEMS (including: loud snoring/obstructive sleep apnea, excessive sleepiness/ narcolepsy, restless legs/periodic leg movements, insomnia, other sleep problems).

Family Member	Type of Sleep Problem
____________________	____________________
____________________	____________________
____________________	____________________
____________________	____________________

17. Has anyone in your family ever had a car accident caused by sleepiness (not due to alcohol or drugs)? Yes ☐ No ☐ Don't know ☐
If yes, whom: ______________________________ At what age: ________________________
Type of accident: ____
18. Please list any family members with a significant mental health condition (such as depression, anxiety, alcoholism/substance abuse).

Family Member	Type of Mental Health Problem
____________________	____________________
____________________	____________________
____________________	____________________

SLEEP HISTORY (GENERAL)

19. What time does your child usually go to bed on school nights? __________

Range: _____ am/pm to _____am/pm

20. What is the main reason your child goes to bed at a particular time? (Check one below)

_____ a. Because it fits best with the family's schedule
_____ b. Because she/he feels sleepy then
_____ c. Because that is when her/his TV shows are over
_____ d. Because that is when her/his brothers and sisters go to bed
_____ e. To "get enough sleep" for the following day's activities
_____ f. Other (describe briefly)____

21. What time does your child usually wake up on school day mornings? ___________

Range: _____ am/pm to _____am/pm

22. What usually wakes up your child in the morning on school days? (Check one below)

_____ a. Alarm clock
_____ b. Parent or other family member
_____ c. Noise
_____ d. Needs to go to the bathroom
_____ e. Spontaneous
_____ f. Other (describe briefly):

23. Which of the following applies to waking your child in the morning on school days? (Check one below)

_____ a. I almost always have great difficulty getting him/her out of bed
_____ b. I sometimes have great difficulty getting him/her our of bed
_____ c. I seldom have great difficulty getting him/her out of bed
_____ d. I never have great difficulty getting him/her out of bed

24. What times does your child usually go to bed on weekend nights? ____________

Range: _____ am/pm to_____am/pm

25. What time does your child usually wake up on weekend mornings? __________

Range: _____ am/pm to _____am/pm

26. What usually wakes up your child in the morning on weekends? (Check one below)

_____ a. Alarm clock
_____ b. Parent or other family member
_____ c. Noise
_____ d. Needs to go to the bathroom
_____ e. Spontaneous
_____ f. Other (describe briefly):

27. Which of the following applies to waking your child in the morning on weekends? (Check one below)

_____ a. I almost always have great difficulty getting him/her out of bed
_____ b. I sometimes have great difficulty getting him/her our of bed
_____ c. I seldom have great difficulty getting him/her out of bed
_____ d. I never have great difficulty getting him/her out of bed

28. IN AN AVERAGE TWO-WEEK PERIOD, HOW OFTEN DOES YOUR CHILD ...
(Check one answer for each question; please feel free to comment)

	Every day/ night	**5-6 times**	**3-4 times**	**1-2 times**	**Never**	**Comments:**
snore?	☐	☐	☐	☐	☐	______
snore loudly and disruptively?	☐	☐	☐	☐	☐	______
sleep restlessly?	☐	☐	☐	☐	☐	______
sleep in an abnormal position?	☐	☐	☐	☐	☐	______
sweat while sleeping?	☐	☐	☐	☐	☐	______
pause in breathing	☐	☐	☐	☐	☐	______
complain of headache on waking?	☐	☐	☐	☐	☐	______
have nightmares?	☐	☐	☐	☐	☐	______
sleepwalk?	☐	☐	☐	☐	☐	______
sleeptalk?	☐	☐	☐	☐	☐	______
cry out during sleep?	☐	☐	☐	☐	☐	______
wake up at night?	☐	☐	☐	☐	☐	______
get out of bed at night?	☐	☐	☐	☐	☐	______
complain about his/her sleep?	☐	☐	☐	☐	☐	______
complain of pain at night?	☐	☐	☐	☐	☐	______
wet the bed?	☐	☐	☐	☐	☐	______

29. Has your child ever used medication (over-the-counter or prescription) including herbal or "natural" remedies to help with sleep?
Yes ☐ No ☐ Don't know ☐

If yes, name of medication and how frequently used: ______________________________

Does your child currently (within the past month) use medications (over-the-counter or prescription) to help with sleep? Yes ☐ No ☐ Don't know ☐

If yes, name of medication and how frequently used: ______________________________

SLEEP HISTORY - DAYTIME SLEEPINESS

30. During the LAST TWO WEEKS, has your child struggled to stay awake (fought sleep) or fallen asleep in the following situations? (Mark one answer for every item)

	No	Struggled to stay awake (fought sleep)	Fallen asleep	Don't Know	Does not Apply
a. in a face-to-face conversation with another person?	☐	☐	☐	☐	☐
b. traveling in a car, bus?	☐	☐	☐	☐	☐
c. at the movies?	☐	☐	☐	☐	☐
d. watching television?	☐	☐	☐	☐	☐
e. listening to the radio or stereo?	☐	☐	☐	☐	☐
f. reading, studying or doing homework?	☐	☐	☐	☐	☐
g. in a class at school?	☐	☐	☐	☐	☐
h. while doing work on a computer?	☐	☐	☐	☐	☐
i. playing video games?	☐	☐	☐	☐	☐
j. eating a meal?	☐	☐	☐	☐	☐

MEDICAL HISTORY:

31. Were there any problems with this pregnancy or delivery (prematurity, high blood pressure, etc.)? ____

____

32. What was the birth weight? __________

33. Was your child ever on an apnea monitor at home? Yes ☐ No ☐

If yes, for how long? ________

34. Does your child have any significant health problems? Yes ☐ No ☐

If so, please describe: ____

____

35. Has your child ever been hospitalized? Yes ☐ No ☐

If yes, when: ______________________ What for? ______________________

______________________ ______________________

______________________ ______________________

36. Has your child ever had any operations (other than tonsils/adenoids removal)?

Yes ☐ No ☐

If yes, type of operation? ______________________ Year __________

______________________ Year __________

______________________ Year __________

37. Have your child's tonsils or adenoids been removed?

a. Tonsils: Yes ☐ At what age?_______

For what reason: ______________________________

b. Adenoids: Yes ☐ At what age?_______

For what reason: ______________________________

c. Describe briefly any changes you noticed in your child's sleep or waking behavior after removal of tonsils or adenoids:

____

38. If NO, do you think the tonsils or adenoids are a problem? Yes ☐ No ☐ Don't know ☐
For how long have they been a problem? ______ years

39. Has your child ever broken his/her nose or other facial bones? Yes ☐ No ☐

40. Does your child have difficulty breathing through his/her nose? Yes ☐ No ☐

41. In the past year, has your child had strep throats/tonsillitis? Yes ☐ No ☐

Frequent colds/respiratory infections? Yes ☐ No ☐

Frequent sinus infections? Yes ☐ No ☐

42. Does your child have allergies? Yes ☐ No ☐ Possibly ☐

If yes, to what?______________________________

43. Does your child have asthma? Yes ☐ No ☐ If "Yes", please answer the following questions:

In the **past year**....
a. How many days has your child missed school due to asthma? _______ None ☐
b. How many days has your child been hospitalized for asthma? _______ None ☐
c. List any medications your child takes for asthma:

Type: ____________________ Frequency: ____________________
Type: ____________________ Frequency: ____________________
Type: ____________________ Frequency: ____________________

44. Does your child frequently complain of heartburn? Yes ☐ No ☐ Don't know ☐

Has he/she ever been diagnosed with gastroesophageal (stomach) reflux?

Yes ☐ No ☐ Only when younger ☐

45. Has your child had any head injuries requiring medical evaluation and/or treatment or loss of consciousness? If yes, please describe:______________________________

46. List any prescription or over-the counter medications your child has taken in the last month:

Type: ____________________ Reason for medication: ____________________

Type: ____________________ Reason for medication: ____________________

Type: ____________________ Reason for medication: ____________________

47. Do you have additional comments about your child's medical history? (Continue on additional sheets if necessary.)

____

____

____

HEALTH HABITS - Please answer the following questions regarding health habits which may impact on sleep. In the past 2 weeks, on average:

48. How much caffeinated soda did your child drink?

- ☐ More than 3 glasses per day
- ☐ Between 1 and 3 glasses per day
- ☐ Less than one glass per day
- ☐ None
- ☐ Don't know

49. How much television and/or videos did your child watch on school days?

☐ 0-2 hours per day	☐ between 2 and 4 hours	☐ between 4 and 6 hours
☐ between 6 and 8 hours	☐ more than 8 hours	☐ don't know

a. How much time does your child spend on the computer on school days?

☐ 0-2 hours per day	☐ between 2 and 4 hours	☐ between 4 and 6 hours
☐ between 6 and 8 hours	☐ more than 8 hours	☐ don't know

How much television and/or videos did your child watch on weekend days?

☐ 0-2 hours per day	☐ between 2 and 4 hours	☐ between 4 and 6 hours
☐ between 6 and 8 hours	☐ more than 8 hours	☐ don't know

a. How much time does your child spend on the computer on weekend days?

☐ 0-2 hours per day	☐ between 2 and 4 hours	☐ between 4 and 6 hours
☐ between 6 and 8 hours	☐ more than 8 hours	☐ don't know

50. Did your child watch TV and/or videos in the 30 minutes before falling asleep?

- ☐ every night
- ☐ 5-6 nights
- ☐ 3-4 nights
- ☐ 1-2 nights
- ☐ not at all

51. Does your child have a television set in his/her bedroom? Yes ☐ No ☐

DEVELOPMENT HISTORY- PART A

52. In what grade is your child currently enrolled? __________ grade

53. What school does your child attend this year?________________________________

54. Has your child been diagnosed with:

	YES	NO	COMMENTS
a. dyslexia	☐	☐	______________
b. a speech impairment	☐	☐	______________
c. mental retardation	☐	☐	______________
d. a behavior disorder	☐	☐	______________
e. attention deficit disorder	☐	☐	______________
f. other learning disorder (please specify)________________	☐	☐	______________

55. Is your child enrolled in any special education (special needs) classes in school?

☐ Yes ☐ No Please describe:

____

56. Does your child have an Individualized Education Plan (I.E.P.) provided by the school?

☐ Yes ☐No If yes, for what reason:

____

57. Generally, how often does your child attend school?
   a. ☐ Every day
   b. ☐ 3-4 days per week
   c. ☐ 1-2 days per week
   d. ☐ Less than once per week

58. Generally, how often is your child late to school?
   a. ☐ Every day
   b. ☐ 3-4 days per week
   c. ☐ 1-2 days per week
   d. ☐ Less than once per week

DEVELOPMENTAL HISTORY- PART B

59. Does your child have any significant behavioral or mental health problems? Yes ☐
No ☐
If yes, please describe ____

____

60. Has your child ever received counseling for behavioral or mental health problems?
Yes ☐ No ☐ If so, for what reason?

____

Please give approximate dates:

____

61. Have <u>you</u> or <u>your spouse</u> ever been seen by a mental health counselor for concerns regarding your child? Yes ☐ No ☐
If yes, for what reason? ____

62. To what organized groups does your child currently belong? (e.g., team sports, scouts, church, groups, etc.) ____

____

SLEEP BELIEFS

In order to better understand your sense of the average child's sleep, please answer the following questions based on your beliefs for an <u>average</u> child (your child's age) who does <u>not</u> have sleep problems?

a. How many hours of sleep per night does the average child need? ______ hours
b. How many hours of sleep per night does the average child get? _______ hours
c. How long does it take the average child to get to sleep? _______ minutes
d. How many times does the average child wake up during the night? ______ times
e. How long does the average child spend awake in bed during the night?
______ minutes or _____ hours
f. Do you think most children get enough sleep? Yes ☐ No ☐ Don't Know ☐

THANK YOU VERY MUCH FOR YOUR TIME!

ADOLESCENT SLEEP HABITS SURVEY
(BOY'S SELF REPORT)

Instructions: This form should be filled out by the adolescent patient himself if at all possible.
Today's Date: _____/_____/_____

1. Name:____ 2. Date of Birth: ____/____/____
3. Please describe your sleep problem(s): ______________________________________
____
____

4. How long have you had difficulty with sleep? (check one)
☐ less than a month ☐ 1-6 months
☐ 6-12 months ☐ 1-5 years
☐ more than 5 years

5. Have your problems with sleep gotten worse? ☐ Yes ☐ No ☐Not sure
If yes, when did you notice that your sleep problems got worse: ____________________

6. What do you think is causing your sleep problem? (check all that apply)
☐ stress at school ☐ relationship problems with parents/family
☐ relationship problems with peers ☐ poor sleep habits
☐ poor eating habits ☐ a physical problem
Other (describe briefly)______________________________________

SLEEP HABITS: This set of questions asks about your usual sleep habits. Please answer as honestly as possible.

7. With whom do you share a bedroom? (check all that apply)

	Yes	No
Mother/step-mother	☐	☐
Father/step-father	☐	☐
Older brother(s)/sister(s)	☐	☐
Younger brother(s)/sister(s)	☐	☐
Other family member(s)..................................	☐	☐

8. In the last two weeks, have you slept in the same bed?
☐ every night ☐ almost every night
☐ a few nights ☐ not at all

The next set of questions has to do with your usual schedule on days when you have school. Please list both the USUAL times or number of hours/minutes, and the RANGE (earliest to latest, lowest to highest). Please check AM or PM for each time.

9. What time do you **usually** go to bed on school days? __________
Range: ______ ☐ AM/ ☐ PM to _______ ☐ AM/ ☐ PM

SLEEP HABITS (continued)

10. There are many reasons for doing things at one time or another. What is the **main reason** you usually go to bed at this time on school days? (check one)

☐ My parents have set my bedtime
☐ I finish my homework
☐ My brother(s) or sister(s) go to bed
☐ I get home from my job
☐ I feel sleepy
☐ My TV shows are over
☐ I finish socializing
☐ Other: ______________________________

11. What time do you **usually** wake up on school days? __________
Range: _____ ☐AM/ ☐PM to ______ ☐AM/ ☐ PM

12. There are many reasons for doing things at one time or another. What is the **main reason** you usually wake up at this time on school days? (check one)

☐ Noises or my pet wakes me up
☐ My parents wake me up
☐ I don't know, I just wake up
☐ My alarm clock wakes me up
☐ I need to go to the bathroom
☐ Other: ______________________________

13. What time do you **usually** leave home on school days? __________
Range: _____ ☐AM/ ☐ PM to ______ ☐AM/ ☐ PM

14. How do you usually get to school? (check one)
☐ Walk
☐ Take the bus
☐ Get a ride with parent
☐ Get a ride with friend(s)
☐ Drive my car

What time do you need to arrive at school? __________

15. Figure out how long you **usually** sleep on a normal school night and fill it in here. (Do not include time you spend awake in bed. Remember to mark hours and minutes, even if minutes are zero.)
Usual amount of sleep: _____ hours and______ minutes
Range: _____ hours and______ minutes to _____ hours and______ minutes

16. On school days, after you go to bed at night, about how long does it usually take you to fall asleep? (If longer than one hour, change to minutes.)
Usual amount: ______ minutes
Range: _____ minutes to ______ minutes

The next set of questions has to do with your usual schedule on days when you DO NOT have school, such as the weekend.

17. What time do you **usually** go to bed on weekends? __________
Range: _____ ☐AM/ ☐PM to ______ ☐AM/ ☐ PM

18. There are many reasons for doing things at one time or another. What is the **main reason** you usually go to bed at this time on **weekends**? (check one)
☐My parents have set my bedtime
☐ I finish my homework
☐ My brother(s) or sister(s) go to bed
☐ I get home from my job
☐ I feel sleepy
☐ My TV shows are over
☐ I finish socializing
☐ Other: ______________________________

Adolescent Sleep Habits-Boys **2 of 12** **Rev. 8/25/05**

SLEEP HABITS (continued)

19. What time do you **usually** wake up on weekends? _______ ☐AM/ ☐PM
Range: ______ ☐ AM/ ☐PM to _______ ☐AM/ ☐ PM

20. What is the **main reason** you usually wake up at this time on weekends? (check one)
☐ Noises or my pet wakes me up
☐ My parents wake me up
☐ I don't know, I just wake up
☐ My alarm clock wakes me up
☐ I need to go to the bathroom
☐ Other: ______________________________

21. Figure out how long you **usually** sleep on a night when you do not have school the next day (such as a weekend night) and fill it in here. (Do not include time you spend awake in bed. Remember to mark hours and minutes, even if minutes are zero.)
Usual amount of sleep: ______ hours and_______ minutes
Range: ______ hours and_______ minutes to ______ hours and_______ minutes

22. On weekends, after you go to bed at night, about how long does it usually take you to fall asleep? (If longer than one hour, change to minutes.)
Range: ______ minutes to _______ minutes

23. Can you figure out how much sleep you need? Fill out how much sleep you think you would need each night to feel your best every day. (Do not include time you spend awake in bed. Remember to mark hours and minutes, even if minutes are zero.)
______ hours _______ minutes

The following questions ask about other sleep habits you may have. Please answer as honestly as possible.

24. In the last two weeks, how often have you done any of the following activities in bed?

	Every day/night	Several times	Twice	Once	Never
Read?	☐	☐	☐	☐	☐
Watch TV?	☐	☐	☐	☐	☐
Eat?...	☐	☐	☐	☐	☐
Do schoolwork?	☐	☐	☐	☐	☐
Worry?	☐	☐	☐	☐	☐

25. When you have difficulty falling asleep or getting back to sleep, what do you do? (check all that apply)
☐ Stay in bed and try to get to sleep
☐ Do something in bed (e.g., read or watch TV)
☐ Get up and watch TV
☐ Get up and drink alcohol
☐ Get up and drink warm milk
☐ Get up and drink something? (circle all that apply: soda/water/coffee/tea)
☐ Get up and have a cigarette
Other (please specify): ____

SLEEP HABITS (continued)

26. Please circle a number from 1-10 to indicate how much difficulty you have relaxing away tension in your body while trying to sleep.

0	1	2	3	4	5	6	7	8	9	10
No Difficulty					Some Difficulty					Great Difficulty

27. Please circle a number from 1-10 to indicate how much difficulty you have in "slowing down" or "turning off" your mind while trying to sleep.

0	1	2	3	4	5	6	7	8	9	10
No Difficulty					Some Difficulty					Great Difficulty

28. Do you currently use medications (over-the-counter or prescription) to help you sleep?
☐Yes ☐ No
If yes, how often (check one):
☐ once a month or less ☐ once a week or less ☐ few times a week ☐ nightly

Please list any medications you are currently using (within the past month) to help you sleep:

Name of Medication	**Amount**	**How long have you used this medicine?**	**Meds make you feel**		
			Better	**No Change**	**Worse**
______			☐	☐	☐
______			☐	☐	☐
______			☐	☐	☐

If you are not currently using medication to help you sleep, have you ever used medication in the past (over-the-counter or prescription) to help you sleep? ☐ Yes ☐ No

If yes, list any medications you used to help you sleep:

Name of Medication	**Amount**	**How long did you use medicine?**	**Meds make you feel**		
			Better	**No Change**	**Worse**
______			☐	☐	☐
______			☐	☐	☐
______			☐	☐	☐

SLEEP HISTORY (GENERAL)

29. In an average 2 week period, how often do you... (Check **ONE** answer for each question)

	Every day/night	5-6 times	3-4 times	1-2 times	Never	Don't know
need more than one reminder to get up in the morning?	☐	☐	☐	☐	☐	☐
arrive late to class because you overslept?	☐	☐	☐	☐	☐	☐
fall asleep in a morning class?	☐	☐	☐	☐	☐	☐
fall asleep in a afternoon class?	☐	☐	☐	☐	☐	☐
feel tired, dragged out, or sleepy during the day?	☐	☐	☐	☐	☐	☐
go to bed because you just could not stay awake any longer?	☐	☐	☐	☐	☐	☐
sleep in past noon?	☐	☐	☐	☐	☐	☐
stay up until at least 3 am?	☐	☐	☐	☐	☐	☐
stay up all night?	☐	☐	☐	☐	☐	☐
have an extremely hard time falling asleep? ...	☐	☐	☐	☐	☐	☐
awaken too early in the morning and couldn't get back to sleep?	☐	☐	☐	☐	☐	☐
have fearful thoughts or images as you are falling asleep?	☐	☐	☐	☐	☐	☐
have nightmares or bad dreams during the night?	☐	☐	☐	☐	☐	☐
walk in your sleep?	☐	☐	☐	☐	☐	☐
have a good night's sleep?	☐	☐	☐	☐	☐	☐
wet your bed?	☐	☐	☐	☐	☐	☐
wake up once during the night?	☐	☐	☐	☐	☐	☐
wake up more than once during the night?	☐	☐	☐	☐	☐	☐
snore?	☐	☐	☐	☐	☐	☐
snore loudly?	☐	☐	☐	☐	☐	☐
stop breathing while you sleep or wake up gasping for breath?	☐	☐	☐	☐	☐	☐
feel satisfied with your sleep?	☐	☐	☐	☐	☐	☐

30. Have you ever been unable to move when falling asleep or immediately upon waking?
☐ Yes ☐ No ☐ Don't know

31. Have you ever had episodes of sudden muscular weakness (paralysis, inability to move) when laughing, angry, or in other emotional situations? ☐ Yes ☐ No ☐ Don't know

DAYTIME SLEEPINESS

32. People sometimes feel sleepy during the daytime. During your daytime activities, how much of a problem do you have with sleepiness (feeling sleepy, struggling to stay awake)?
☐ no problem at all ☐ a little problem ☐ more than a little problem
☐ a big problem ☐ a very big problem

33. Some people take naps in the daytime every day, others never do. When do you nap? (check all that apply)
☐ I never nap ☐ I nap every day ☐ I sometimes nap on school days
☐ I sometimes nap on weekends ☐I never nap unless I am sick

34. During the last two weeks, have you struggled to stay awake (fought sleep) and/or fallen asleep in the following situations? (Check one answer for every item)

	No	Struggled to stay awake (fount sleep)	Fallen asleep	Does not apply
In a face-to-face conversation with another person?...	☐	☐	☐	☐
Traveling in a bus, train, place or car?........................	☐	☐	☐	☐
Attending a performance (movie, concert, play)?........	☐	☐	☐	☐
Watching television?...	☐	☐	☐	☐
Reading, studying, or doing homework?	☐	☐	☐	☐
During a test?..	☐	☐	☐	☐
Driving a car?...	☐	☐	☐	☐
In a class at school?	☐	☐	☐	☐
While doing work on a computer or typewriter?	☐	☐	☐	☐
Playing video games?...	☐	☐	☐	☐
Riding a bicycle?..	☐	☐	☐	☐
Eating a meal?	☐	☐	☐	☐

35. **Complete only if you have a driver's license:**
Have you ever had a car accident(s) caused by your sleepiness (not due to alcohol or drugs)?
☐ Yes ☐ No ☐ Don't know

Have you ever had a near car accident(s) ("close calls") caused by your sleepiness (not due to alcohol or drugs)? ☐ Yes ☐ No ☐ Don't know

In the past month, how often have you driven while sleepy?
☐ never ☐ 1-2 times ☐ 3-4 times ☐ 5 or more times

SLEEP/WAKE RHYTHMS: For items 36-45, please check the response for each item that best describes you.

36. Considering only your own "feeling best" rhythm, at what time would you get up if you were entirely free to plan your day?
☐ 5:00-6:30 AM ☐ 6:30-7:45 AM ☐7:45-9:45 AM
☐ 9:45-11 AM ☐ 11:00 AM-12:00 PM (noon)

37. Considering only your own "feeling best" rhythm, at what time would you go to bed if you were entirely free to plan your evening?
☐ 8:00-9:00 PM ☐ 9:00-10:15 PM ☐ 10:15 PM-12:30 AM
☐ 12:30-1:45 AM ☐ 1:45-3:00 AM

38. Assuming normal circumstances, how easy do you find getting up in the morning? (check one)
☐ Not at all easy ☐ Slightly easy
☐ Fairly easy ☐ Very easy

39. How alert do you feel during the first half hour after having awakened in the morning? (check one)
☐ Not at all alert ☐ Slightly alert
☐ Fairly alert ☐ Very alert

40. During the first half hour after having awakened in the morning, how tired do you feel? (check one)
☐ Not at all tired ☐ Fairly tired
☐ Fairly refreshed ☐ Very refreshed

41. At what time in the evening do you feel tired and as a result in need of sleep?
☐ 8:00-9:00 PM ☐ 9:00-10:15 PM ☐ 10:15 PM-12:30 AM
☐ 12:30-1:45 AM ☐ 1:45-3:00 AM

42. The bad news: you have to take a two-hour test. The good news: you can take it when you think you'll do your best. What time is that? Considering only your own "feeling best" rhythm, at what time would you go to bed if you were entirely free to plan your evening?
☐ 8:00-10:00 AM ☐ 11:00 AM-1:00 PM
☐ 3:00-5:00 PM ☐ 7:00-9:00 PM

43. One hears about "morning" and "evening" types of people. Which ONE of these types do you consider yourself to be? (check one)
☐ Definitely a morning type ☐ More a morning type than evening type
☐ More an evening type than morning type ☐ Definitely an evening type

44. If you always had to rise at 6:00 AM, what do you think it would be like? (check one)
☐ Very difficult and unpleasant ☐ Rather difficult and unpleasant
☐ A little unpleasant but no great problem ☐ Easy and not unpleasant

45. How long does it usually take before you "recover your senses" in the morning after rising from a night's sleep? (check one)
☐ 0-10 minutes ☐ 11-20 minutes
☐ 21-40 minutes ☐ More than 40 minutes

SCHOOL INFORMATION: The next set of questions are about school and other activities.
46. What grade are you in?
☐ 4 ☐5 ☐ 6 ☐ 7 ☐ 8 ☐ 9 ☐ 10 ☐ 11 ☐12

47. Are your grades in school mostly?
☐ A's ☐ A's & B's ☐ B's
☐ B's & C's ☐ C's ☐ C's & D's
☐ D's ☐ D's and F's

48. What is the highest grade in school you expect to complete? (check one)
☐ may not finish high school ☐ will finish high school
☐ will get a college degree ☐ will get a degree beyond college

49. During the last 2 weeks, did you work at a job for pay? ☐ Yes ☐ No (If no skip to item 50)
What kind of job? ______________________________

On average, how many hours did you work at your paying job per week:
during school week: ________ hours during the weekend: ________ hours

50. During the last 2 weeks, did you engage in organized sports or a regularly scheduled physical activity?
☐ Yes ☐ No (If no skip to item 51)

What kind of sport or activity? ____

On average, how many hours did you practice per week:
during school week: _______ hours during the weekend: _______ hours

51. During the last 2 weeks, did you participate in organized extracurricular activities? (For example, committees, clubs, volunteer work, musical groups, church groups, etc.)
☐ Yes ☐ No (If no skip to item 52)
What kind of sport or activity? ____

On average, how many hours did you work at your paying job per week:
during school week: _______ hours during the weekend: _______ hours

52. During the last 2 weeks, did you study/do homework? ☐ Yes ☐ No

On average, how many hours per week:
during school week: _______ hours during the weekend: _______ hours

53. Generally, how often do you attend school?
a. ☐ Every day
b. ☐ 3-4 days per week
c. ☐ 1-2 days per week
d. ☐ Less than once per week

54. Generally, how often are you late to school?
a. ☐ Every day
b. ☐ 3-4 days per week
c. ☐ 1-2 days per week
d. ☐ Less than once per week

HEALTH INFORMATION

(Questions 54-58 are about changes that may be happening to your body. These changes normally happen to different young people at different ages. If you do not understand a question or do not know the answer, just check "I don't know".)

55. Would you say that your growth in height? (check one)
☐ has not begun to spurt ("spurt" means faster growth than usual) ☐ has barely started
☐ is definitely underway ☐ seems complete
☐ I don't know

56. And how about the growth of your body hair? ("Body hair" means hair any place other than your head, such as under your arms). Would you say that your body hair grown: (check one)
☐ has not yet started to grow ☐ has barely started to grow
☐ is definitely underway ☐ seems completed
☐ I don't know

57. Have you noticed any skin changes, especially pimples: (check one)
☐ skin has not yet started changing ☐ skin has barely started changing
☐ skin changes are definitely underway ☐ skin changes seem complete
☐ I don't know

58. Compared to other people your age, would you say that your health is:
☐ poor ☐ fair ☐ good ☐ excellent

59. During the last 2 weeks, how many days did you stay home from school because you were:
sick?: ☐ 1 ☐ 2 ☐ 3 ☐ 4 ☐ 5 ☐ 6 ☐ 7 ☐ 8 ☐ 9 ☐ 10 ☐ Does not apply
other?: ☐ 1 ☐ 2 ☐ 3 ☐ 4 ☐ 5 ☐ 6 ☐ 7 ☐ 8 ☐ 9 ☐ 10 ☐ Does not apply

Why did you stay home from school? ______________________________

HEALTH HABITS: Please answer the following questions about health habits that can have effects on sleep.

60. During the LAST MONTH

How much did you use tobacco products?
☐ More than 1 pack (20 cigarettes) per day ☐ Between 5 and 20 cigarettes per day
☐ Between 1 and 5 cigarettes per day ☐ Less than 1 cigarette per day
☐ None

If you smoke, at what time do you usually have your last cigarette of the day ______☐ AM/ ☐ PM

How much coffee did you drink?
☐ More than 3 glasses per day ☐ Between 1 and 3 glasses per day
☐ Less than one glass per day None

How much caffeinated soda did you drink?
☐ More than 3 glasses per day ☐ Between 1 and 3 glasses per day
☐ Less than one glass per day None

SLEEP BELIEFS

61. In order to better understand your sense of the average teenager's sleep, please answer the following questions based on your beliefs for an **average** adolescent who does **not** have sleep problems?
How many hours of sleep per night does the average teenager get? ______ hours
How long does it take the average teenager to get to sleep? ______ minutes
How many times does the average teenager wake up during the night? ______ times

How long does the average teenager spend awake in bed during the night?
____minutes **OR** ____hours
Do you think most teenagers get enough sleep? ☐ Yes ☐ No ☐ Don't Know

Please indicate how important the **average** teenager **thinks** the following health habits are:
(Please put an X on the line)

using sun screen

Not Important | Somewhat important | Very important

avoiding high fat foods

Not Important | Somewhat important | Very important

not driving after drinking alcohol

Not Important | Somewhat important | Very important

not driving while drowsy

Not Important | Somewhat important | Very important

getting a good night's sleep

Not Important | Somewhat important | Very important

not smoking cigarettes

Not Important | Somewhat important | Very important

exercising regularly

Not Important | Somewhat important | Very important

SLEEP BELIEFS (continued)
Please indicate how likely the **average** teenager is to **do** the following are: (Please put an X on the line)

use sun screen

Not Important	Somewhat important	Very important

avoid high fat foods

Not Important	Somewhat important	Very important

not driving after drinking alcohol

Not Important	Somewhat important	Very important

not driving while drowsy

Not Important	Somewhat important	Very important

getting a good night's sleep

Not Important	Somewhat important	Very important

not smoking cigarettes

Not Important	Somewhat important	Very important

not using drugs

Not Important	Somewhat important	Very important

exercising regularly

Not Important	Somewhat important	Very important

THANK YOU VERY MUCH FOR YOUR TIME!

ADOLESCENT SLEEP HABITS SURVEY
(GIRL'S SELF REPORT)

Instructions: This form should be filled out by the adolescent patient herself if at all possible.
Today's Date: _____/_____/_____

1. Name:____2. Date of Birth: ____/____/____
3. Please describe your sleep problem(s): ____
____
____

4. How long have you had difficulty with sleep? (check one)
☐ less than a month ☐ 1-6 months
☐ 6-12 months ☐ 1-5 years
☐ more than 5 years

5. Have your problems with sleep gotten worse? ☐ Yes ☐ No ☐Not sure
If yes, when did you notice that your sleep problems got worse: _______________________

6. What do you think is causing your sleep problem? (check all that apply)
☐ stress at school ☐ relationship problems with parents/family
☐ relationship problems with peers ☐ poor sleep habits
☐ poor eating habits ☐ a physical problem
Other (describe briefly)____

SLEEP HABITS: This set of questions asks about your usual sleep habits. Please answer as honestly as possible.

7. With whom do you share a bedroom? (check all that apply)

	Yes	**No**
Mother/step-mother	☐	☐
Father/step-father	☐	☐
Older brother(s)/sister(s)	☐	☐
Younger brother(s)/sister(s)	☐	☐
Other family member(s).................................	☐	☐

8. In the last two weeks, have you slept in the same bed?
☐ every night ☐ almost every night
☐ a few nights ☐ not at all

The next set of questions has to do with your usual schedule on days when you have school. Please list both the USUAL times or number of hours/minutes, and the RANGE (earliest to latest, lowest to highest). Please check AM or PM for each time.

9. What time do you **usually** go to bed on school days? __________
Range: ______ ☐ AM/ ☐ PM to ______ ☐ AM/ ☐ PM

SLEEP HABITS (continued)

10. There are many reasons for doing things at one time or another. What is the **main reason** you usually go to bed at this time on school days? (check one)

☐ My parents have set my bedtime
☐ I finish my homework
☐ My brother(s) or sister(s) go to bed
☐ I get home from my job
☐ I feel sleepy
☐ My TV shows are over
☐ I finish socializing
☐ Other: ______________________________

11. What time do you **usually** wake up on school days? __________
Range: ______ ☐AM/ ☐PM to ______ ☐AM/ ☐ PM

12. There are many reasons for doing things at one time or another. What is the **main reason** you usually wake up at this time on school days? (check one)

☐ Noises or my pet wakes me up
☐ My parents wake me up
☐ I don't know, I just wake up
☐ My alarm clock wakes me up
☐ I need to go to the bathroom
☐ Other: ______________________________

13. What time do you **usually** leave home on school days? __________
Range: ______ ☐AM/ ☐ PM to ______ ☐AM/ ☐ PM

14. How do you usually get to school? (check one)
☐ Walk
☐ Take the bus
☐ Get a ride with parent
☐ Get a ride with friend(s)
☐ Drive my car

What time do you need to arrive at school? __________

15. Figure out how long you **usually** sleep on a normal school night and fill it in here. (Do not include time you spend awake in bed. Remember to mark hours and minutes, even if minutes are zero.)
Usual amount of sleep: ______ hours and______ minutes
Range: ______ hours and______ minutes to ______ hours and______ minutes

16. On school days, after you go to bed at night, about how long does it usually take you to fall asleep? (If longer than one hour, change to minutes.)
Usual amount: ______ minutes
Range: ______ minutes to ______ minutes

The next set of questions has to do with your usual schedule on days when you DO NOT have school, such as the weekend.

17. What time do you **usually** go to bed on weekends? __________
Range: ______ ☐AM/ ☐PM to ______ ☐AM/ ☐ PM

18. There are many reasons for doing things at one time or another. What is the **main reason** you usually go to bed at this time on **weekends**? (check one)
☐My parents have set my bedtime
☐ I finish my homework
☐ My brother(s) or sister(s) go to bed
☐ I get home from my job
☐ I feel sleepy
☐ My TV shows are over
☐ I finish socializing
☐ Other: ______________________________

SLEEP HABITS (continued)

19. What time do you **usually** wake up on weekends? _______ ☐AM/ ☐PM
Range: ______ ☐ AM/ ☐PM to _______ ☐AM/ ☐ PM

20. What is the **main reason** you usually wake up at this time on weekends? (check one)
☐ Noises or my pet wakes me up
☐ My parents wake me up
☐ I don't know, I just wake up
☐ My alarm clock wakes me up
☐ I need to go to the bathroom
☐ Other: ______________________________

21. Figure out how long you **usually** sleep on a night when you do not have school the next day (such as a weekend night) and fill it in here. (Do not include time you spend awake in bed. Remember to mark hours and minutes, even if minutes are zero.)
Usual amount of sleep: ______ hours and_______ minutes
Range: ______ hours and_______ minutes to ______ hours and_______ minutes

22. On weekends, after you go to bed at night, about how long does it usually take you to fall asleep? (If longer than one hour, change to minutes.)
Range: ______ minutes to _______ minutes

23. Can you figure out how much sleep you need? Fill out how much sleep you think you would need each night to feel your best every day. (Do not include time you spend awake in bed. Remember to mark hours and minutes, even if minutes are zero.)
______ hours _______ minutes

The following questions ask about other sleep habits you may have. Please answer as honestly as possible.

24. In the last two weeks, how often have you done any of the following activities in bed?

	Every day/night	Several times	Twice	Once	Never
Read?	☐	☐	☐	☐	☐
Watch TV?	☐	☐	☐	☐	☐
Eat?	☐	☐	☐	☐	☐
Do schoolwork?	☐	☐	☐	☐	☐
Worry?	☐	☐	☐	☐	☐

25. When you have difficulty falling asleep or getting back to sleep, what do you do? (check all that apply)
☐ Stay in bed and try to get to sleep
☐ Do something in bed (e.g., read or watch TV)
☐ Get up and watch TV
☐ Get up and drink alcohol
☐ Get up and drink warm milk
☐ Get up and drink something? (circle all that apply: soda/water/coffee/tea)
☐ Get up and have a cigarette
Other (please specify): ______________________________

SLEEP HABITS (continued)

26. Please circle a number from 1-10 to indicate how much difficulty you have relaxing away tension in your body while trying to sleep.

0	1	2	3	4	5	6	7	8	9	10
No Difficulty					Some Difficulty					Great Difficulty

27. Please circle a number from 1-10 to indicate how much difficulty you have in "slowing down" or "turning off" your mind while trying to sleep.

0	1	2	3	4	5	6	7	8	9	10
No Difficulty					Some Difficulty					Great Difficulty

28. Do you currently use medications (over-the-counter or prescription) to help you sleep?

☐Yes ☐ No

If yes, how often (check one):

☐ once a month or less ☐ once a week or less ☐ few times a week ☐ nightly

Please list any medications you are currently using (within the past month) to help you sleep:

Name of Medication	Amount	How long have you used this medicine?	Meds make you feel: Better	No Change	Worse
			☐	☐	☐
			☐	☐	☐
			☐	☐	☐

If you are not currently using medication to help you sleep, have you ever used medication in the past (over-the-counter or prescription) to help you sleep? ☐ Yes ☐ No

If yes, list any medications you used to help you sleep:

Name of Medication	Amount	How long did you use medicine?	Meds make you feel: Better	No Change	Worse
			☐	☐	☐
			☐	☐	☐
			☐	☐	☐

SLEEP HISTORY (GENERAL)

29. In an average 2 week period, how often do you... (Check **ONE** answer for each question)

	Every day/night	5-6 times	3-4 times	1-2 times	Never	Don't know
need more than one reminder to get up in the morning?	☐	☐	☐	☐	☐	☐
arrive late to class because you overslept?	☐	☐	☐	☐	☐	☐
fall asleep in a morning class?	☐	☐	☐	☐	☐	☐
fall asleep in a afternoon class?	☐	☐	☐	☐	☐	☐
feel tired, dragged out, or sleepy during the day?	☐	☐	☐	☐	☐	☐
go to bed because you just could not stay awake any longer?	☐	☐	☐	☐	☐	☐
sleep in past noon?	☐	☐	☐	☐	☐	☐
stay up until at least 3 am?	☐	☐	☐	☐	☐	☐
stay up all night?	☐	☐	☐	☐	☐	☐
have an extremely hard time falling asleep?	☐	☐	☐	☐	☐	☐
awaken too early in the morning and couldn't get back to sleep?	☐	☐	☐	☐	☐	☐
have fearful thoughts or images as you are falling asleep?	☐	☐	☐	☐	☐	☐
have nightmares or bad dreams during the night?	☐	☐	☐	☐	☐	☐
walk in your sleep?	☐	☐	☐	☐	☐	☐
have a good night's sleep?	☐	☐	☐	☐	☐	☐
wet your bed?	☐	☐	☐	☐	☐	☐
wake up once during the night?	☐	☐	☐	☐	☐	☐
wake up more than once during the night?	☐	☐	☐	☐	☐	☐
snore?	☐	☐	☐	☐	☐	☐
snore loudly?	☐	☐	☐	☐	☐	☐
stop breathing while you sleep or wake up gasping for breath?	☐	☐	☐	☐	☐	☐
feel satisfied with your sleep?	☐	☐	☐	☐	☐	☐

30. Have you ever been unable to move when falling asleep or immediately upon waking?
☐ Yes ☐ No ☐ Don't know

31. Have you ever had episodes of sudden muscular weakness (paralysis, inability to move) when laughing, angry, or in other emotional situations? ☐ Yes ☐ No ☐ Don't know

DAYTIME SLEEPINESS

32. People sometimes feel sleepy during the daytime. During your daytime activities, how much of a problem do you have with sleepiness (feeling sleepy, struggling to stay awake)?
☐ no problem at all ☐ a little problem ☐ more than a little problem
☐ a big problem ☐ a very big problem

33. Some people take naps in the daytime every day, others never do. When do you nap? (check all that apply)
☐ I never nap ☐ I nap every day ☐ I sometimes nap on school days
☐ I sometimes nap on weekends ☐ I never nap unless I am sick

34. During the last two weeks, have you struggled to stay awake (fought sleep) and/or fallen asleep in the following situations? (Check one answer for every item)

	No	Struggled to stay awake (fount sleep)	Fallen asleep	Does not apply
In a face-to-face conversation with another person?...	☐	☐	☐	☐
Traveling in a bus, train, place or car?........................	☐	☐	☐	☐
Attending a performance (movie, concert, play)?........	☐	☐	☐	☐
Watching television?..	☐	☐	☐	☐
Reading, studying, or doing homework?	☐	☐	☐	☐
During a test?...	☐	☐	☐	☐
Driving a car?...	☐	☐	☐	☐
In a class at school?	☐	☐	☐	☐
While doing work on a computer or typewriter?	☐	☐	☐	☐
Playing video games?..	☐	☐	☐	☐
Riding a bicycle?...	☐	☐	☐	☐
Eating a meal?	☐	☐	☐	☐

35. **Complete only if you have a driver's license:**
Have you ever had a car accident(s) caused by your sleepiness (not due to alcohol or drugs)?
☐ Yes ☐ No ☐ Don't know

Have you ever had a near car accident(s) ("close calls") caused by your sleepiness (not due to alcohol or drugs)? ☐ Yes ☐ No ☐ Don't know

In the past month, how often have you driven while sleepy?
☐ never ☐ 1-2 times ☐ 3-4 times ☐ 5 or more times

SLEEP/WAKE RHYTHMS: For items 36-45, please check the response for each item that best describes you.

36. Considering only your own "feeling best" rhythm, at what time would you get up if you were entirely free to plan your day?
☐ 5:00-6:30 AM ☐ 6:30-7:45 AM ☐7:45-9:45 AM
☐ 9:45-11 AM ☐ 11:00 AM-12:00 PM (noon)

37. Considering only your own "feeling best" rhythm, at what time would you go to bed if you were entirely free to plan your evening?
☐ 8:00-9:00 PM ☐ 9:00-10:15 PM ☐ 10:15 PM-12:30 AM
☐ 12:30-1:45 AM ☐ 1:45-3:00 AM

38. Assuming normal circumstances, how easy do you find getting up in the morning? (check one)
☐ Not at all easy ☐ Slightly easy
☐ Fairly easy ☐ Very easy

39. How alert do you feel during the first half hour after having awakened in the morning? (check one)
☐ Not at all alert ☐ Slightly alert
☐ Fairly alert ☐ Very alert

40. During the first half hour after having awakened in the morning, how tired do you feel? (check one)
☐ Not at all tired ☐ Fairly tired
☐ Fairly refreshed ☐ Very refreshed

41. At what time in the evening do you feel tired and as a result in need of sleep?
☐ 8:00-9:00 PM ☐ 9:00-10:15 PM ☐ 10:15 PM-12:30 AM
☐ 12:30-1:45 AM ☐ 1:45-3:00 AM

42. The bad news: you have to take a two-hour test. The good news: you can take it when you think you'll do your best. What time is that? Considering only your own "feeling best" rhythm, at what time would you go to bed if you were entirely free to plan your evening?
☐ 8:00-10:00 AM ☐ 11:00 AM-1:00 PM
☐ 3:00-5:00 PM ☐ 7:00-9:00 PM

43. One hears about "morning" and "evening" types of people. Which ONE of these types do you consider yourself to be? (check one)
☐ Definitely a morning type ☐ More a morning type than evening type
☐ More an evening type than morning type ☐ Definitely an evening type

44. If you always had to rise at 6:00 AM, what do you think it would be like? (check one)
☐ Very difficult and unpleasant ☐ Rather difficult and unpleasant
☐ A little unpleasant but no great problem ☐ Easy and not unpleasant

45. How long does it usually take before you "recover your senses" in the morning after rising from a night's sleep? (check one)
☐ 0-10 minutes ☐ 11-20 minutes
☐ 21-40 minutes ☐ More than 40 minutes

SCHOOL INFORMATION: The next set of questions are about school and other activities.
46. What grade are you in?
☐ 4 ☐ 5 ☐ 6 ☐ 7 ☐ 8 ☐ 9 ☐ 10 ☐ 11 ☐ 12

47. Are your grades in school mostly?
☐ A's ☐ A's & B's ☐ B's
☐ B's & C's ☐ C's ☐ C's & D's
☐ D's ☐ D's and F's

48. What is the highest grade in school you expect to complete? (check one)
☐ may not finish high school ☐ will finish high school
☐ will get a college degree ☐ will get a degree beyond college

49. During the last 2 weeks, did you work at a job for pay? ☐ Yes ☐ No (If no skip to item 50)
What kind of job? ______________________________

On average, how many hours did you work at your paying job per week:
during school week: ________ hours during the weekend: ________ hours

50. During the last 2 weeks, did you engage in organized sports or a regularly scheduled physical activity?
☐ Yes ☐ No (If no skip to item 51)

What kind of sport or activity? ____

On average, how many hours did you practice per week:
during school week: _______ hours during the weekend: _______ hours

51. During the last 2 weeks, did you participate in organized extracurricular activities? (For example, committees, clubs, volunteer work, musical groups, church groups, etc.)
☐ Yes ☐ No (If no skip to item 52)
What kind of sport or activity? ____

On average, how many hours did you work at your paying job per week:
during school week: _______ hours during the weekend: _______ hours

52. During the last 2 weeks, did you study/do homework? ☐ Yes ☐ No

On average, how many hours per week:
during school week: _______ hours during the weekend: _______ hours

53. Generally, how often do you attend school?
a. ☐ Every day
b. ☐ 3-4 days per week
c. ☐ 1-2 days per week
d. ☐ Less than once per week

54. Generally, how often are you late to school?
a. ☐ Every day
b. ☐ 3-4 days per week
c. ☐ 1-2 days per week
d. ☐ Less than once per week

HEALTH INFORMATION

(Questions 54-58 are about changes that may be happening to your body. These changes normally happen to different young people at different ages. If you do not understand a question or do not know the answer, just check "I don't know".)

55. Would you say that your growth in height? (check one)
☐ has not begun to spurt ("spurt" means faster growth than usual) ☐ has barely started
☐ is definitely underway ☐ seems complete
☐ I don't know

56. And how about the growth of your body hair? ("Body hair" means hair any place other than your head, such as under your arms). Would you say that your body hair grown: (check one)
☐ has not yet started to grow ☐ has barely started to grow
☐ is definitely underway ☐ seems completed
☐ I don't know

57. Have you noticed any skin changes, especially pimples: (check one)
☐ skin has not yet started changing ☐ skin has barely started changing
☐ skin changes are definitely underway ☐ skin changes seem complete
☐ I don't know

58. Have you noticed that your breasts have begun to grow: (check one)
☐ have not yet started growing ☐ have barely started changing
☐ breast growth is definitely underway ☐ breast growth seems completed
☐ I don't know

59. Have you begun to menstruate (started your period)? ☐ Yes ☐ No
If yes how old were you (years):
☐ 8 ☐ 9 ☐ 10 ☐ 11 ☐ 12 ☐ 13 ☐ 14 ☐ 15 ☐ 16 ☐ Older than 16 ☐ I don't know

60. Compared to other people your age, would you say that your health is:
☐ poor ☐ fair ☐ good ☐ excellent

61. During the last 2 weeks, how many days did you stay home from school because you were:
sick?: ☐ 1 ☐ 2 ☐ 3 ☐ 4 ☐ 5 ☐ 6 ☐ 7 ☐ 8 ☐ 9 ☐ 10 ☐ Does not apply
other?: ☐ 1 ☐ 2 ☐ 3 ☐ 4 ☐ 5 ☐ 6 ☐ 7 ☐ 8 ☐ 9 ☐ 10 ☐ Does not apply

Why did you stay home from school? ______________________________

HEALTH HABITS: Please answer the following questions about health habits that can have effects on sleep.

62. During the LAST MONTH

How much did you use tobacco products?
☐ More than 1 pack (20 cigarettes) per day ☐ Between 5 and 20 cigarettes per day
☐ Between 1 and 5 cigarettes per day ☐ Less than 1 cigarette per day
☐ None

If you smoke, at what time do you usually have your last cigarette of the day ______☐ AM/ ☐ PM

How much coffee did you drink?
☐ More than 3 glasses per day ☐ Between 1 and 3 glasses per day
☐ Less than one glass per day None

How much caffeinated soda did you drink?
☐ More than 3 glasses per day ☐ Between 1 and 3 glasses per day
☐ Less than one glass per day None

SLEEP BELIEFS

63. In order to better understand your sense of the average teenager's sleep, please answer the following questions based on your beliefs for an **average** adolescent who does **not** have sleep problems?
How many hours of sleep per night does the average teenager get? ______ hours
How long does it take the average teenager to get to sleep? ______ minutes
How many times does the average teenager wake up during the night? ______ times

How long does the average teenager spend awake in bed during the night?
____minutes **OR** ____hours
Do you think most teenagers get enough sleep? ☐ Yes ☐ No ☐ Don't Know

Please indicate how important the **average** teenager **thinks** the following health habits are:
(Please put an X on the line)

using sun screen

Not Important | Somewhat important | Very important

avoiding high fat foods

Not Important | Somewhat important | Very important

not driving after drinking alcohol

Not Important | Somewhat important | Very important

not driving while drowsy

Not Important | Somewhat important | Very important

getting a good night's sleep

Not Important | Somewhat important | Very important

not smoking cigarettes

Not Important | Somewhat important | Very important

exercising regularly

Not Important | Somewhat important | Very important

SLEEP BELIEFS (continued)
Please indicate how likely the **average** teenager is to **do** the following are: (Please put an X on the line)

use sun screen

Not Important	Somewhat important	Very important

avoid high fat foods

Not Important	Somewhat important	Very important

not driving after drinking alcohol

Not Important	Somewhat important	Very important

not driving while drowsy

Not Important	Somewhat important	Very important

getting a good night's sleep

Not Important	Somewhat important	Very important

not smoking cigarettes

Not Important	Somewhat important	Very important

not using drugs

Not Important	Somewhat important	Very important

exercising regularly

Not Important	Somewhat important	Very important

THANK YOU VERY MUCH FOR YOUR TIME!

ADOLESCENT SLEEP HABITS SURVEY (PARENT VERSION)

1. Name of Patient: ______________________________2. Date of Birth:___/___/___
3. Name of person completing questionnaire_____________________________________
Relationship to child ______________________________
Referred by ____
Pediatrician ____
4. A copy of the sleep clinic evaluation will be sent to you, your pediatrician, and any referring physician. Please indicate anyone else who should receive a copy:
Name: ______________________________ Address: ______________________________
____
5. What are your major concerns about your adolescent's sleep?___________________
____
____
6. What do you think is causing your adolescent's sleep problem?__________________
____
7. When did your adolescent's sleep problems start? ____________________________
____

FAMILY INFORMATION

8. Please list all members of the households in which your adolescent lives full or part-time:

Name/Relationship to Adolescent	Age	Adolescent lives with (please indicate full-time or part-time)
______________________	__________	______________________
______________________	__________	______________________
______________________	__________	______________________
______________________	__________	______________________
______________________	__________	______________________
______________________	__________	______________________

9. Mother's Marital Status: Married Divorced Separated Widowed Single
If divorced, adolescent custody with: ________________________
10. Mother's education: ______________________________
11. Mother's occupation: ______________________________
Does mother work outside of home? ☐ yes ☐ no
If yes, mark each label that best describes her work:

☐ day shift	☐ full time
☐ evening shift	☐ part time
☐ night shift (graveyard)	☐ one job
☐ changing shifts	☐ more than one job

12. Father's Marital Status: Married Divorced Separated Widowed Single
If divorced, adolescent custody with: ________________________
13. What is father's education: __________________________

14. Father's occupation: ______________________________

Does father work outside of home? Yes No

If yes, mark each label that best describes his work:

☐day shift ☐ full time

☐evening shift ☐ part time

☐ night shift (graveyard) ☐ one job

☐ changing shifts ☐ more than one job

15. What best describes your adolescent's racial/ethnic background?

White/Caucasian____________ Asian/Asian American _____________

Black/African American __________ Native American ___________________

Hispanic/Latino ________________ Multiracial (Please specify)___________

Other (Please specify)____

16. Please list family members (parents, grandparents, siblings, aunts/uncles) with a history of any SLEEP PROBLEMS (including: loud snoring/obstructive sleep apnea, excessive sleepiness/narcolepsy, restless legs/periodic leg movements, insomnia, other sleep problems).

Family Member	Type of Sleep Problem
______________________	____________________________
______________________	____________________________
______________________	____________________________
______________________	____________________________

17. Has anyone in your family ever had a car accident caused by sleepiness (not due to alcohol or drugs)? ☐Yes ☐No ☐Don't know

If yes, whom: ________________________At what age:______________________

Type of accident: ____

18. Please list any family members with a significant mental health condition (such as depression, anxiety, alcoholism/substance abuse).

Family Member	Type of Mental Health Problem
______________________	___________________________________
______________________	___________________________________
______________________	___________________________________

SLEEP HISTORY (GENERAL)

19. What time does your adolescent usually go to bed on school nights? __________

Range: _____ am/pm to _____am/pm

20. What is the main reason your adolescent goes to bed at a particular time? (Check one below)

_____ a. Because it fits best with the family's schedule

_____ b. Because she/he feels sleepy then

_____ c. Because that is when her/his TV shows are over

_____ d. Because that is when her/his brothers and sisters go to bed

_____ e. To "get enough sleep" for the following day's activities

_____ f. Other (describe briefly) ____

21. What time does your adolescent usually wake up on school day mornings? ________

Range: _____ am/pm to _____am/pm

22. What usually wakes up your adolescent in the morning on school days? (Check one below)

_____ a. Alarm clock
_____ b. Parent or other family member
_____ c. Noise
_____ d. Needs to go to the bathroom
_____ e. Spontaneous
_____ f. Other (describe briefly):

23. Which of the following applies to waking your adolescent in the morning on school days?
(Check one below)

_____ a. I almost always have great difficulty getting him/her out of bed
_____ b. I sometimes have great difficulty getting him/her our of bed
_____ c. I seldom have great difficulty getting him/her out of bed
_____ d. I never have great difficulty getting him/her out of bed

24. What times does your adolescent usually go to bed on weekend nights? ___________
Range: _____ am/pm to_____am/pm

25. What time does your adolescent usually wake up on weekend mornings? ___________
Range: _____ am/pm to _____am/pm

26. What usually wakes up your adolescent in the morning on weekends? (Check one below)

_____ a. Alarm clock
_____ b. Parent or other family member
_____ c. Noise
_____ d. Needs to go to the bathroom
_____ e. Spontaneous
_____ f. Other (describe briefly):

27. Which of the following applies to waking your adolescent in the morning on weekends?
(Check one below)

_____ a. I almost always have great difficulty getting him/her out of bed
_____ b. I sometimes have great difficulty getting him/her our of bed
_____ c. I seldom have great difficulty getting him/her out of bed
_____ d. I never have great difficulty getting him/her out of bed

28. IN AN AVERAGE TWO-WEEK PERIOD, HOW OFTEN DOES YOUR ADOLESCENT...
(Check one answer for each question; please feel free to comment)

	Every day/ night	**5-6 times**	**3-4 times**	**1-2 times**	**Never**	**Comments:**
snore?	☐	☐	☐	☐	☐	__________
snore loudly and disruptively?	☐	☐	☐	☐	☐	__________
sleep restlessly?	☐	☐	☐	☐	☐	__________
sleep in an abnormal position?	☐	☐	☐	☐	☐	__________
sweat while sleeping?	☐	☐	☐	☐	☐	__________
pause in breathing?	☐	☐	☐	☐	☐	__________
complain of headache on waking?	☐	☐	☐	☐	☐	__________
have nightmares?	☐	☐	☐	☐	☐	__________
sleepwalk?	☐	☐	☐	☐	☐	__________
sleeptalk?	☐	☐	☐	☐	☐	__________

29. Has your adolescent ever used medication (over-the-counter or prescription) including herbal or "natural" remedies to help with sleep?
□ Yes □ No □ Don't know
If yes, name of medication and how frequently used: ____________________

30. Does your adolescent currently (within the past month) use medications (over-the-counter or prescription) to help with sleep? □ Yes □ No □ Don't know
If yes, name of medication and how frequently used: ____________________

SLEEP HISTORY - DAYTIME SLEEPINESS

31. During the LAST TWO WEEKS, has your adolescent struggled to stay awake (fought sleep) or fallen asleep in the following situations? (Mark one answer for every item)

	No	**Struggled to stay awake (fought sleep)**	**Fallen asleep**	**Don't Know**	**Does not Apply**
a. in a face-to-face conversation with another person?	□	□	□	□	□
b. traveling in a car, bus?	□	□	□	□	□
c. at the movies?	□	□	□	□	□
d. watching television?	□	□	□	□	□
e. listening to the radio or stereo?	□	□	□	□	□
f. reading, studying or doing homework?	□	□	□	□	□
g. in a class at school?	□	□	□	□	□
h. while doing work on a computer or typewriter?	□	□	□	□	□
i. playing video games?	□	□	□	□	□
j. eating a meal?	□	□	□	□	□

MEDICAL HISTORY:

32. Were there any problems with this pregnancy or delivery (prematurity, high blood pressure, etc.)?
____
____

33. What was the birth weight? __________

34. Was your adolescent ever on an apnea monitor at home? □ Yes □ No
If yes, for how long? ________

35. Does your adolescent have any significant health problems? □ Yes □ No
If so, please describe:
____
____

36. Has your adolescent ever been hospitalized? □ Yes □ No
If yes, when: ____________________ What for? ____________________
____________________ ____________________
____________________ ____________________

37. Has your adolescent ever had any operations (other than tonsils/adenoids removal)?
☐ Yes ☐ No
If yes, type of operation?____________________ Year ____________
____________________ Year ____________
____________________ Year ____________

38. Have your adolescent's tonsils or adenoids been removed?
a. Tonsils: ☐ Yes At what age?_______
For what reason: ____________________________
b. Adenoids: ☐ Yes At what age?_______
For what reason: ____________________________
c. Describe briefly any changes you noticed in your adolescent's sleep or waking behavior after removal of tonsils or adenoids: ____________________

39. If NO, do you think the tonsils or adenoids are a problem?
☐ Yes ☐ No ☐ Don't know
For how long have they been a problem? ______ years

40. Has your adolescent ever broken his/her nose or other facial bones? ☐ Yes ☐ No

41. Does your adolescent have difficulty breathing through his/her nose? ☐ Yes ☐ No

42. In the past year, has your adolescent had strep throats/tonsillitis? ________________
☐ Yes ☐ No
Frequent colds/respiratory infections? ☐ Yes ☐ No
Frequent sinus infections? ☐ Yes ☐ No

43. Does your adolescent have allergies? ☐ Yes ☐ No ☐ Possibly
If yes, to what?________________________________

44. Does your adolescent have asthma? ☐ Yes ☐ No If "Yes", please answer the following questions:

In the **past year**....
a. How many days has your adolescent missed school due to asthma? _______ None
b. How many days has your adolescent been hospitalized for asthma? _______ None
c. List any medications your adolescent takes for asthma:

Type: ____________________ Frequency: ____________________
Type: ____________________ Frequency: ____________________
Type: ____________________ Frequency: ____________________

45. Does your adolescent frequently complain of heartburn? ☐ Yes ☐ No ☐ Don't know
Has he/she ever been diagnosed with gastroesophageal (stomach) reflux?
☐ Yes ☐ No ☐ Only when younger

46. Has your adolescent had any head injuries requiring medical evaluation and/or treatment or loss of consciousness? If yes, please describe:____________________

47. List any prescription or over-the counter medications your adolescent has taken in the last month:
Type: ____________________ Reason for medication: ________________
Type: ____________________ Reason for medication: ________________
Type: ____________________ Reason for medication: ________________

48. Menstrual history (Girls only):
a. Age she started menstruating ________ years
b. Regularity of her menstrual periods:
- ☐ About one per month (28 days)
- ☐ Usually much longer than one month between periods
- ☐ Usually shorter than one month between periods
- ☐ Very irregular; no apparent pattern
- ☐ Do not know

c. Number of days since her last menstrual period ________

49. Do you have additional comments about your adolescent's medical history? (Continue on additional sheets if necessary.)

____

____

____

HEALTH HABITS - Please answer the following questions regarding health habits which may
impact on sleep.

50. In the past month, how much did your adolescent use tobacco products?
- ☐ More than one pack (20 cigarettes) per day
- ☐ Between 5 and 20 cigarettes per day
- ☐ Between 1 and 5 cigarettes per day
- ☐ Less than 1 cigarette per day
- ☐ None
- ☐ Don't know

51. How much coffee did your adolescent drink?
- ☐ More than 3 cups glasses per day
- ☐ Between 1 and 3 cups per day
- ☐ Less than one cup per day
- ☐ None
- ☐ Don't know

52. How much caffeinated soda did your adolescent drink?
- ☐ More than 3 glasses per day
- ☐ Between 1 and 3 per day
- ☐ Less than one per day
- ☐ None
- ☐ Don't know

53. How much time does your adolescent spend on the computer on school days?

☐ 0-2 hours per day ☐ between 2 and 4 hours ☐ between 4 and 6 hours
☐ between 6 and 8 hours ☐ more than 8 hours ☐ don't know

54. How much time does your adolescent spend on the computer on weekend days?

☐ 0-2 hours per day ☐ between 2 and 4 hours ☐ between 4 and 6 hours
☐ between 6 and 8 hours ☐ more than 8 hours ☐ don't know

DEVELOPMENT HISTORY- PART A

55. In what grade is your adolescent currently enrolled? __________ grade
56. What school does your adolescent attend this year?______________________________
57. Has your adolescent been diagnosed with:

	YES	NO	COMMENTS
a. dyslexia	☐	☐	____________________
b. a speech impairment	☐	☐	____________________
c. mental retardation	☐	☐	____________________
d. a behavior disorder	☐	☐	____________________
e. attention deficit disorder	☐	☐	____________________
f. other learning disorder (please specify)____________________	☐	☐	____________________

58. Is your adolescent enrolled in any special education (special needs) classes in school?
☐ Yes ☐ No Please describe: ____

59. Does your adolescent have an Individualized Education Plan (I.E.P.) provided by the school? ☐ Yes ☐ No If yes, for what reason: ______________________________

60. Generally, how often does your adolescent attend school?
   a. ☐ Every day
   b. ☐ 3-4 days per week
   c. ☐ 1-2 days per week
   d. ☐ Less than once per week

61. Generally, how often is your adolescent late to school?
   a. ☐ Every day
   b. ☐ 3-4 days per week
   c. ☐ 1-2 days per week
   d. ☐ Less than once per week

DEVELOPMENTAL HISTORY- PART B

62. Does your adolescent have any significant behavioral or mental health problems
☐ Yes ☐ No
If yes, please describe ____
____

63. Has your adolescent ever received counseling for behavioral or mental health problems?
☐ Yes ☐ No If so, for what reason? ____
Please give approximate dates:
____

64. Have you or your spouse ever been seen by a mental health counselor for concerns regarding your adolescent? ☐ Yes ☐ No
If yes, for what reason?____

65. To what organized groups does your adolescent currently belong? (e.g., team sports, scouts, church, groups, etc.)

____

____

SLEEP BELIEFS

In order to better understand your sense of the average teenager's sleep, please answer the following questions based on your beliefs for an average teenager (your adolescent's age) who does not have sleep problems?

a. How many hours of sleep per night does the average teenager get? _______ hours
b. How long does it take the average teenager to get to sleep? _______ minutes
c. How many times does the average teenager wake up during the night? ______ times
d. How long does the average teenager spend awake in bed during the night?
_____ minutes or _____ hours
e. Do you think most teenagers get enough sleep? □ Yes □ No □ Don't Know

THANK YOU VERY MUCH FOR YOUR TIME!

Reference

1. KIDZZZSLEEP Pediatric Sleep Disorders Program. (April 3, 2009). *Clinical tools*. Retrieved June 17, 2009, from http://www.kidzzzsleep.org/clinicaltools.htm.

Representative Studies Using Scale

None.

2 Adolescent Sleep-Wake Scale

Purpose A modified version of the Children's Sleep-Wake Scale, this questionnaire was developed by LeBourgeois and colleagues [1] in order to address the unique needs of an older testing population. The instrument is designed to assess overall sleep quality by measuring the adolescent's responses along five behavioral dimensions: going to bed, falling asleep, maintaining sleep, reinitiating sleep, and returning to wakefulness. A six-point, Likert-type scale asks respondents to indicate how often they have exhibited certain sleep behaviors during the last month (with 1 meaning "always," and 6 meaning "never").

Population for Testing Adolescents between 12 and 18 years of age.

Administration All 28 items are self-reported using a pencil-and-paper instrument. Requires 10–15 min for testing.

Reliability and Validity LeBourgeois et al. [1] found good internal consistency across its samples (Cronbach's α for the instrument's subscales ranged from .60 to .81), while the full scale possessed a reliability of $\alpha = .80$.

Obtaining a Copy A published copy can be found in a study by LeBourgeois and colleagues [1].

Direct correspondence to:
Dr. M. LeBourgeois
Sleep and Chronobiology Research Laboratory
E.P. Bradley Hospital/Brown Medical School
1011 Veterans Memorial Pkwy, East Providence, RI 02915, USA
Email: monique_lebourgeois@brown.edu

Scoring Calculating mean scores for each subscale allows for individual assessment of the five sleep-behavior domains examined by the questionnaire, while an overall sleep-quality score (the mean of the five subscales) can also be obtained. LeBourgeois and colleagues [1] offer few guidelines for interpreting questionnaire results, and suggest only that higher scores are indicative of better sleep quality. Thus, the instrument may be more valuable when scores can be compared across research participants or over the course of multiple clinical visits.

Reference

1. LeBourgeois, M. K., Giannotti, F., Cortesi, F., Wolfson, A. R., & Harsh, J. (2005). The relationship between reported sleep quality and sleep hygiene in Italian and American adolescents. *Pediatrics, 115*(1), 257–259.

Representative Studies Using Scale

Palermo, T., Toliver-Sokol, M., Fonareva, I., & Koh, J. (2007). Objective and subjective assessment of sleep in adolescents with chronic pain compared to healthy adolescents. *Clinical Journal of Pain, 23*(9), 812–820.

A. Shahid et al. (eds.), *STOP, THAT and One Hundred Other Sleep Scales*,
DOI 10.1007/978-1-4419-9893-4_2, © Springer Science+Business Media, LLC 2012

3 Apnea Beliefs Scale

Purpose Consisting of 24 statements regarding obstructive sleep apnea (OSA), the instrument targets nine different dimensions of belief about the disorder, including: perceived impact of OSA, outcome expectations, continuous positive airway pressure (CPAP) acceptance, and willingness to ask for help. Smith and colleagues [1] designed the questionnaire as a tool for investigating treatment compliance in apneic individuals. As some have postulated that more positive beliefs and attitudes about OSA treatment are associated with improved compliance, higher scores on the test may be linked to a greater commitment to the treatment process. Further research will hopefully illuminate this potential relationship more clearly. For a similar tool, see the Apnea Knowledge Test (Chap. 4).

Population for Testing The test's developers did not specify an age range for administration. However, in a study evaluating the tool's psychometric properties, most participants were middle aged (mean age, 52.6 ± 12.6 SD). A reading ability at approximately the sixth grade level is required for comprehension.

Administration The pencil-and-paper scale requires approximately 5–10 min for completion by patient respondents.

Reliability and Validity Smith et al. [1] conducted an initial evaluation of the test's psychometric properties and found it had modest internal reliability (Cronbach's $\alpha = .75$).

Obtaining a Copy A published copy can be found in the original study conducted by Smith and colleagues [1].

Direct correspondence to:
S. Smith
Telephone: +617-3365-6408
Fax: +6173365-4466
Email: s.smith@psy.uq.edu.au

Scoring On a Likert-type scale, respondents are asked to indicate the extent to which they agree with certain statements. The scale ranges from 1 ("strongly agree") to 5 ("strongly disagree"), with half of the items worded negatively in order to prevent a response bias. To evaluate results, negative items are reversed and a total score is calculatead. Higher totals indicate more positive treatment beliefs and attitudes, which may be a marker of improved compliance.

A. Shahid et al. (eds.), *STOP, THAT and One Hundred Other Sleep Scales*,
DOI 10.1007/978-1-4419-9893-4_3, © Springer Science+Business Media, LLC 2012

ABS

Answer each of these questions by shading the number that best represents your answer.

①	②	③	④	⑤
Strongly disagree	Disagree	Not sure / neutral	Agree	Strongly agree

Sleep apnea has no effect on my life	① ② ③ ④ ⑤
If things become too much I generally don't go through with them	① ② ③ ④ ⑤
CPAP is "the answer" to my sleep apnea	① ② ③ ④ ⑤
Sleep apnea gets in the way of my friendships	① ② ③ ④ ⑤
I intend to use the CPAP machine all night every night.	① ② ③ ④ ⑤
I believe using the CPAP mask will be a nuisance	① ② ③ ④ ⑤
I am willing to ask for help when it is required	① ② ③ ④ ⑤
CPAP is the best treatment for my health problems	① ② ③ ④ ⑤
I am willing to follow the directions of medical staff "to the letter"	① ② ③ ④ ⑤
I believe that using CPAP is very confusing	① ② ③ ④ ⑤
Wearing the CPAP mask will make falling asleep hard	① ② ③ ④ ⑤
Once I make a decision, I stick with that decision	① ② ③ ④ ⑤
Wearing the CPAP mask will improve the quality of my sleep	① ② ③ ④ ⑤
I find it stressful to use new machinery or technology	① ② ③ ④ ⑤
Good health is secondary to being able to do what I want in life	① ② ③ ④ ⑤
I enjoy trying new things, like snorkelling	① ② ③ ④ ⑤
I don't believe I have a sleep problem	① ② ③ ④ ⑤
I find it embarrassing to ask for help	① ② ③ ④ ⑤
Sleep apnea is my major health problem	① ② ③ ④ ⑤
I believe that CPAP will make little difference to my sleep	① ② ③ ④ ⑤
I want to improve my health	① ② ③ ④ ⑤
I am confident that I will be able to use the CPAP machine as taught	① ② ③ ④ ⑤
I would try anything that I thought might help my sleep apnea	① ② ③ ④ ⑤
I believe that I know what is the best treatment for me	① ② ③ ④ ⑤

Reference

1. Smith, S. S., Lang, C. P., Sullivan, K. A., & Warren, J. (2004). Two new tools for assessing obstructive sleep apnea and continuous positive airway pressure therapy. *Sleep Medicine, 5*, 359–367.

Representative Studies Using Scale

Smith, S. S., Lang, C. P., Sullivan, K. A., & Warren, J. (2004). A preliminary investigation of the effectiveness of a sleep apnea education program. *Journal of Psychosomatic Research, 56*(2), 245–249.

4 Apnea Knowledge Test

Purpose A multiple-choice questionnaire designed to assess the respondent's knowledge of obstructive sleep apnea and Continuous Positive Airway Pressure (CPAP). Developed by Smith and colleagues [1], the questionnaire was initially intended to be administered before and after patient education programs. A significant difference between the knowledge scores achieved pre- and post-program would indicate an effective intervention. Though findings thus far have been inconclusive, the questionnaire's developers suggest that CPAP compliance may be related to patient knowledge and beliefs – a standardized tool for measuring education level will allow future studies to investigate this claim. For a similar tool, see the Apnea Beliefs Scale (Chap. 3).

Population for Testing No age range was specified by developers, but their study investigating the tool's psychometric properties used a sample of predominantly middle-aged (mean age, 52.6 ± 12.6 SD) obstructive sleep apnea patients. The test was found to be comprehensible at about a fourth grade reading level.

Administration Self-report, pencil-and-paper test. Requires 5–10 min for testing.

Reliability and Validity In an initial study evaluating the tool's psychometric properties, Smith et al. [1] found a low-to-modest internal consistency (Cronbach's $\alpha = .60$).

Obtaining a Copy A published copy can be found in the original study conducted by Smith and colleagues [1].

Direct correspondence to:
S. Smith
Telephone: +617-3365-6408
Fax: +617-3365-4466
Email: s.smith@psy.uq.edu.au

Scoring Correct responses on multiple-choice questions are given one point. For the two open-ended questions at the close of the test, respondents are awarded one point per correct element, allowing for a maximum of four points for question 16 and three points for question 17. Higher scores indicate a greater knowledge of obstructive sleep apnea and CPAP titration, while lower scores may suggest the need for educational intervention, particularly if later findings indicate a relationship between apnea-related knowledge and treatment outcomes. Until conclusive evidence has been found linking CPAP compliance to patient education, this tool is better suited to research purposes rather than clinical use.

A. Shahid et al. (eds.), *STOP, THAT and One Hundred Other Sleep Scales*,
DOI 10.1007/978-1-4419-9893-4_4, © Springer Science+Business Media, LLC 2012

Apnea Knowledge Test

1. The type of sleep apnea that causes a patient to forget to breathe is:

① central sleep apnea ② obstructive sleep apnea

③ mixed sleep apnea ④ none of the above

2. CPAP stands for:

① continues to push air past your nose ② closed passages and pressures

③ continuous positive airway pressure ④ central pauses and pressures

3. To diagnose sleep apnea, lab testing is usually held:

① in the morning ② at night

③ in the afternoon ④ none of the above

4. Air leakages can occur:

① from the mouth area ② into the eyes

③ from the nostril region ④ all of the above

5. The type of sleep apnea that is caused when air passages in or near the throat become blocked, is called:

① central sleep apnea ② obstructive sleep apnea

③ mixed sleep apnea ④ none of the above

6. CPAP works by:

① keeping your airways open ② administering medication to help you sleep

③ encouraging sleep at a subconscious level ④ none of the above

7. During the CPAP trial in hospital

① you will have to get up every hour to adjust the CPAP system ② you will be allowed to sleep as if at home, unattached to machines/computers

③ you will be asked to wear a CPAP mask ④ none of the above

8. What is (are) the general rule(s) sleep apnea patients should remember?

① reduce weight ② reduce alcohol intake

③ exercise more ④ all of the above

9. Possible problems with using the CPAP system include:

① blocked nose ② pressure sores

③ dry mouth ④ all of the above

10. CPAP equipment should be washed using

① bleach ② antiseptic solution

③ dishwashing detergent ④ all of the above

11. The mask and frame should be washed

① every morning	② every mouth
③ every week	④ when necessary

12. CPAP works best when used

① whenever you sleep	② every second night
③ every night	④ weekdays only

13. CPAP should NOT be used

① in winter	② when you have a head cold
③ in summer	④ none of the above

16. What is sleep apnea? ______________________________

17. Name three symptoms of sleep apnea? ______________________________

Reference

1. Smith, S. S., Lang, C. P., Sullivan, K. A., & Warren, J. (2004). Two new tools for assessing obstructive sleep apnea and continuous positive airway pressure therapy. *Sleep Medicine, 5*, 359–367.

Representative Studies Using Scale

Smith, S. S., Lang, C. P., Sullivan, K. A., & Warren, J. (2004). A preliminary investigation of the effectiveness of a sleep apnea education program. *Journal of Psychosomatic Research, 56*(2), 245–249.

Note: There are no items '14' and '15' in the original publication.

5 Athens Insomnia Scale (AIS)

Purpose The scale assesses the severity of insomnia using diagnostic criteria set forth by the International Classification of Diseases (ICD-10). The eight-item questionnaire evaluates sleep onset, night and early-morning waking, sleep time, sleep quality, frequency and duration of complaints, distress caused by the experience of insomnia, and interference with daily functioning. A shorter version of the questionnaire, consisting of the first five items alone, may also be used.

Population for Testing The instrument has been validated in patients with insomnia and with control participants aged 18–79 years.

Administration Requiring between 3 and 5 min for administration, the scale is a self-report, pencil-and-paper measure.

Reliability and Validity An initial study evaluating the psychometric properties of both the long and shorter versions of the scale [1] found an internal consistency ranging from .87 to .89 and a test-retest reliability of .88 – .89. In terms of the instrument's validity, results on the AIS correlated highly with scores obtained on the Sleep Problems Scale (.85–.90).

Obtaining a Copy A copy can be found in the developers' original article [1].

Direct correspondence to:
C.R. Soldatos
Eginition Hospital
72-74 Vas. Sophias Ave.
11528 Athens, Greece
Telephone: +30-301-7289324
Email: egslelabath@hol.gr

Scoring Respondents use Likert-type scales to show how severely certain sleep difficulties have affected them during the past month. Scores range from 0 (meaning that the item in question has not been a problem) to 3 (indicating more acute sleep difficulties). Developers Soldatos and colleagues [2] suggest a cutoff score of 6, which correctly distinguished between insomnia patients and controls in 90% of cases.

A. Shahid et al. (eds.), *STOP, THAT and One Hundred Other Sleep Scales*,
DOI 10.1007/978-1-4419-9893-4_5, © Springer Science+Business Media, LLC 2012

Athens Insomnia Scale

Instructions: This scale is intended to record your own assessment of any sleep difficulty you might have experienced. Please, check (by circling the appropriate number) the items below to indicate your estimate of any difficulty, provided that it occurred at least three times per week during the last month.

Sleep induction (time it takes you to fall asleep after turning-off the lights)
0: No problem 1: Slightly delayed 2: Markedly delayed 3: Very delayed or did not sleep at all

Awakenings during the night
0: No problem 1: Minor problem 2: Considerable problem 3: Serious problem or did not sleep all

Final awakening earlier than desired
0: Not earlier 1: A little earlier 2: Markedly earlier 3: Much earlier or did not sleep at all

Total sleep duration
0: Sufficient 1: Slightly insufficient 2: Markedly insufficient 3: Very insufficient or did not sleep at all

Overall quality of sleep (no matter how long you slept)
0: Satisfactory 1: Slightly unsatisfactory 2: Markedly unsatisfactory 3: Very unsatisfactory or did not sleep at all

Sense of well-being during the day
0: Normal 1: Slightly decreased 2: Markedly decreased 3: Very decreased

Functioning (physical and mental) during the day
0: Normal 1: Slightly decreased 2: Markedly decreased 3: Very decreased

Sleepiness during the day
0: None 1: Mild 2: Considerable 3: Intense

References

1. Soldatos, C. R., Dikeos, D.G., & Paparrigopoulos, T.J. (2000). Athens insomnia scale: validation of an instrument based on ICD-10 criteria. *Journal of Psychosomatic Research, 48*(6), 555–560.
2. Soldatos, C. R., Dimitris, G. D., & Paparrigopoulos, T.J. (2003). The diagnostic validity of the Athens insomnia scale. *Journal of Psychosomatic Research, 55*, 263–267.

Representative Studies Using Scale

Szelenberger, W., & Niemcewicz, S. (2000). Severity of insomnia correlates with cognitive impairment. *Acta Neurobiologiae Experimentalis, 60*(3), 373.

Novak, M., Molnar, M., Ambrus, C., Kovacs, A., Koczy, A., Remport, A., Szeifert, L., Szentkiralyi, A., Shapiro, C. M., Kopp, M. S., & Mucsi, I. (2006). Chronic insomnia in transplant recipients. *American Journal of Kidney Diseases, 47*(4), 655–665.

6 Basic Nordic Sleep Questionnaire (BNSQ)

Purpose A standardized questionnaire to assess a variety of sleep complaints, the BNSQ consists of 27 items in 21 different questions and queries a wide range of sleep complaints, including difficulties initiating and maintaining sleep, subjective sleep quality, the use of medication to induce sleep, excessive daytime sleepiness, napping, snoring, and general sleep habits [1].

Population for Testing The scale was designed for use with adults and has been applied to a variety of patient populations, ranging from young adults with asthma [2] to women undergoing menopause [3].

Administration The BNSQ is a self-report, measure requiring between 5 and 10 min for administration. The scale can be administered either by interview or using paper and pencil.

Reliability and Validity No reliability or validity data has been made available.

Obtaining a Copy A copy can be found in the original article published by Partinen and Gislason [1].

Direct correspondence to:
Markku Partinen
Department of Neurology, University of Helsinki
FIN00-290 Helsinki, Finland

Scoring The BNSQ incorporates a number of different question types, with most items scored on a scale ranging from 1 (indicating that the complaint is mild or infrequently present) to 5 (denoting a problem that occurs very frequently or severely). Other questions ask for specific durations or times, and these items should be interpreted differently depending on the researcher's purposes. As the scale's psychometric properties have not been evaluated, standard cutoff scores are not available and individual researchers and clinicians will need to decide how to apply results as they are obtained.

A. Shahid et al. (eds.), *STOP, THAT and One Hundred Other Sleep Scales*,
DOI 10.1007/978-1-4419-9893-4_6, © Springer Science+Business Media, LLC 2012

Basic Nordic Sleep Questionnaire

1. Have you had difficulties to fall asleep during the past three months?
   1 never or less than once per month
   2 less than once per week
   3 on 1-2 days per week
   4 on 3-5 days per week
   5 daily or almost daily

2. How long time (how many minutes as an average) do you stay awake in bed before you fall asleep (after lights off)?
   a. During working days: it takes about _____ minutes before I fall asleep
   b. During freetime: it takes about _____ minutes

3. How often have you awakened at night during the past three months?
   1 never or less than once per month
   2 less than once per week
   3 on 1-2 nights per week
   4 on 3-5 nights per week
   5 every night or almost every night

4. If you use to wake up during night, how many times do you usually wake up during one night (during the past three months)?
   1 usually I don't wake up at night
   2 once per night
   3 2 times
   4 3-4 times
   5 at least 5 times per night

5. How often have you awakened too early in the morning without being able to fall asleep again during the past three months?
   1 never or less than once per month
   2 less than once per week
   3 on 1-2 days per week
   4 on 3-5 days per week
   5 daily or almost daily

6. How well have you been sleeping during the past three months?
   1 well
   2 rather well
   3 neither well nor badly
   4 rather badly
   5 badly

7. Have you used some sleeping pills (by prescription) during the past three months?
   1 never or less than once per month
   2 less than once per week
   3 on 1-2 days per week
   4 on 3-5 days per week
   5 daily or almost daily

Which sleeping pill(s): ____

8. Do you feel excessively sleepy in the morning after awakening?
   1 never or less than once per month
   2 less than once per week
   3 on 1-2 days per week
   4 on 3-5 days per week
   5 daily or almost daily

9. Do you feel excessively sleepy during daytime?
   1 never or less than once per month
   2 less than once per week
   3 on 1-2 days per week
   4 on 3-5 days per week
   5 daily or almost daily

10. Have you suffered from irresistible tendency to fall asleep while <u>at work</u> during the past three months?
   1 never or less than once per month
   2 less than once per week
   3 on 1-2 days per week
   4 on 3-5 days per week
   5 daily or almost daily

11. Have you suffered from irresistible tendency to fall asleep during <u>free time</u> (leisure time) during the past three months?
   1 never or less than once per month
   2 less than once per week
   3 on 1-2 days per week
   4 on 3-5 days per week
   5 daily or almost daily

12. How many hours do you usually sleep per night?
   I sleep about ___ hours per night

13. At what time do you usually go to bed (in order to sleep)?
   a. during working week: at _____
   b. during free days: at _____

14. At what time do you usually wake up?
   a. during working week: at _____
   b. during free days: at _____

15a. How often to you sleep naps at daytime?
   1 never or less than once per month
   2 less than once per week
   3 on 1-2 days per week
   4 on 3-5 days per week
   5 daily or almost daily

15b. If you sleep a nap, how long does it usually last for?
   My naps usually last for about _____ h _____ min

(continued)

16. Do you snore while sleeping (ask other people if you are not sure)?
    1 never or less than once per month
    2 less than once per week
    3 on 1-2 days per week
    4 on 3-5 days per week
    5 daily or almost daily
17. How do you snore (ask other people about the quality of your snoring)?
    1 I don't snore
    2 My snoring sounds regular and it is of low voice
    3 It sounds regular but rather loud
    4 It sounds regular but it is very loud (other people hear my snoring in the next Room)
    5 I snore very loudly and intermittently (there are silent breathing pauses when snoring is not heard and at times very loud snorts with gasping)
18. Have you had breathing pauses (sleep apnea) at sleep (have other people noticed that you have pauses in respiration when you sleep)?
    1 never or less than once per month
    2 less than once per week
    3 on 1-2 days per week
    4 on 3-5 days per week
    5 daily or almost daily
19. If you snore at least 1-2 times per week, how many years have you been snoring (ask other people if you don't know)?
    I have been snoring for about _____years. I was about _____ years old when I Started to snore
20. How many hours of sleep do you need per night (how many hours would you sleep if you had possibility to sleep as long as you need to)?
    I need _____ hours and _____ min of sleep per night.
21. If you have problems with your sleep, what kind of problems do you have (describe your problems with your own words):

References

1. Partinen, M., & Gislason, T. (1995). Basic Nordic sleep questionnaire (BNSQ): a quantitated measure of subjective sleep complaints. *Journal of Sleep Research, 4*(S1), 150–155.
2. Janson, C., De Backer, W., Gislason, T., Plaschke, P., Bjornsson, E., Hetta, J., Kristbjarnarson, H., Vermeire, P., & Boman, G. (1996). Increased prevalence of sleep disturbances and daytime sleepiness in subjects with bronchial asthma: a population study of young adults in three European countries. *European Respiratory Journal, 9*, 2132–2138.
3. Sarti, C. D., Chiantera, A., Graziottin, A., Ognisanti, F., Sidoli, C., Mincigrucci, M., & Parazzini, F. (2005). Hormone therapy and sleep quality in women around menopause. *Menopause, 12*(5), 545–551.

Representative Studies Using Scale

Durán, J., Esnaola, S., Rubio, R., & Iztueta, Á. (2001). Obstructive sleep apnea-hypopnea and related clinical features in a population-based sample of subjects aged 30 to 70 yr. *American Journal of Respiratory and Critical Care Medicine, 163*(3), 685–689.

Budh, C. N., Hultling, C., & Lundeberg, T. (2005). Quality of sleep in individuals with spinal cord injury: a comparison between patients with and without pain. *Spinal Cord, 43*, 85–95.

7 BEARS Sleep Screening Tool

Purpose The BEARS is a quick 5-item screening tool to be used with children in a primary care setting. In order to make the instrument "user-friendly" for families and easy to remember for clinicians, each letter of the test's acronym represents one of the five items for query: Bedtime issues, Excessive daytime sleepiness, night Awakenings, Regularity and duration of sleep, and Snoring. Parents are asked about possible problems in each domain: a "yes" response prompts physicians to solicit further information (e.g., frequency and nature of problem). Though the tool is not likely to improve a clinician's ability to diagnose sleep difficulties in children, it has been shown to increase the amount of sleep information that physicians request from patients and families, improving the likelihood that disordered sleep will receive attention and treatment in a general care setting.

Population for Testing The survey is designed for use with children between the ages of 2 and 12.

Administration Delivered in a clinical interview format by a primary care physician, the test is not particularly structured and administration times will vary depending on specific patient needs.

Reliability and Validity Though not yet evaluated for its psychometric properties, the instrument has been shown to increase the amount of sleep information collected by physicians by a twofold to tenfold difference (Owens and Dalzell 2005).

Obtaining a Copy A published copy can be obtained in the original study conducted by Owens and Dalzell [1].

Direct correspondence to:
J.A. Owens
Telephone: 401 444-8280
Fax: 401 444-6218
Email: owensleep@aol.com

Scoring Results depend on the interpretation of trained clinicians – identified problems should be addressed with recommendations or referrals where appropriate.

A. Shahid et al. (eds.), *STOP, THAT and One Hundred Other Sleep Scales*,
DOI 10.1007/978-1-4419-9893-4_7, © Springer Science+Business Media, LLC 2012

BEARS Sleep Screening Tool

	Preschool (2-5 years)	School-aged (6-12 years)	Adolescent (13-18 years)
***B**edtime problems*	Does your child have any problems going to bed? Falling asleep?	Does your child have any problems at bedtime? (P) Do you have any problems going to bed? (C)	Do you have any problems falling asleep at bedtime? (C)
***E**xcessive daytime sleepiness*	Does your child seem over tired or sleepy a lot during the day? Does she still take Naps?	Does your child have difficulty waking in the morning, seem sleepy during the day or take naps? (P) Do you feel tired a lot? (C)	Do you feel sleepy a lot during the day? in school? while driving? (C)
***A**wakenings during the night*	Does your child wake up a lot at night?	Does your child seem to wake up a lot at night? Any sleepwalking or nightmares? (P) Do you wake up a lot at night? Have trouble getting back to sleep? (C)	Do you wake up a lot at night? Have trouble getting back to sleep? (C)
***R**egularity and duration of sleep*	Does your child have a regular bedtime and wake time? What are they?	What time does your child go to bed and get up on school days? weekends? Do you think s/he is getting enough sleep? (P)	What time do you usually go to bed on school nights? Weekends? How much sleep do you usually get? (C)
***S**leep-disordered Breathing*	Does your child snore a lot or have difficulty breathing at night?	Does your child have loud or nightly snoring or any breathing difficulties at night? (P)	Does your teenager snore loudly or or nightly? (P)

B bedtime problems; *E* excessive daytime sleepiness; *A* awakenings during the night; *R* regularity and duration of sleep; *S* sleep-disordered breathing; *P* Parent; *C* Child

Reference

1. Owens, J. A., & Dalzell, V. (2005). Use of the "BEARS" sleep screening tool in a pediatric residents' community clinic: a pilot study. *Sleep Medicine, 6*(1), 63–69.

Representative Studies Using Scale

Beebe, D. W. (2006). Neural and neurobehavioral dysfunction in children with obstructive sleep apnea. *PLoS Medicine, 3*(8), e323.

Valrie, C. R., Gil, K. M., Redding-Lallinger, R., & Daeschner, C. (2007). The influence of pain and stress on sleep in children with sickle cell disease. *Children's Health Care, 36*(4), 335–353.

Beck Depression Inventory

8

Purpose All three versions of the Beck Depression Inventory (BDI-I, BDI-IA, and BDI-II) are designed to rate the severity of respondents' depression in the weeks preceding questionnaire completion. Suited to both clinical and research populations, the 21-item instrument evaluates a variety of cognitive and physical symptoms of depression. One question in each version relates directly to sleep concerns: Question 16 asks respondents to indicate if they have experienced a recent disturbance in their sleeping habits. However, depression appears to be especially prevalent among patients diagnosed with sleep disorders; thus, some researchers have suggested that administration of a depression scale like the BDI should be a routine step in the diagnosis and treatment of sleep disorders [1]. The 28 items of the scale are drawn from the 111 items shown on the following pages.

Population for Testing Patients between 13 and 80 years of age.

Administration A self-report, paper-and-pencil format; the questionnaire can be completed by respondents unaided, or can be administered by interview. Requires 5–10 min for testing. The most recent version, the BDI-II, is particularly recommended for use with patients who may have sleeping difficulties, as it has been updated to reflect the fact that sleep can both increase and decrease as a result of depression.

Reliability and Validity On revising the original BDI, Beck and colleagues [2] performed a study analyzing the psychometric properties of the BDI-II and found an internal consistency of $\alpha=.91$.

Obtaining a Copy Published by Pearson
Authors: Aaron T. Beck, Robert A. Steer, & Gregory K. Brown
Visit the publisher's Web site at: http://pearson-assess.com/HAIWEB/Cultures/en-us/default

Scoring Each of the 21 questions presents four different statements and asks respondents to select the option that best represents them. Statements refer to depressive states in varying degrees of severity (from "I do not feel sad" to "I am so sad or unhappy that I can't stand it"), and this is reflected in the scoring process which

A. Shahid et al. (eds.), *STOP, THAT and One Hundred Other Sleep Scales*,
DOI 10.1007/978-1-4419-9893-4_8, © Springer Science+Business Media, LLC 2012

Beck Depression Inventory®–II (BDI®-II) Simulated Items

Unhappiness

0	I do not feel unhappy.
1	I feel unhappy.
2	I am unhappy.
3	I am so unhappy that I can't stand it.

Changes in Activity Level

0	I have not experienced any change in activity level.
1a	I am somewhat more active than usual.
1b	I am somewhat less active than usual.
2a	I am a lot more active than usual.
2b	I am a lot less active than usual.
3a	I am not active most of the day.
3b	I am active all of the day.

Information concerning the *BDI®-II* is available from:
NCS Pearson, Inc. Attn: Customer Service
19500 Bulverde Road San Antonio, TX 78259
Phone: (800) 627.7271 Fax: (800) 232-1223
Web site: www.psychcorp.com
Email: clinicalcustomersupport@pearson.com

assigns higher values to responses indicating more acute symptoms of depression.

References

1. Vandeputte, M., & de Weerd, A. (2003). Sleep disorders and depressive feelings: a global survey with the Beck depression scale. *Sleep Medicine, 4*(4), 343–345.
2. Beck, A. T., Steer, R. A., Ball, R., & Ranieri, W. F. (1996). Comparison of Beck depression inventories-IA and –II in psychiatric outpatients. *Journal of Personality Assessment, 67*(3), 588–597.

Representative Studies Using Scale

Beck, A. T., Brown, G., Berchick, R. J., Stewart, B. L., & Steer, R. A. (1990). Relationship between hopelessness and ultimate suicide: a replication with psychiatric outpatients. *American Journal of Psychiatry, 147*(2), 190–195.

Perlis, M. L., Giles, D. E., Buysse, D. J., Tu, X., & Kupfer, D. J. (1997). Self-reported sleep disturbance as a prodromal symptom in recurrent depression. *Journal of Affective Disorders, 42*(2–3), 209–212.

9 Behavioral Evaluation of Disorders of Sleep (BEDS)

Purpose Developed as a 28-item questionnaire, the BEDS scale evaluates the presence of four different types of sleep problems in elementary-school-aged children: expressive sleep disturbances (e.g., screaming, sleep-walking), sensitivity to the environment, disoriented awakening, and apnea/bruxism. As these factors do not necessarily relate to specific sleep disorder diagnoses, the tool is recommended by its developers for research purposes and not as "an instrument to replace a qualified clinical diagnosis" [1].

Population for Testing The scale has been validated for children between the ages of 5 and 12 years.

Administration A paper-and-pencil format, parents respond to a collection of descriptive statements based on their child's sleep behavior within the past 6 months. Requires between 5 and 10 min for administration.

Reliability and Validity Initial analyses conducted by Schreck and colleagues [1] demonstrated an internal consistency of $\alpha = .82$.

Obtaining a Copy A published copy can be found by contacting the authors.

Direct correspondence to:
Kimberly A. Schreck, Penn State University
777 W Harrisburg Pike
Middletown, PA 17057, USA
Email: kas24@psu.edu

Scoring Parents are asked to use a five-point scale to rate the frequency of certain sleep behaviors exhibited by their child (0 is "never," while 5 is "always"). Higher scores indicate more severe sleep issues.

A. Shahid et al. (eds.), *STOP, THAT and One Hundred Other Sleep Scales*,
DOI 10.1007/978-1-4419-9893-4_9, © Springer Science+Business Media, LLC 2012

BEDS 1

Behavioral Evaluation of Disorders of Sleep

Child's name: ______________________
Age: ________ *Sex*: ________
Parent's Name: ______________________
Date Completed ________________

BEDS Scores

	Score	Mean	Standard Dev.
Expressive Awakening		1.57	3.39
Sensitivity to the Environment		4.31	3.84
Disoriented Awakening		4.15	3.28
Apnea		.22	.74
Total Score		11.45	8.63

BEDS 2

Instructions for completing the BEDS

Please answer the following statements about how often the child you care for does or has done the following behaviors in the last six months. If the child never experiences the sleep problem, circle "0". If the child always experiences the problem, circle "4". If the statement does not apply, answer "0".

(0) Never (1) Rarely (2) Sometimes (3) Frequently (4) Always

My child:

0 1 2 3 4 1. wakes up screaming during the night for more than 1 minute
0 1 2 3 4 2. is sluggish when awakened
0 1 2 3 4 3. sleeps more than other children his/her age
0 1 2 3 4 4. is disoriented when awakened
0 1 2 3 4 5. has trouble falling asleep
0 1 2 3 4 6. has a sudden leg jerk when falling asleep
0 1 2 3 4 7. plays with toys in bedroom at bed time
0 1 2 3 4 8. has headaches
0 1 2 3 4 9. can't move body when waking up or going to sleep
0 1 2 3 4 10. doesn't remember crying or screaming during the night
0 1 2 3 4 11. gets less than 6 hours sleep in a 24 hour period
0 1 2 3 4 12. complains that bed is uncomfortable
0 1 2 3 4 13. plays video games less than 1 hour before going to bed
0 1 2 3 4 14. sleeps in my room now

0 1 2 3 4 15. watches horror and/or action movies/TV show before bed
0 1 2 3 4 16. wakes up screaming during the night and cannot be calmed down
0 1 2 3 4 17. engages in violent behaviors while asleep (hits, kicks, punches, tackles)
0 1 2 3 4 18. takes frequent naps during the day
0 1 2 3 4 19. stops breathing during sleep
0 1 2 3 4 20. needs me to read before falling asleep
0 1 2 3 4 21. takes a day to "catch-up" on sleep
0 1 2 3 4 22. needs something to eat before falling asleep
0 1 2 3 4 23. can not be awakened when sleep walking
0 1 2 3 4 24. needs a night light to fall asleep
0 1 2 3 4 25. sleeps better in a place other than own bed
0 1 2 3 4 26. talks in sleep without knowing it
0 1 2 3 4 27. complains of jaw pain
0 1 2 3 4 28. requires medicine to help sleep
0 1 2 3 4 29. has no problem sleeping, when it is quiet outside
0 1 2 3 4 30. will stay in bed unless I get him/her up
0 1 2 3 4 31. has frequent skin rashes
0 1 2 3 4 32. is sleepy during the day

BEDS 3

(0) Never (1) Rarely (2) Sometimes (3) Frequently (4) Always

0 1 2 3 4 33. sleeps longer or shorter on weekends than weekdays
0 1 2 3 4 34. complains that room is not dark enough to sleep
0 1 2 3 4 35. wakes up screaming and sweating during the night
0 1 2 3 4 36. needs a pacifier to fall asleep
0 1 2 3 4 37. walks in sleep
0 1 2 3 4 38. goes to bed at different times
0 1 2 3 4 39. has nightmares
0 1 2 3 4 40. acts out dreams
0 1 2 3 4 41. screams during the 2nd half of the night
0 1 2 3 4 42. wakes up crying at night
0 1 2 3 4 43. watches TV in bedroom
0 1 2 3 4 44. wakes up screaming approximately two hours after going to sleep
0 1 2 3 4 45. drinks soda/caffeine before bed
0 1 2 3 4 46. rocks body in sleep
0 1 2 3 4 47. has problems/been upset since a new adult moved into the home
0 1 2 3 4 48. sleep walks about 2 hours after going to sleep
0 1 2 3 4 49. does homework less than 1 hour before going to bed or in bed
0 1 2 3 4 50. has problems/been upset since a divorce or separation in the family
0 1 2 3 4 51. eats 1 hour before going to sleep
0 1 2 3 4 52. sees flashes of light when first going to sleep
0 1 2 3 4 53. does not remember walking in sleep
0 1 2 3 4 54. slept in my room as an infant
0 1 2 3 4 55. is afraid of falling, at bedtime
0 1 2 3 4 56. bangs head in sleep
0 1 2 3 4 57. stalls at bedtime
0 1 2 3 4 58. exercises before bed
0 1 2 3 4 59. looks at books or reads in bed
0 1 2 3 4 60. seems depressed
0 1 2 3 4 61. complains that room is uncomfortable
0 1 2 3 4 62. has problems/been upset since moving to a new home or school
0 1 2 3 4 63. wakes up during violent behaviors
0 1 2 3 4 64. throws temper tantrums at bedtime
0 1 2 3 4 65. has problems/been upset since the death of a family member, friend, or pet
0 1 2 3 4 66. frequently has an upset stomach
0 1 2 3 4 67. rocks head in sleep
0 1 2 3 4 68. wets bed
0 1 2 3 4 69. is not awake when screaming at night

(continued)

BEDS 4

(0) Never (1) Rarely (2) Sometimes (3) Frequently (4) Always

0 1 2 3 4	70. sleeps worse after eating certain foods/beverages
0 1 2 3 4	71. is irritable
0 1 2 3 4	72. reacts slowly when awakened
0 1 2 3 4	73. will sleep for 6 hours or longer at a time
0 1 2 3 4	74. cries easily
0 1 2 3 4	75. needs something to drink before falling asleep
0 1 2 3 4	76. is awakened by loud noises (trains, traffic, etc.)
0 1 2 3 4	77. speaks slowly when awakened
0 1 2 3 4	78. chooses own bedtime
0 1 2 3 4	79. is under emotional stress
0 1 2 3 4	80. is sad
0 1 2 3 4	81. complains of aches, pains, or sore eyes
0 1 2 3 4	82. has difficulty breathing during sleep
0 1 2 3 4	83. wakes up screaming in the 2nd half of the night
0 1 2 3 4	84. is afraid of noises in the night
0 1 2 3 4	85. actively plays before bed
0 1 2 3 4	86. sleeps in inappropriate places
0 1 2 3 4	87. grinds teeth at night
0 1 2 3 4	88. takes medicine during the day that makes him/her sleep worse
0 1 2 3 4	89. wakes up during the night to eat
0 1 2 3 4	90. needs to rock to sleep
0 1 2 3 4	91. seems anxious or scared
0 1 2 3 4	92. needs a toy, stuffed animal or doll to go to sleep
0 1 2 3 4	93. needs a blanket to fall asleep
0 1 2 3 4	94. sleeps poorly without medicine at night
0 1 2 3 4	95. is afraid to fall asleep
0 1 2 3 4	96. takes naps without being told
0 1 2 3 4	97. snores
0 1 2 3 4	98. eats in bed
0 1 2 3 4	99. has a new sibling
0 1 2 3 4	100. sleeps less than other children his/her age
0 1 2 3 4	101. drinks more than 1 glass of water awakening
0 1 2 3 4	102. teeth are smooth
0 1 2 3 4	103. falls asleep before being put to bed
0 1 2 3 4	104. rubs eyes
0 1 2 3 4	105. becomes pale or blue during sleep
0 1 2 3 4	106. is limp or stiff during sleep
0 1 2 3 4	107. sleeps on a mattress that is less than 3 inches thick

BEDS 5

Supplementary Questions

108. How many hours does your child typically sleep per night? ____________________

109. How many hours has your child slept in the last 24 hours? ____________________

110. How many hours does your child typically nap during the day? ____________________

111. Do you think your child has a sleeping problem? YES NO

Reference

1. Schreck, K. A., Mulick, J. A., & Rojahn, J. (2003). Development of the behavioral evaluation of disorders of sleep scale. *Journal of Child and Family Studies, 12*(3), 349–359.

Representative Studies Using Scale

Polimeni, M. A., Richdale, A. L., & Francis, A. J. P. (2005). A survey of sleep problems in autism, Asperger's disorder and typically developing children. *Journal of Intellectual Disability Research,* 49(4), 260–268.

Schreck, K. A., Mulick, J. A., & Smith, A. F. (2004). Sleep problems as possible predictors of intensified symptoms of autism. *Research in Developmental Disabilities,* 25(1), 57–66.

10 Berlin Questionnaire

Purpose Designed to identify individuals at high risk for sleep apnea, the short survey (11 questions) focuses on three categories of apnea signs and symptoms: snoring, daytime sleepiness, and obesity/high blood pressure. The instrument may be indicated for use in both research, and as a screening tool for clinicians hoping to quickly establish apnea risk factors in their patients.

Population for Testing Validated in patients 18 years old and over.

Administration Questions are self-reported in a paper-and-pencil format: Administration should require about 5–10 min, though possibly longer as blood pressure may need to be taken and recent weight and height measurements are necessary for the calculation of body mass index. For a similar measure, see the STOP-Bang (Chap. 91).

Reliability and Validity A number of studies have examined the psychometric properties of the instrument, and findings suggest that the kind of patient population being examined has some bearing on the sensitivity and efficacy of the measure. Though Chung and colleagues [1] found the tool to be moderately sensitive in a surgical patient population, a second study examining patients at a sleep clinic [2] discovered a sensitivity of only 62%, making it unlikely to benefit clinicians during diagnosis. In almost all of the literature, the tool appears to be more valuable when apnea is moderate or severe.

Obtaining a Copy A number of adapted versions are available without copyright. See the original article [3] and that published by Chung and colleagues [1].

Scoring As the scoring process tends to be rather complex in comparison to other apnea scales, the instrument is often recommended for use by sleep specialists or individuals with similarly relevant training. The survey evaluates "yes or no" responses and multiple-choice selections, and includes space for calculating Body Mass Index (BMI) based on respondent measurements. Points are given to responses that indicate more acute symptoms. For "yes or no" questions, one point is given to an answer of "yes." In the case of multiple-choice questions, the two answers that correspond with the highest severity of apnea both receive one point. Categories one and two are considered high risk if the individual receives two or more points. Category three questions (obesity and blood pressure). The respondent is considered high risk when blood pressure is found to be high or when BMI is greater than 30 kg/m^2.

A. Shahid et al. (eds.), *STOP, THAT and One Hundred Other Sleep Scales*,
DOI 10.1007/978-1-4419-9893-4_10, © Springer Science+Business Media, LLC 2012

BERLIN QUESTIONNAIRE

Height (m) ________ Weight (kg)________ Age______ Male / Female

Please choose the correct response to each question.

CATEGORY 1

1. Do you snore?

☐ a. Yes
☐ b. No
☐ c. Don't know

If you snore:

2. Your snoring is:

☐ a. Slightly louder than breathing
☐ b. As loud as talking
☐ c. Louder than talking
☐ d. Very loud – can be heard in adjacent rooms

3. How often do you snore

☐ a. Nearly every day
☐ b. 3-4 times a week
☐ c. 1-2 times a week
☐ d. 1-2 times a month
☐ e. Never or nearly never

4. Has your snoring ever bothered other people?

☐ a. Yes
☐ b. No
☐ c. Don't Know

5. Has anyone noticed that you quit breathing during your sleep?

☐ a. Nearly every day
☐ b. 3-4 times a week
☐ c. 1-2 times a week
☐ d. 1-2 times a month
☐ e. Never or nearly never

CATEGORY 2

6. How often do you feel tired or fatigued after you sleep?

☐ a. Nearly every day
☐ b. 3-4 times a week
☐ c. 1-2 times a week
☐ d. 1-2 times a month
☐ e. Never or nearly never

7. During your waking time, do you feel tired, fatigued or not up to par?

☐ a. Nearly every day
☐ b. 3-4 times a week
☐ c. 1-2 times a week
☐ d. 1-2 times a month
☐ e. Never or nearly never

8. Have you ever nodded off or fallen asleep while driving a vehicle?

☐ a. Yes
☐ b. No

If yes:

9. How often does this occur?

☐ a. Nearly every day
☐ b. 3-4 times a week
☐ c. 1-2 times a week
☐ d. 1-2 times a month
☐ e. Never or nearly never

CATEGORY 3

10. Do you have high blood pressure?

☐ Yes
☐ No
☐ Don't know

Please mark "X" as appropriate:	Almost Daily	Often	Rarely	Not at all
Do you typically awaken with a dry mouth?	☐	☐	☐	☐
Do you typically awaken with a sore throat?	☐	☐	☐	☐
Do you drool on your pillow during the night?	☐	☐	☐	☐
Men: Do you have problems with penile erections (i.e. impotence)?	☐	☐	☐	☐
Do you frequently awaken during the night to void urine?	☐	☐	☐	☐
Do you experience frequent heartburn or reflux during the night?	☐	☐	☐	☐
Do you wake up with headaches in the morning?	☐	☐	☐	☐
Did you ever have a fractured jaw, broken nose or oral problems?	☐	☐	☐	☐
Have you ever done heavy exercise or manual labour?	☐	☐	☐	☐

References

1. Chung, F., Yegneswaran, B, Liao, P, Chung, S. A., Vairavanathan, S., Islam, S., Khajehdehi, A., Shapiro, C. (2008). Validation of the Berlin questionnaire and American Society of Anesthesiologists checklist as screening tools for obstructive sleep apnea in surgical patients. *Anesthesiology, 108*(5), 822–830.
2. Ahmadi, N., Chung, S. A., Gibbs, A., & Shapiro, C. (2008).The Berlin questionnaire for sleep apnea in a sleep clinic population: relationship to polysomnographic measurement of respiratory disturbance. *Sleep and Breathing, 12*(1), 39–45.
3. Netzer NC, Stoohs RA, Netzer CM, Clark K, Strohl KP (1999). Using the Berlin Questionnaire to identify patients at risk for the sleep apnea syndrome. *Ann Intern Med*, 131(7):485–491.

Representative Studies Using Scale

Chung, F., Ward, B., Ho, J., Yuan, H., Kayumov, L., & Shapiro, C. (2007). Preoperative identification of sleep apnea risk in elective surgical patients, using the Berlin questionnaire. *Journal of Clinical Anesthesia, 19*(2), 130–134.

Hiestand, D. M., Britz, P., Goldman, M., & Phillips, B. (2006). Prevalence of symptoms of obstructive sleep apnea in the US population: results from the National Sleep Foundation sleep in America 2005 poll. *Chest, 130*(3), 780–786.

11 Brief Fatigue Inventory

Purpose The instrument is used to quickly assess the severity of fatigue experienced by cancer patients, as well as its impact on their ability to function over the previous 24 h. It can be administered in a clinical setting as part of patient screening processes, and may also be useful for clinical trials. As a short scale that can be rapidly administered and easily understood, the BFI is designed to be well tolerated by patients suffering even the most severe degrees of fatigue.

Population for Testing Patients experiencing fatigue as a result of cancer and cancer treatment.

Administration A pencil-and-paper scale, patients provide self-report ratings either orally through an interview, or in written form. With only nine items, the instrument was designed to be completed rapidly and relatively painlessly. Approximately 2–3 min should be sufficient for administration.

Reliability and Validity Following instrument development, Mendoza and colleagues [1] conducted a study to evaluate the scale's psychometric properties. To find concurrent validity, they compared BFI to two previously validated fatigue scales: the Fatigue Assessment of Cancer Therapy ($r=0.88$, $p<.001$) and the Profile of Mood States ($r=0.84$, $p<.001$). Internal consistency was measured as Cronbach's $\alpha=.96$.

Obtaining a Copy A published copy can be found in an article by Mendoza and colleagues [1].

Direct correspondence to:
Charles S. Cleeland, Ph.D.
Pain Research Group
Box 221, 1100 Holcombe Blvd.
Houston, TX 77030, USA

Scoring Respondents rate each item on a 0–10 numeric scale, with 0 meaning "no fatigue" and 10 meaning "fatigue as bad as you can imagine." Scores are categorized as Mild (1–3), Moderate (4–6), and Severe (7–10). Finally, a global fatigue score can be found by averaging the score obtained on each test item.

A. Shahid et al. (eds.), *STOP, THAT and One Hundred Other Sleep Scales*,
DOI 10.1007/978-1-4419-9893-4_11, © Springer Science+Business Media, LLC 2012

Brief Fatigue Inventory

STUDY ID# ____________ HOSPITAL # ____________

Date: ____/____/____ Time: ____________

Name ______________ ______________ ______________
Last First Middle Initial

Throughout our lives, most of us have times when we feel very tired or fatigued. Have you felt unusually tired or fatigued in the last week? Yes ☐ No ☐

1. Please rate your fatigue (weariness, tiredness) by circling the one number that best describes your fatigue right NOW.

0 1 2 3 4 5 6 7 8 9 10
No Fatigue — As bad as you can imagine

2. Please rate your fatigue (weariness, tiredness) by circling the one number that best describes your USUAL level of fatigue during past 24 hours.

0 1 2 3 4 5 6 7 8 9 10
No Fatigue — As bad as you can imagine

3. Please rate your fatigue (weariness, tiredness) by circling the one number that best describes your WORST level of fatigue during past 24 hours.

0 1 2 3 4 5 6 7 8 9 10
No Fatigue — As bad as you can imagine

4. Circle the one number that describes how, during the past 24 hours, fatigue has interfered with your:

A. General activity
0 1 2 3 4 5 6 7 8 9 10
Does not interfere — Completely Interferes

B. Mood
0 1 2 3 4 5 6 7 8 9 10
Does not interfere — Completely Interferes

C. Walking ability
0 1 2 3 4 5 6 7 8 9 10
Does not interfere — Completely Interferes

D. Normal work (includes both work outside the home and daily chores)
0 1 2 3 4 5 6 7 8 9 10
Does not interfere — Completely Interferes

E. Relations with other people
0 1 2 3 4 5 6 7 8 9 10
Does not interfere — Completely Interferes

F. Enjoyment of life
0 1 2 3 4 5 6 7 8 9 10
Does not interfere — Completely Interferes

Reference

1. Mendoza, T. R., Wang, X. S., Cleeland, C. S., Morrissey, M., Johnson, B. A., Wendt, J. K., & Huber, S. L. (1999). The rapid assessment of fatigue severity in cancer patients. *Cancer, 85*(5), 1186–1196.

Representative Studies Using Scale

Anderson, K.O., Getto, C. J., Mendoza, C. R., Palmer, S. N., Wang, X. S., Reyes-Gibby, C. C., & Cleeland, C. S. (2003). Fatigue and sleep disturbance in patients with cancer, patients with clinical depression, and community-dwelling adults. *Journal of Pain and Symptom Management, 25*(4), 307–318.

Dimeo, F., Schwartz, S., Wesel, N., Voigt, A., & Thiel, E. (2008). Effects of an endurance and resistance exercise program on persistent cancer-related fatigue after treatment. *Annals of Oncology, 19*(8), 1495–1499.

Brief Infant Sleep Questionnaire (BISQ)

12

Purpose The instrument is intended to serve as a screening tool in a variety of pediatric settings. Consisting of only a few items, the survey asks parents about their child's sleeping location, position, and schedule during the past week. The tool can be used for both clinical and research purposes.

Population for Testing The test is designed for infants between 0 and 3 years of age.

Administration Completion of the pencil-and-paper form should require about 5–10 min, and is performed by the child's parent or guardian.

Reliability and Validity Sadeh [1] conducted a study in which high test-retest correlations were found (r>.82). Additionally, items asking about number of night-wakings and nocturnal sleep duration both appear to be especially relevant to assessing differences between clinical and control groups: Based on these measures, participants were assigned to the correct group at a rate of 85%.

Obtaining a Copy A published copy can be found in an article by Sadeh [1].

Direct correspondence to:
Avi Sadeh, Department of Psychology –
Tel Aviv University Ramat Aviv,
Tel Aviv 69978,
Israel
Email: sadeh@post.tau.ac.il

Scoring Based on comparative analyses performed between the BISQ and other infant sleep measures, developer Sadeh [1] suggests several clinical cutoffs: If the child wakes more than three times a night, spends more than 1 h in wakefulness each night, or receives less than 9 h of sleep during each 24-h period, a further clinical referral should be considered.

Reference

1. Sadeh, A. (2004). A brief screening questionnaire for infant sleep problems: validation and findings for an internet sample. *Pediatrics, 113*(6), e570–e577.

Representative Studies Using Scale

Mindell, J. A., Telofski, L. S., Wiegand, B., & Kurtz, E. S. (2009). A nightly bedtime routine: impact on sleep in young children and maternal mood. *Sleep, 32*(5), 599–606.

A. Shahid et al. (eds.), *STOP, THAT and One Hundred Other Sleep Scales*,
DOI 10.1007/978-1-4419-9893-4_12, © Springer Science+Business Media, LLC 2012

13 Brief Pain Inventory (BPI)

Purpose Given the bidirectional link between sleep and pain, we have included this instrument. Both long and short versions of the BPI have been developed, with the long version including additional descriptive items that may help with assessment. The shorter version consists of 12 items that assess two factors: the severity of pain and its impact on daily life. The severity factor queries current symptoms, symptoms on average, and the range of pain intensity that they experience. The impact factor asks respondents how pain interferes with their general activity, mood, mobility, work, relationships, sleep, and enjoyment of life.

Population for Testing The BPI has been designed for use with adults, and has been validated for the assessment of pain in a variety of patient populations including those with cancer [1] and individuals with arthritis and lower back pain [2].

Administration The scale is a self-report measure that can be administered by interview or by paper and pencil. It requires approximately 5 min for completion.

Reliability and Validity Several studies have been conducted to evaluate the psychometric properties of the BPI. In a study of surgical cancer patients, Tittle and colleagues [1] found an internal reliability ranging from .95 to .97. Similarly, Keller and colleagues [2] have demonstrated that the scale possesses an internal reliability ranging from .82 to .95 in patients with lower back pain and arthritis. Additionally, researchers found that scores on the BPI were highly correlated with scores on other condition-specific scales and were sensitive to changes in health [3].

Obtaining a Copy The scale is under copyright and can be obtained through The University of Texas MD Anderson Cancer Center.
Web site: http://www.mdanderson.org/education-and-research/departments-programs-and-labs/departments-and-divisions/symptom-research/symptom-assessment-tools/brief-pain-inventory.html

Scoring Patients are asked to rate their current symptoms, their average experiences of pain, and the minimum and maximum intensities of their symptoms on scales that range from 0 to 10. A total pain severity score can be found by averaging these items or a single item can be treated as the primary outcome measure. A score relating to impact on daily life can be calculated by averaging scores on each of the seven items, which also use scales from 0 to 10. Higher scores indicate greater severity and more interference.

A. Shahid et al. (eds.), *STOP, THAT and One Hundred Other Sleep Scales*,
DOI 10.1007/978-1-4419-9893-4_13, © Springer Science+Business Media, LLC 2012

PROTOCOL # ____________ INSTITUTION ____________

PATIENT SEQUENCE # ____________ HOSPITAL CHART # ____________

DO NOT WRITE ABOVE THIS LINE

Brief Pain Inventory

Date: ___/___/___

Name: ____________ Last ____________ First ____________ Middle Initial

Phone: (___) ____________ Sex: ☐ Female ☐ Male

Date of Birth: ___/___/___

1) Marital Status (at present)

1. ☐ Single
2. ☐ Married
3. ☐ Widowed
4. ☐ Separated/Divorced

2) Education (Circle only the highest grade or degree completed)

Grade	0	1	2	3	4	5	6	7	8	9
	10	11	12	13	14	15	16	M.A./M.S.		

Professional degree (please specify) ____________

3) Current occupation ____________
(specify titles; if you are not working, tell us your previous occupation)

4) Spouse's occupation ____________

5) Which of the following best describes your current job status?

1. ☐ Employed outside the home, full-time
2. ☐ Employed outside the home, part-time
3. ☐ Homemaker
4. ☐ Retired
5. ☐ Unemployed
6. ☐ Other

6) How long has it been since you first learned your diagnosis? ______ months

7) Have you ever had pain due to your present disease?

1. ☐ Yes
2. ☐ No
3. ☐ Uncertain

8) When you first received your diagnosis, was pain one of your symptoms?

1. ☐ Yes 2. ☐ No 3. ☐ Uncertain

9) Have you had surgery in the past month? 1. ☐ Yes 2. ☐ No

If YES, what kind? ____________________

10) Throughout our lives, most of us have had pain from time to time (such as minor headaches, sprains, toothaches). Have you had pain other than these everyday kinds of pain during the last week?

1. ☐ Yes 2. ☐ No

10a) Did you take pain medications in the last 7 days?

1. ☐ Yes 2. ☐ No

10b) I feel I have some form of pain now that requires medication each and every day.

1. ☐ Yes 2. ☐ No

IF YOUR ANSWERS TO 10, 10a, AND 10b WERE ALL NO, PLEASE STOP HERE AND GO TO THE LAST PAGE OF THE QUESTIONNAIRE AND SIGN WHERE INDICATED ON THE BOTTOM OF THE PAGE.
IF ANY OF YOUR ANSWERS TO 10, 10a, AND 10b WERE YES, PLEASE CONTINUE.

11) On the diagram, shade in the areas where you feel pain. Put an X on the area that hurts the most.

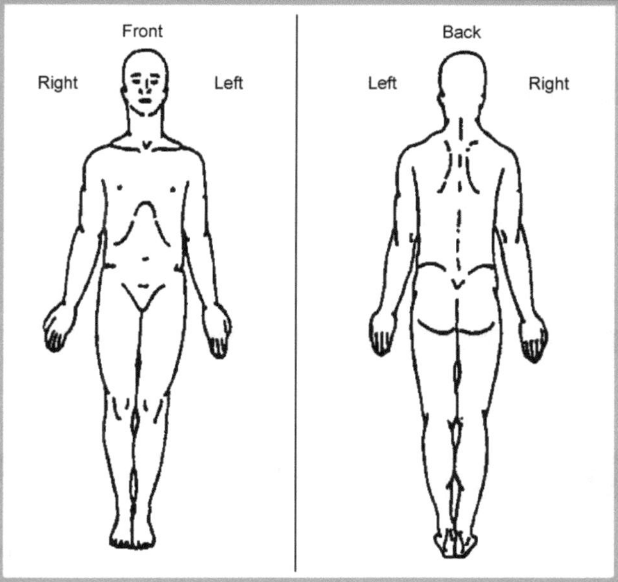

12) Please rate your pain by circling the one number that best describes your pain at its **worst** in the last week.

0	1	2	3	4	5	6	7	8	9	10
No Pain										Pain as bad as you can imagine

13) Please rate your pain by circling the one number that best describes your pain at its **least** in the last week.

0	1	2	3	4	5	6	7	8	9	10
No Pain										Pain as bad as you can imagine

14) Please rate your pain by circling the one number that best describes your pain on the **average.**

0	1	2	3	4	5	6	7	8	9	10
No Pain										Pain as bad as you can imagine

15) Please rate your pain by circling the one number that tells how much pain you have **right now.**

0	1	2	3	4	5	6	7	8	9	10
No Pain										Pain as bad as you can imagine

16) What kinds of things make your pain feel better (for example, heat, medicine, rest)?

____

____

17) What kinds of things make your pain worse (for example, walking, standing, lifting)?

____

____

18) What treatments or medications are you receiving for pain?

____

____

19) In the last week, how much relief have pain treatments or medications provided? Please circle the one percentage that most shows how much relief you have received.

0%	10%	20%	30%	40%	50%	60%	70%	80%	90%	100%
No Relief										Complete Relief

20) If you take pain medication, how many hours does it take before the pain returns?

1. ☐ Pain medication doesn't help at all
2. ☐ One hour
3. ☐ Two hours
4. ☐ Three hours
5. ☐ Four hours
6. ☐ Five to twelve hours
7. ☐ More than twelve hours
8. ☐ I do not take pain medication

**21) Check the appropriate answer for each item.
I believe my pain is due to:**

☐ Yes ☐ No 1. The effects of treatment (for example, medication, surgery, radiation, prosthetic device).

☐ Yes ☐ No 2. My primary disease (meaning the disease currently being treated and evaluated).

☐ Yes ☐ No 3. A medical condition unrelated to my primary disease (for example, arthritis).
Please describe condition: ______________________

22) For each of the following words, check Yes or No if that adjective applies to your pain.

Aching	☐ Yes	☐ No
Throbbing	☐ Yes	☐ No
Shooting	☐ Yes	☐ No
Stabbing	☐ Yes	☐ No
Gnawing	☐ Yes	☐ No
Sharp	☐ Yes	☐ No
Tender	☐ Yes	☐ No
Burning	☐ Yes	☐ No
Exhausting	☐ Yes	☐ No
Tiring	☐ Yes	☐ No
Penetrating	☐ Yes	☐ No
Nagging	☐ Yes	☐ No
Numb	☐ Yes	☐ No
Miserable	☐ Yes	☐ No
Unbearable	☐ Yes	☐ No

23) Circle the one number that describes how, during the past week, pain has interfered with your:

A. General Activity

0	1	2	3	4	5	6	7	8	9	10
Does not interfere										Completely interferes

B. Mood

0	1	2	3	4	5	6	7	8	9	10
Does not interfere										Completely interferes

C. Walking Ability

0	1	2	3	4	5	6	7	8	9	10
Does not interfere										Completely interferes

D. Normal Work (includes both work outside the home and housework)

0	1	2	3	4	5	6	7	8	9	10
Does not interfere										Completely interferes

E. Relations with other people

0	1	2	3	4	5	6	7	8	9	10
Does not interfere										Completely interferes

F. Sleep

0	1	2	3	4	5	6	7	8	9	10
Does not interfere										Completely interferes

G. Enjoyment of life

0	1	2	3	4	5	6	7	8	9	10
Does not interfere										Completely interferes

24) I prefer to take my pain medicine:

1. ☐ On a regular basis
2. ☐ Only when necessary
3. ☐ Do not take pain medicine

25) I take my pain medicine (in a 24 hour period):

1. ☐ Not every day
2. ☐ 1 to 2 times per day
3. ☐ 3 to 4 times per day
4. ☐ 5 to 6 times per day
5. ☐ More than 6 times per day

26) Do you feel you need a stronger type of pain medication?

1. ☐ Yes 2. ☐ No 3. ☐ Uncertain

27) Do you feel you need to take more of the pain medication than your doctor has prescribed?

1. ☐ Yes 2. ☐ No 3. ☐ Uncertain

28) Are you concerned that you use too much pain medication?

1. ☐ Yes 2. ☐ No 3. ☐ Uncertain

If Yes, why? ______________________________

____

29) Are you having problems with side effects from your pain medication?

1. ☐ Yes 2. ☐ No

Which side effects? ______________________________

30) Do you feel you need to receive further information about your pain medication?

1. ☐ Yes 2. ☐ No

31) Other methods I use to relieve my pain include: (Please check all that apply)

Warm compresses ☐	Cold compresses ☐	Relaxation techniques ☐
Distraction ☐	Biofeedback ☐	Hypnosis ☐
Other ☐	Please specify ______________________________	

32) Medications not prescribed by my doctor that I take for pain are:

____

____

Please sign the back of this questionnaire.

Patient's Signature ______________________________

Thank you for your participation.

References

1. Tittle, M. B., McMillan, S. C., & Hagan, S. (2003). Validating the brief pain inventory for use with surgical patients with cancer. *Oncology Nursing Forum, 30*(2), 325–330.
2. Keller, S., Bann, C. M., Dodd, S. L., Schein, J., & Mendoza, T. R. (2004). Validity of the brief pain inventory for use in documenting the outcomes of patients with noncancer pain. *Clinical Journal of Pain, 20*(5), 309–318.
3. Tan, G., Jensen, M. P., Thornby, J. I., & Shanti, B. F. (2004). Validation of the brief pain inventory for chronic nonmalignant pain. *Journal of Pain, 5*(2), 133–137.

Representative Studies Using Scale

Beck, S. L., Dudley, W. N., Barsevick, A. (2005). Pain, sleep disturbance, and fatigue in patients with cancer: using a mediation model to test a symptom cluster. *Oncology Nursing Forum, 32*(3), E48–E55.

Davison, S. N., & Jhangri, G. S. (2005). The impact of chronic pain on depression, sleep, and the desire to withdraw from dialysis in hemodialysis patients. *Journal of Pain and Symptom Management, 30*(5), 465–473.

Calgary Sleep Apnea Quality of Life Index (SAQLI)

14

Purpose A 35-item, interview-administered scale, the SAQLI evaluates four domains of quality of life associated with sleep apnea: daily functioning, social interactions, emotional functioning, and symptoms. A fifth domain – treatment-related symptoms – was developed for use with individuals currently undergoing therapeutic intervention. With its excellent responsiveness to change, the scale is ideal for monitoring the effectiveness of different apnea treatments.

Population for Testing In a validation study conducted by developers Flemons and Reimer [1], participants had a mean age of 52.1 years ± 10.4.

Administration The scale is a self-report measure intended for administration by a trained interviewer. Time requirements for the SAQLI fall between 10 and 15 min.

Reliability and Validity The scale has been subjected to a number of psychometric evaluations, indicating good reliability and validity. At its inception, the scale was tested by developers Flemons and Reimer [2] and was found to have an internal consistency ranging from .88 to .92. The scale was responsive to mean change scores of 1.0 in patients undergoing treatment for apnea. Finally, changes in quality of life scores as measured by the SAQLI were correlated with scores obtained on most domains of a similar measure, the SF-36 (Chap. 76).

Obtaining a Copy A copy can be found in the original article published by developers [2].

Direct correspondence:
W. Ward Flemons
Alberta Lung Association Sleep Disorders Centre, Foothills Hospital
1403 29th Street N. W., Calgary, AB, Canada
T2N 2T9

Scoring The processes involved in both scoring and administering the scale are relatively complex, limiting its use to those who have been specifically trained. For the first three domains (daily functioning, social interactions, and emotional functioning), respondents are queried about the frequency and severity of certain quality-of-life-related issues, and the degree to which they have been concerned about these issues. Individuals respond to these items using seven-point, Likert-type scales that range from 1 to 7, with higher scores indicating a decreased quality of life. The fourth and fifth domains offer respondents lists of symptoms (both treatment-related and not) and ask whether or not they have experienced those symptoms. Following this, individuals are required to select the five most important symptoms and to rate how much of a problem they have been on a scale from 1 to 7. A final visual analogue rating scale is offered, which respondents use to rate the changes treatment has made in their lives (both in improved quality of life and in treatment-related symptoms).

A. Shahid et al. (eds.), *STOP, THAT and One Hundred Other Sleep Scales*,
DOI 10.1007/978-1-4419-9893-4_14, © Springer Science+Business Media, LLC 2012

If domain five has not been endorsed, scoring is performed by finding the mean scores for each of the first four domains, summing them, and dividing by four to obtain an overall mean score. However, if treatment is underway and the fifth domain has been used, symptom scores are reversed, summed, and a mean score is found by dividing by five. This value is then weighted and applied to the overall score in order to obtain an accurate measure of both the benefits and costs of treatment.

References

1. Flemons, W. W., & Reimer, M. A. (2002). Measurement properties of the Calgary sleep apnea quality of life index. *American Journal of Respiratory and Critical Care Medicine, 165*, 159–164.
2. Flemons, W. W., & Reimer, M. A. (1998). Development of a disease-specific health-related quality of life questionnaire for sleep apnea. *American Journal of Respiratory and Clinical Care Medicine, 158*(2), 494–503.

Representative Studies Using Scale

Parish, J. M., & Lyng, P. J. (2003). Quality of life in bed partners of patients with obstructive sleep apnea or hypopnea after treatment with continuous positive airway pressure. *Chest, 124*(3), 942–947.

Whitelaw, W. A., Brant, R. F., & Flemons, W. W. (2005). Clinical usefulness of home oximetry compared with polysomnography for assessment of sleep apnea. *American Thoracic Society, 171*, 188–193.

15 Cataplexy Emotional Trigger Questionnaire (CETQ)

Purpose The CETQ was designed by Moore and colleagues [1] to be a very brief measure of cataplexy. The 55-item scale was inspired by the observation that self-reported muscle weakness during laughter, anger, and joking is the best method for identifying individuals with cataplexy [2]. Respondents are asked a single screening question regarding muscle weakness during laughter. If such a symptom is present, several follow-up questions are posed regarding physical symptoms (slurring of speech, trouble hearing, and location of symptoms).

Population for Testing The scale has been validated among patients with narcolepsy aged 20–84 years.

Administration The CETQ is a self-report measure that can be administered through interview or with paper and pencil. It requires approximately 2 min for completion.

Reliability and Validity The CETQ is based on a larger 51-item scale. During validation of this initial cataplexy questionnaire, researchers found that as few as 3 of those 51 items were generally sufficient to distinguish cataplexy from other forms of muscle weakness [2]. The CETQ represents a less cumbersome version of the original scale, reducing the number of items to a mere five. In a study validating the CETQ, Moore and colleagues [1] found that the first item of the scale possessed a sensitivity of .94 and a specificity of .99, while the second item had a sensitivity of .90 and a specificity of .99. As question 1 was found to carry almost no risk of false positive, the scale's additional four items do not improve its sensitivity, specificity, or predictive value. However, they may help to confirm findings and provide valuable information for the purposes of diagnosis.

Obtaining a Copy A copy of the scale can be found in the original article published by developers [1].

Direct correspondence to:
Wendy Moore
Mayo Sleep Disorders Center, Eisenberg 8 G
200 1st Street SW
Rochester, MN 55905, USA
Email: moore.wendy@mayo.edu

Scoring Consisting of only a single screening question, scoring is simple: Symptoms of cataplexy are either present or absent. Thus, follow-up screening is either indicated or ruled out based on the results of the first question. Questions 2 through 5 are included only to aid in confirmation.

A. Shahid et al. (eds.), *STOP, THAT and One Hundred Other Sleep Scales*,
DOI 10.1007/978-1-4419-9893-4_15, © Springer Science+Business Media, LLC 2012

Cataplexy Emotional Trigger Questionnaire (CETQ)

Please place an X in the grey boxes below		No	Yes
1.	Have you **EVER** experienced sudden muscle weakness when you laugh?		

If NO, thank you for answering. You do not need to continue.

If YES, please continue.

During your episodes of muscle weakness, ⇩		**No**	**Yes**
2.	Can you hear?		
3.	Does your speech ever become slurred?		
4.	Is your head affected ?		
5.	Is your whole body affected?		

References

1. Moore, W. R., Silber, M. H., Decker, P. A., Heim-Penokie, R. N., Sikkink, V. K., Slocumb, N., Richardson, J. W., & Krahn, L. E. (2007). Cataplexy emotional trigger questionnaire (CETQ) – a brief patient screen to identify cataplexy in patients with narcolepsy. *Journal of Clinical Sleep Medicine, 3*(1), 37–40.
2. Anic-Labat, S., Guilleminault, C., Kraemer, H. C., Meehan, J., Arrigoni, J.., & Mignot, E. (1999). Validation of a cataplexy questionnaire in 983 sleep-disorders patients. *Sleep, 22*(1), 77–87.

Representative Studies Using Scale

None.

16 Center for Epidemiological Studies Depression Scale for Children (CES-DC)

Purpose Consisting of 20 items, the scale is a modified version of the Center for Epidemiological Studies Depression Scale and was developed to screen for depression in children. Youth respondents are asked to indicate how strongly they have felt a certain way during the past week using a Likert-type scale that ranges from "not at all" to "a lot." Only two items on the questionnaire relate specifically to sleep or fatigue: item 7, "I was too tired to do things;" and item 11, "I didn't sleep as well as I usually sleep." However, research suggests there may be a biological link between sleep and depression in children [1], and clinicians may find that screening for both issues allows for more effective diagnosis and treatment.

Population for Testing The scale has been validated with youth aged 6–23 years old.

Administration This self-report, pencil-and-paper test requires approximately 5 min for completion. Younger children may require help.

Reliability and Validity In a study conducted by Fendrich and colleagues [2], internal consistency was $\alpha = .89$, effect size was estimated at .72, and sensitivity was 80%.

Obtaining a Copy Copies are available free at: www.brightfutures.org/mentalhealth/.

Scoring For the majority of questions, an answer of "not at all" receives a score of 0, "a little" receives 1, "some" receives 2, and "a lot" receives 3. However, items 4, 8, 12, and 16 are worded positively and scores are reversed, ensuring that respondents attend to questions and answer honestly. Higher scores represent greater depressive symptoms, and developers recommend a score of 15 as a cutoff for screening.

A. Shahid et al. (eds.), *STOP, THAT and One Hundred Other Sleep Scales*,
DOI 10.1007/978-1-4419-9893-4_16, © Springer Science+Business Media, LLC 2012

BRIGHT FUTURES TOOL FOR PROFESSIONALS

INSTRUCTIONS FOR USE

Center for Epidemiological Studies Depression Scale for Children (CES-DC)

The Center for Epidemiological Studies Depression Scale for Children (CES-DC) is a 20-item self-report depression inventory with possible scores ranging from 0 to 60. Each response to an item is scored as follows:

0 = "Not At All"

1 = "A Little"

2 = "Some"

3 = "A Lot"

However, items 4, 8, 12, and 16 are phrased positively, and thus are scored in the opposite order:

3 = "Not At All"

2 = "A Little"

1 = "Some"

0 = "A Lot"

Higher CES-DC scores indicate increasing levels of depression. Weissman et al. (1980), the developers of the CES-DC, have used the cutoff score of 15 as being suggestive of depressive symptoms in children and adolescents. That is, scores over 15 can be indicative of significant levels of depressive symptoms.

Remember that screening for depression can be complex and is only an initial step. Further evaluation is required for children and adolescents identified through a screening process. Further evaluation is also warranted for children or adolescents who exhibit depressive symptoms but who do not screen positive.

See also

Tool for Families: Symptoms of Depression in Adolescents, p. 126.

Tool for Families: Common Signs of Depression in Children and Adolescents, p. 147.

REFERENCES

Weissman MM, Orvaschel H, Padian N. 1980. Children's symptom and social functioning self-report scales: Comparison of mothers' and children's reports. *Journal of Nervous Mental Disorders* 168(12):736–740.

Faulstich ME, Carey MP, Ruggiero L, et al. 1986. Assessment of depression in childhood and adolescence: An evaluation of the Center for Epidemiological Studies Depression Scale for Children (CES-DC). *American Journal of Psychiatry* 143(8):1024–1027.

BRIGHT FUTURES TOOL FOR PROFESSIONALS

Center for Epidemiological Studies Depression Scale for Children (CES-DC)

Number ____________

Score ____________

INSTRUCTIONS

Below is a list of the ways you might have felt or acted. Please check how *much* you have felt this way during the *past week*.

DURING THE PAST WEEK	Not At All	A Little	Some	A Lot
1. I was bothered by things that usually don't bother me.	___	___	___	___
2. I did not feel like eating, I wasn't very hungry.	___	___	___	___
3. I wasn't able to feel happy, even when my family or friends tried to help me feel better.	___	___	___	___
4. I felt like I was just as good as other kids.	___	___	___	___
5. I felt like I couldn't pay attention to what I was doing.	___	___	___	___

DURING THE PAST WEEK	Not At All	A Little	Some	A Lot
6. I felt down and unhappy.	___	___	___	___
7. I felt like I was too tired to do things.	___	___	___	___
8. I felt like something good was going to happen.	___	___	___	___
9. I felt like things I did before didn't work out right.	___	___	___	___
10. I felt scared.	___	___	___	___

DURING THE PAST WEEK	Not At All	A Little	Some	A Lot
11. I didn't sleep as well as I usually sleep.	___	___	___	___
12. I was happy.	___	___	___	___
13. I was more quiet than usual.	___	___	___	___
14. I felt lonely, like I didn't have any friends.	___	___	___	___
15. I felt like kids I know were not friendly or that they didn't want to be with me.	___	___	___	___

DURING THE PAST WEEK	Not At All	A Little	Some	A Lot
16. I had a good time.	___	___	___	___
17. I felt like crying.	___	___	___	___
18. I felt sad.	___	___	___	___
19. I felt people didn't like me.	___	___	___	___
20. It was hard to get started doing things.	___	___	___	___

Note: For sleep researches dealing with depression in children and adolescents, we have put a booklet we developed for parents, teaches, medical, paramedical professionals and psychologists on our website. This book entitled "Detecting Depression in Children and Adolescents" is (we believe) helpful in general and specifically for dealing with children and parents referred to a sleep clinic and who are then "confronted" with a diagnosis of depression. The website is www.sleepontario.com

References

1. Ivanenko, A., Crabtree, V. M., & Gozal, David. (2005). Sleep and depression in children and adolescents. *Sleep Medicine Reviews, 9*(2), 115–129.
2. Fendrich, M., Weissman, M. M., & Warner, V. (1990). Screening for depressive disorder in children and adolescents: validating the center for epidemiologic studies depression scale for children. *American Journal of Epidemiology, 131*(3), 538–551.

Representative Studies Using Scale

Iwata, N, & Buka, S. (2002). Race/ethnicity and depressive symptoms: a cross-cultural/ethnic comparison among university students in East Asia, North and South America. *Social Science and Medicine, 55*(12), 2243–2252.

17 Chalder Fatigue Scale

Purpose Designed to measure the severity of fatigue in adults, the 14-item instrument is indicated for use in both clinical and research settings. Symptoms examined by the scale can be divided into two categories: physical and mental.

Population for Testing The scale was validated using a sample of participants aged 18–45.

Administration The instrument is a self-report measure that can be administered both by interview and through the use of a pencil-and-paper test. Requires 3–5 min for completion.

Reliability and Validity Chalder and colleagues [1] analyzed the scale for its psychometric properties, demonstrating an internal consistency ranging from .88 to .90 and a validity of .85.

Obtaining a Copy A copy can be found in the developers' original published article [1].

Direct correspondence to:
Trudie Chalder
Academic Department of Psychological Medicine
King's College Hospital, Denmark Hill
Camberwell, London SE5 9RS, U.K.

Scoring Respondents are asked to answer questions pertaining to fatigue with one of four response choices: "better than usual," "no more than usual," "worse than usual," or "much worse than usual." In terms of scoring, the scale can accommodate two different methods. The first weights the individual's responses as Likert-type items and uses those scores to interpret results. The second ignores the severity of responses and uses a bimodal system to categorize each answer as either problematic or not. Thus, responses of "worse than usual" and "much worse than usual" become equivalent. The benefit of such an approach is that it eliminates error caused by individuals who are inclined to select the most or least extreme options.

A. Shahid et al. (eds.), *STOP, THAT and One Hundred Other Sleep Scales*,
DOI 10.1007/978-1-4419-9893-4_17, © Springer Science+Business Media, LLC 2012

Chalder Fatigue Scale

Physical Symptoms

1. Do you have problems with tiredness?
   (a) Better than usual (b) No more than usual (c) Worse than usual
   (d) Much worse than usual
2. Do you need to rest more?
   (a) Better than usual (b) No more than usual (c) Worse than usual
   (d) Much worse than usual
3. Do you feel sleepy or drowsy?
   (a) Better than usual (b) No more than usual (c) Worse than usual
   (d) Much worse than usual
4. Do you have problems starting things?
   (a) Better than usual (b) No more than usual (c) Worse than usual
   (d) Much worse than usual
5. Do you start things without difficulty but get weak as you go on?
   (a) Better than usual (b) No more than usual (c) Worse than usual
   (d) Much worse than usual
6. Are you lacking in energy?
   (a) Better than usual (b) No more than usual (c) Worse than usual
   (d) Much worse than usual
7. Do you have less strength in your muscles?
   (a) Better than usual (b) No more than usual (c) Worse than usual
   (d) Much worse than usual
8. Do you feel weak?
   (a) Better than usual (b) No more than usual (c) Worse than usual
   (d) Much worse than usual

Mental Symptoms

9. Do you have difficulty concentrating?
   (a) Better than usual (b) No more than usual (c) Worse than usual
   (d) Much worse than usual
10. Do you have problems thinking clearly?
    (a) Better than usual (b) No more than usual (c) Worse than usual
    (d) Much worse than usual
11. Do you make slips of the tongue when speaking?
    (a) Better than usual (b) No more than usual (c) Worse than usual
    (d) Much worse than usual
12. Do you find it more difficult to find the correct word?
    (a) Better than usual (b) No more than usual (c) Worse than usual
    (d) Much worse than usual
13. How is your memory?
    (a) Better than usual (b) No more than usual (c) Worse than usual
    (d) Much worse than usual
14. Have you lost interest in the things you used to do?
    (a) Better than usual (b) No more than usual (c) Worse than usual
    (d) Much worse than usual

Reference

1. Chalder, T., Berelowitz, G., Pawlikowska, T., Watts, L., Wessely, S., Wright, D., & Wallace, E. P. (1993). Development of a fatigue scale. *Journal of Psychometric Research, 37*(2), 147–153.

Representative Studies Using Scale

Roberts, A. D. L., Wessely, S., Chalder, T., Papadopoulos, A., & Cleare, A. J. (2004). Salivary cortisol response to awakening in chronic fatigue syndrome. *British Journal of Psychiatry, 184*(2), 136–141.

Jerjes, W. K., Taylor, N. F., Wood, P. J., & Cleare, A. J. (2007). Enhanced feedback sensitivity to prednisolone in chronic fatigue syndrome. *Psychoneuroendocrinology, 32*(2), 192–198.

Child Behavior Checklist (CBCL), 1½–5

18

Purpose Completed from the perspective of the child's parent or guardian, the questionnaire evaluates a variety of behavioral problems and competencies in young children. Parents respond to 99 Likert-type items by selecting the option that best represents their child's behavior over the past 6 months (0 = "Not true (as far as you know)," 1 = "Somewhat or sometimes true," and 2 = "Very true or often true"). The questionnaire classifies individuals across a range of syndromes and DSM-oriented diagnoses, including emotionally reactive, somatic complaints, aggressive behavior, pervasive developmental problems, and attention deficit/hyperactivity problems. Though the scale is designed to measure overall behavioral competence, several items relate directly to sleep issues and combine to create a separate syndrome category for sleep problems:

22. Doesn't want to sleep alone
38. Has trouble getting to sleep
48. Nightmares
64. Resists going to bed at night
74. Sleeps less than most kids during the day and/or night
84. Talks or cries out in sleep
94. Wakes up often at night

The scale is by no means a diagnostic measure of sleep disorders in children. Questions that might specifically screen for a well-recognized disorder such as sleep apnea, for example, are conspicuously absent. However, the questionnaire allows clinicians and researchers to obtain a general overview of sleep behaviors – one that could potentially lead to further screening where relevant. The scale also collects information on a variety of other measures that may also be relevant to sleep, including inattention and hyperactivity [1].

Population for Testing Designed for children 1½–5, a version for older youth between the ages of 6 and 18 has also been created.

Administration Responses are solicited from a parent or guardian, and the scale can be administered in the form of a clinical interview or as a pencil-and-paper questionnaire. Administration time ranges from 15 to 20 min. In order to purchase the scale, clinicians and researchers must complete a "Test User Qualification Form" to be reviewed by the distributor. While those administering the questionnaire do not need to possess any particular qualifications, those supervising the testing and interpreting results must have completed at least two courses in tests and measurements at a university level. Exceptions are dealt with on a case-by-case basis, but generally, one must have achieved a relevant background in testing through other means. For this age range, developers also offer a Caregiver-Teacher Report Form (C-TRF), which may be useful in understanding the child's behavior in a different context.

Reliability and Validity Studies assessing the psychometric properties of the CBCL have been numerous and include evaluations of its efficacy

A. Shahid et al. (eds.), *STOP, THAT and One Hundred Other Sleep Scales*,
DOI 10.1007/978-1-4419-9893-4_18, © Springer Science+Business Media, LLC 2012

in different cultural settings and its potential uses in discriminating a variety of patient populations. According to research conducted by the developers [2], the scale has an average test-retest reliability of .85, and an average cross-informant correlation of .61.

Obtaining a Copy The scale was developed and refined by Thomas Achenbach and colleagues for the Achenbach System of Empirically Based Assessment (ASEBA). To find a distributor in your area, visit the publisher's Web site: http://www.aseba.org/index.html

Scoring Though the test can be scored by hand, the ASEBA also sells a computer scoring program called the Assessment Data Manager. *T*-scores and percentiles of the normative sample are found by plotting raw scores for each of the test's eight syndrome constructs on a scale. Each *T*-score falls into one of three ranges: normal (below 67), borderline (between 67 and 70), and clinical (above 70). Children also receive Internalizing, Externalizing, and Total Problem scores. While the CBCL is often treated as the gold standard in research and clinical questionnaires, it is important to remember that it is not a substitute for a full clinical evaluation. Some have criticized the test for its lack of subtlety in detecting certain problems and others have suggested that its length may be unnecessary [3].

ASEBA *Please print.* **CHILD BEHAVIOR CHECKLIST FOR AGES 1½-5**

For office use only
ID #

CHILD'S FULL NAME First Middle Last

CHILD'S GENDER ☐ Boy ☐ Girl

CHILD'S AGE

CHILD'S ETHNIC GROUP OR RACE

TODAY'S DATE Mo______ Day______ Year______

CHILD'S BIRTHDATE Mo______ Day______ Year______

Please fill out this form to reflect *your* view of the child's behavior even if other people might not agree. Feel free to write additional comments beside each item and in the space provided on page 2. ***Be sure to answer all items.***

PARENTS' USUAL TYPE OF WORK, even if not working now. *Please be specific — for example, auto mechanic, high school teacher, homemaker, laborer, lathe operator, shoe salesman, army sergeant*

FATHER'S TYPE OF WORK ______________________

MOTHER'S TYPE OF WORK ______________________

THIS FORM FILLED OUT BY: (print your full name)

____

Your relationship to child:

☐ Mother ☐ Father ☐ Other (specify):

Below is a list of items that describe children. For each item that describes the child ***now or within the past 2 months***, please circle the ***2*** if the item is ***very true or often true*** of the child. Circle the ***1*** if the item is ***somewhat or sometimes true*** of the child. If the item is ***not true*** of the child, circle the ***0***. Please answer all items as well as you can, even if some do not seem to apply to the child.

0 = Not True (as far as you know) **1 = Somewhat or Sometimes True** **2 = Very True or Often True**

0 1 2 1. Aches or pains (without medical cause; ***do not*** include stomach or headaches)
0 1 2 2. Acts too young for age
0 1 2 3. Afraid to try new things
0 1 2 4. Avoids looking others in the eye
0 1 2 5. Can't concentrate, can't pay attention for long
0 1 2 6. Can't sit still, restless, or hyperactive
0 1 2 7. Can't stand having things out of place
0 1 2 8. Can't stand waiting; wants everything now
0 1 2 9. Chews on things that aren't edible
0 1 2 10. Clings to adults or too dependent
0 1 2 11. Constantly seeks help
0 1 2 12. Constipated, doesn't move bowels (when not sick)
0 1 2 13. Cries a lot
0 1 2 14. Cruel to animals
0 1 2 15. Defiant
0 1 2 16. Demands must be met immediately
0 1 2 17. Destroys his/her own things
0 1 2 18. Destroys things belonging to his/her family or other children
0 1 2 19. Diarrhea or loose bowels (when not sick)
0 1 2 20. Disobedient
0 1 2 21. Disturbed by any change in routine
0 1 2 22. Doesn't want to sleep alone
0 1 2 23. Doesn't answer when people talk to him/her
0 1 2 24. Doesn't eat well (describe): ______________________
0 1 2 25. Doesn't get along with other children
0 1 2 26. Doesn't know how to have fun; acts like a little adult
0 1 2 27. Doesn't seem to feel guilty after misbehaving
0 1 2 28. Doesn't want to go out of home
0 1 2 29. Easily frustrated
0 1 2 30. Easily jealous
0 1 2 31. Eats or drinks things that are not food—***don't*** include sweets (describe): ______________________
0 1 2 32. Fears certain animals, situations, or places (describe): ______________________
0 1 2 33. Feelings are easily hurt
0 1 2 34. Gets hurt a lot, accident-prone
0 1 2 35. Gets in many fights
0 1 2 36. Gets into everything
0 1 2 37. Gets too upset when separated from parents
0 1 2 38. Has trouble getting to sleep
0 1 2 39. Headaches (without medical cause)
0 1 2 40. Hits others
0 1 2 41. Holds his/her breath
0 1 2 42. Hurts animals or people without meaning to
0 1 2 43. Looks unhappy without good reason
0 1 2 44. Angry moods
0 1 2 45. Nausea, feels sick (without medical cause)
0 1 2 46. Nervous movements or twitching (describe): ______________________
0 1 2 47. Nervous, highstrung, or tense
0 1 2 48. Nightmares
0 1 2 49. Overeating
0 1 2 50. Overtired
0 1 2 51. Shows panic for no good reason
0 1 2 52. Painful bowel movements (without medical cause)
0 1 2 53. Physically attacks people
0 1 2 54. Picks nose, skin, or other parts of body (describe): ______________________

Be sure you answered all items. Then see other side.

7-28-00 Edition-601

Please print your answers. Be sure to answer all items.

0 = Not True (as far as you know) **1 = Somewhat or Sometimes True** **2 = Very True or Often True**

0 1 2 55. Plays with own sex parts too much
0 1 2 56. Poorly coordinated or clumsy
0 1 2 57. Problems with eyes (without medical cause) (describe): ______________________
0 1 2 58 Punishment doesn't change his/her behavior
0 1 2 59 Quickly shifts from one activity to another
0 1 2 60 Rashes or other skin problems (without medical cause)
0 1 2 61. Refuses to eat
0 1 2 62. Refuses to play active games
0 1 2 63. Repeatedly rocks head or body
0 1 2 64. Resists going to bed at night
0 1 2 65. Resists toilet training (describe): ______________________
0 1 2 66. Screams a lot
0 1 2 67. Seems unresponsive to affection
0 1 2 68. Self-conscious or easily embarrassed
0 1 2 69. Selfish or won't share
0 1 2 70. Shows little affection toward people
0 1 2 71. Shows little interest in things around him/her
0 1 2 72. Shows too little fear of getting hurt
0 1 2 73 Too shy or timid
0 1 2 74 Sleeps less than most kids during day and/or night (describe): ______________________
0 1 2 75. Smears or plays with bowel movements
0 1 2 76. Speech problem (describe): ______________________
0 1 2 77. Stares into space or seems preoccupied
0 1 2 78. Stomachaches or cramps (without medical cause)

0 1 2 79. Rapid shifts between sadness and excitement
0 1 2 80. Strange behavior (describe): ______________________
0 1 2 81. Stubborn, sullen, or irritable
0 1 2 82. Sudden changes in mood or feelings
0 1 2 83 Sulks a lot
0 1 2 84 Talks or cries out in sleep
0 1 2 85. Temper tantrums or hot temper
0 1 2 86. Too concerned with neatness or cleanliness
0 1 2 87 Too fearful or anxious
0 1 2 88 Uncooperative
0 1 2 89. Underactive, slow moving, or lacks energy
0 1 2 90. Unhappy, sad, or depressed
0 1 2 91 Unusually loud
0 1 2 92. Upset by new people or situations (describe): ______________________
0 1 2 93 Vomiting, throwing up (without medical cause)
0 1 2 94 Wakes up often at night
0 1 2 95. Wanders away
0 1 2 96. Wants a lot of attention
0 1 2 97. Whining
0 1 2 98. Withdrawn, doesn't get involved with others
0 1 2 99. Worries
0 1 2 100. Please write in any problems the child has that were not listed above
0 1 2 ______________________
0 1 2 ______________________
0 1 2 ______________________

Please be sure you have answered all items. Underline any you are concerned about.

Does the child have any illness or disability (either physical or mental)? ☐ **No** ☐ **Yes—Please describe:**

What concerns you most about the child?

Please describe the best things about the child:

Language Development Survey for Ages 18-35 Months

For office use only
ID #

The Language Development Survey assesses children's word combinations and vocabulary. By carefully completing the Language Development Survey, you can help us obtain an accurate picture of the child's developing language. ***Please print your answers. Be sure to answer all items.***

I. Was the child born earlier than the usual 9 months after conception?

☐ No ☐ Yes—how many weeks early? ________weeks early.

II. How much did the child weigh at birth? ________ pounds ________ounces; or ________ grams.

III. How many ear infections did the child have before age 24 months?

☐ 0-2 ☐ 3-5 ☐ 6-8 ☐ 9 or more

IV. Is any language beside English spoken in the child's home?

☐ No ☐ Yes—please list the languages: ______________ ______________

______________ ______________

V. Has anyone in the child's family been slow in learning to talk?

☐ No ☐ Yes—please list their relationships to the child; for example, brother, father:

____

VI. Are you worried about the child's language development?

☐ No ☐ Yes—why? ____

____

VII. Does the child spontaneously say words in any language? (not just imitates or understands words)?

☐ No ☐ Yes—if yes, please complete item VIII and page 4.

VIII. Does the child combine 2 or more words into phrases? For example: "more cookie," "car bye-bye."

☐ No ☐ Yes—please print 5 of the child's longest and best phrases or sentences.

For each phrase that is not in English, print the name of the language.

1. ____
2. ____
3. ____
4. ____
5. ____

Be sure you answered all items. Then see other side.

Please circle each word that the child says SPONTANEOUSLY (not just imitates or understands). If your child says non-English versions of words on the list, circle the English word and write the first letter of the language (e.g., S for Spanish). Please include words even if they are not pronounced clearly or are in "baby talk" (for example: "baba" for bottle).

FOODS
1. apple
2. banana
3. bread
4. butter
5. cake
6. candy
7. cereal
8. cheese
9. coffee
10. cookie
11. crackers
12. drink
13. egg
14. food
15. grapes
16. gum
17. hamburger
18. hotdog
19. ice cream
20. juice
21. meat
22. milk
23. orange
24. pizza
25. pretzel
26. raisins
27. soda
28. soup
29. spaghetti
30. tea
31. toast
32. water

TOYS
33. ball
34. balloon
35. blocks
36. book
37. crayons
38. doll
39. picture
40. present
41. slide
42. swing
43. teddy bear

OUTDOORS
44. flower
45. house
46. moon
47. rain
48. sidewalk
49. sky
50. snow
51. star
52. street
53. sun
54. tree

ANIMALS
55. bear
56. bee
57. bird
58. bug
59. bunny
60. cat
61. chicken
62. cow
63. dog
64. duck
65. elephant
66. fish
67. frog
68. horse
69. monkey
70. pig
71. puppy
72. snake
73. tiger
74. turkey
75. turtle

BODY PARTS
76. arm
77. belly button
78. bottom
79. chin
80. ear
81. elbow
82. eye
83. face
84. finger
85. foot
86. hair
87. hand
88. knee
89. leg
90. mouth
91. neck
92. nose
93. teeth
94. thumb
95. toe
96. tummy

VEHICLES
97. bike
98. boat
99. bus
100. car
101. motorcycle
102. plane
103. stroller
104. train
105. trolley
106. truck

ACTIONS
107. bath
108. breakfast
109. bring
110. catch
111. clap
112. close
113. come
114. cough
115. cut
116. dance
117. dinner
118. doodoo
119. down
120. eat
121. feed
122. finish
123. fix
124. get
125. give
126. go
127. have
128. help
129. hit
130. hug
131. jump
132. kick
133. kiss
134. knock
135. look
136. love
137. lunch
138. make
139. nap
140. open
141. outside
142. pattycake
143. peekaboo
144. peepee
145. push
146. read
147. ride
148. run
149. see
150. show
151. shut
152. sing
153. sit
154. sleep
155. stop
156. take
157. throw
158. tickle
159. up
160. walk
161. want
162. wash

HOUSEHOLD
163. bathtub
164. bed
165. blanket
166. bottle
167. bowl
168. chair
169. clock
170. crib
171. cup
172. door
173. floor
174. fork
175. glass
176. knife
177. light
178. mirror
179. pillow
180. plate
181. potty
182. radio
183. room
184. sink
185. soap
186. spoon
187. stairs
188. table
189. telephone
190. towel
191. trash
192. T.V.
193. window

PERSONAL
194. brush
195. comb
196. glasses
197. key
198. money
199. paper
200. pen
201. pencil
202. penny
203. pocketbook
204. tissue
205. tooth brush
206. umbrella
207. watch

PLACES
208. church
209. home
210. hospital
211. library
212. park
213. school
214. store
215. zoo

MODIFIERS
216. all gone
217. all right
218. bad
219. big
220. black
221. blue
222. broken
223. clean
224. cold
225. dark
226. dirty
227. dry
228. good
229. happy
230. heavy
231. hot
232. hungry
233. little
234. mine
235. more
236. nice
237. pretty
238. red
239. stinky
240. that
241. this
242. tired
243. wet
244. white
245. yellow
246. yucky

CLOTHES
247. belt
248. boots
249. coat
250. diaper
251. dress
252. gloves
253. hat
254. jacket
255. mittens
256. pajamas
257. pants
258. shirt
259. shoes
260. slippers
261. sneakers
262. socks
263. sweater

OTHER
264. any letter
265. away
266. booboo
267. byebye
268. excuse me
269. here
270. hi, hello
271. in
272. me
273. meow
274. my
275. myself
276. nightnight
277. no
278. off
279. on
280. out
281. please
282. Sesame St
283. shut up
284. thank you
285. there
286. under
287. welcome
288. what
289. where
290. why
291. woofwoof
292. yes
293. you
294. yumyum
295. any number

PEOPLE
296. aunt
297. baby
298. boy
299. daddy
300. doctor
301. girl
302. grandma
303. grandpa
304. lady
305. man
306. mommy
307. own name
308. pet name
309. uncle
310. name of TV or story character

Other words your child says, including non-English words:

____

____

____

____

References

1. Chervin, R. D., Dillon, J. E., Bassetti, C., Ganoczy, D. A., & Pituch, K. J. (1997). Symptoms of sleep disorders, inattention, and hyperactivity in children. *Sleep, 20*(12), 1185–1192.
2. Achenbach, T. M., & Rescorla, L. A. (2001). *Manual for the ASEBA School-Age Forms & Profiles*. Burlington, VT: University of Vermont.
3. Goodman, R., & Scott, S. (1999). Comparing the Strengths and Difficulties Questionnaire and the Child Behavior Checklist: is small beautiful? *Journal of Abnormal Child Psychology, 27*(1), 17–24.

Representative Studies Using Scale

Van Zejil, J., Mesman, J., Van IJzendoorn, M. H., Bakermans-Kranenburg, M. J., Juffer, F., Stolk, M. N., Koot, H. M., & Alink, L. R. A. (2006). Attachment-based intervention for enhancing sensitive discipline in mothers of 1- to 3-year-old children at risk for externalizing behavior problems: a randomized controlled trial. *Journal of Consulting and Clinical Psychology, 74*(6), 994–1005.

Weaver, C. M., Shaw, D. S., Dishion, T. J., & Wilson, M. N. (2008). Parenting self-efficacy and problem behavior in children at high risk for early conduct problems: the mediating role of maternal depression. *Infant Behavior and Development, 31*(4), 594–605.

Child Behavior Checklist (CBCL), 6–18

19

Purpose The questionnaire examines a wide range of childhood behaviors detailed from the perspective of the parent or guardian. In the test's first section, parents are asked to report briefly on several aspects of their child's day-to-day functioning, including involvement with groups and activities, relationships with peers, and performance in school. The second section consists of 118 Likert-type items which require parents to indicate how well the statement represents their child's behaviors during the past 6 months (0="Not true (as far as you know)," 1="Somewhat or sometimes true," and 2="Very true or often true"). Children receive scores across a variety of syndromes and DSM-oriented scales, including aggressive behavior, attention problems, somatic complaints, anxiety problems, attention deficit/hyperactivity problems, and conduct problems. As the questionnaire is intended to measure overall behavioral competence, only a few items relate directly to sleep issues:

47. Nightmares
54. Overtired without good reason
76. Sleeps less than most kids
77. Sleeps more than most kids during day and/or night (describe)
92. Talks or walks in sleep (describe)
100. Trouble sleeping (describe)
108. Wets the bed

However, some research suggests that sleep issues are frequently comorbid with mental disorders [1]. Thus, while clinicians interested in sleep may choose to focus primarily on these seven items of the CBCL, a more general measure of behavioral issues could also be considered valuable, particularly when plotting a course for treatment.

Population for Testing The questionnaire is designed for youth aged 6–18. A second version has also been developed for children aged 1½–5.

Administration Parents provide responses either through interview with an administrator or by completing the pencil-and-paper form themselves. The test requires between 15 and 20 min for completion. Though administrators do not need to possess any specific qualifications, distributors ask individuals attempting to purchase test products to complete a "Test User Qualification Form." In order to be considered qualified to interpret results or supervise use of the test, an individual must have completed at least two university-level courses in tests and measurements (exceptions may be made for those who can demonstrate sufficient background in psychometric measures). Along with this parental response questionnaire, developers have designed a Teacher Report Form (6–18) and a Youth Self-Report form (11–18). These additional measures may be used when a researcher or clinician wishes to understand a child's behavior in a variety of contexts and from several perspectives.

Reliability and Validity Studies assessing the psychometric properties of the CBCL have been numerous and include evaluations of its efficacy

A. Shahid et al. (eds.), *STOP, THAT and One Hundred Other Sleep Scales*,
DOI 10.1007/978-1-4419-9893-4_19, © Springer Science+Business Media, LLC 2012

in different cultural settings and its potential uses in discriminating a variety of patient populations. According to research performed by the developers [2], the test has an inter-rater reliability ranging from .93 to .96, a test-retest reliability of .95–1.00, and an internal consistency of .72 – .97 – all quite high.

Obtaining a Copy The scale was developed and refined by Thomas Achenbach and colleagues for the Achenbach System of Empirically Based Assessment (ASEBA). To find a distributor in your area, visit the publisher's Web site: http://www.aseba.org/index.html.

Scoring Test scoring can be performed by hand or can be conducted through the use of computer software sold by the publisher. In either case, raw scores for each of the test's eight syndrome constructs are tallied and plotted on a scale that converts them to *T*-scores and to percentiles of the normative sample. Each *T*-score falls into one of three ranges: normal (below 67), borderline (between 67 and 70), and clinical (above 70). Children are also given Internalizing, Externalizing, and total problem scores for which borderline and clinical ranges are slightly lower. While the CBCL is often treated as the gold standard in research and clinical questionnaires, it is important to remember that it is no substitute for a full clinical evaluation. Some have criticized the test for its lack of subtlety in detecting certain problems and others have suggested that its length may be unnecessary [3].

Please print. **CHILD BEHAVIOR CHECKLIST FOR AGES 1½-5**

For office use only
ID #

CHILD'S FULL NAME First Middle Last

CHILD'S GENDER ☐ Boy ☐ Girl | CHILD'S AGE | CHILD'S ETHNIC GROUP OR RACE

TODAY'S DATE Mo______Day______Year________ | CHILD'S BIRTHDATE Mo______Day______Year________

Please fill out this form to reflect *your* view of the child's behavior even if other people might not agree. Feel free to write additional comments beside each item and in the space provided on page 2. ***Be sure to answer all items.***

PARENTS' USUAL TYPE OF WORK, even if not working now. *Please be specific — for example, auto mechanic, high school teacher, homemaker, laborer, lathe operator, shoe salesman, army sergeant*

FATHER'S TYPE OF WORK ______________________

MOTHER'S TYPE OF WORK ______________________

THIS FORM FILLED OUT BY: (print your full name)

____

Your relationship to child:

☐ Mother ☐ Father ☐ Other (specify):

Below is a list of items that describe children. For each item that describes the child ***now or within the past 2 months***, please circle the **2** if the item is ***very true or often true*** of the child. Circle the **1** if the item is ***somewhat or sometimes true*** of the child. If the item is ***not true*** of the child, circle the **0**. Please answer all items as well as you can, even if some do not seem to apply to the child.

0 = Not True (as far as you know) **1 = Somewhat or Sometimes True** **2 = Very True or Often True**

0 1 2 1. Aches or pains (without medical cause; ***do not*** include stomach or headaches)
0 1 2 2. Acts too young for age
0 1 2 3. Afraid to try new things
0 1 2 4. Avoids looking others in the eye
0 1 2 5. Can't concentrate, can't pay attention for long
0 1 2 6. Can't sit still, restless, or hyperactive
0 1 2 7. Can't stand having things out of place
0 1 2 8. Can't stand waiting; wants everything now
0 1 2 9. Chews on things that aren't edible
0 1 2 10. Clings to adults or too dependent
0 1 2 11. Constantly seeks help
0 1 2 12. Constipated, doesn't move bowels (when not sick)
0 1 2 13. Cries a lot
0 1 2 14. Cruel to animals
0 1 2 15. Defiant
0 1 2 16. Demands must be met immediately
0 1 2 17. Destroys his/her own things
0 1 2 18. Destroys things belonging to his/her family or other children
0 1 2 19. Diarrhea or loose bowels (when not sick)
0 1 2 20. Disobedient
0 1 2 21. Disturbed by any change in routine
0 1 2 22. Doesn't want to sleep alone
0 1 2 23. Doesn't answer when people talk to him/her
0 1 2 24. Doesn't eat well (describe): ______________________
0 1 2 25. Doesn't get along with other children
0 1 2 26. Doesn't know how to have fun; acts like a little adult
0 1 2 27. Doesn't seem to feel guilty after misbehaving
0 1 2 28. Doesn't want to go out of home
0 1 2 29. Easily frustrated
0 1 2 30. Easily jealous
0 1 2 31. Eats or drinks things that are not food—***don't*** include sweets (describe): ______________________
0 1 2 32. Fears certain animals, situations, or places (describe): ______________________
0 1 2 33. Feelings are easily hurt
0 1 2 34. Gets hurt a lot, accident-prone
0 1 2 35. Gets in many fights
0 1 2 36. Gets into everything
0 1 2 37. Gets too upset when separated from parents
0 1 2 38. Has trouble getting to sleep
0 1 2 39. Headaches (without medical cause)
0 1 2 40. Hits others
0 1 2 41. Holds his/her breath
0 1 2 42. Hurts animals or people without meaning to
0 1 2 43. Looks unhappy without good reason
0 1 2 44. Angry moods
0 1 2 45. Nausea, feels sick (without medical cause)
0 1 2 46. Nervous movements or twitching (describe): ______________________
0 1 2 47. Nervous, highstrung, or tense
0 1 2 48. Nightmares
0 1 2 49. Overeating
0 1 2 50. Overtired
0 1 2 51. Shows panic for no good reason
0 1 2 52. Painful bowel movements (without medical cause)
0 1 2 53. Physically attacks people
0 1 2 54. Picks nose, skin, or other parts of body (describe): ______________________

Be sure you answered all items. Then see other side.

7-28-00 Edition-601

Please print your answers. Be sure to answer all items.

0 = Not True (as far as you know) **1 = Somewhat or Sometimes True** **2 = Very True or Often True**

0 1 2 55. Plays with own sex parts too much

0 1 2 56. Poorly coordinated or clumsy

0 1 2 57. Problems with eyes (without medical cause) (describe): ______________________

0 1 2 58. Punishment doesn't change his/her behavior

0 1 2 59. Quickly shifts from one activity to another

0 1 2 60. Rashes or other skin problems (without medical cause)

0 1 2 61. Refuses to eat

0 1 2 62. Refuses to play active games

0 1 2 63. Repeatedly rocks head or body

0 1 2 64. Resists going to bed at night

0 1 2 65. Resists toilet training (describe): ______________________

0 1 2 66. Screams a lot

0 1 2 67. Seems unresponsive to affection

0 1 2 68. Self-conscious or easily embarrassed

0 1 2 69. Selfish or won't share

0 1 2 70. Shows little affection toward people

0 1 2 71. Shows little interest in things around him/her

0 1 2 72. Shows too little fear of getting hurt

0 1 2 73. Too shy or timid

0 1 2 74. Sleeps less than most kids during day and/or night (describe): ______________________

0 1 2 75. Smears or plays with bowel movements

0 1 2 76. Speech problem (describe): ______________________

0 1 2 77. Stares into space or seems preoccupied

0 1 2 78. Stomachaches or cramps (without medical cause)

0 1 2 79. Rapid shifts between sadness and excitement

0 1 2 80. Strange behavior (describe): ______________________

0 1 2 81. Stubborn, sullen, or irritable

0 1 2 82. Sudden changes in mood or feelings

0 1 2 83. Sulks a lot

0 1 2 84. Talks or cries out in sleep

0 1 2 85. Temper tantrums or hot temper

0 1 2 86. Too concerned with neatness or cleanliness

0 1 2 87. Too fearful or anxious

0 1 2 88. Uncooperative

0 1 2 89. Underactive, slow moving, or lacks energy

0 1 2 90. Unhappy, sad, or depressed

0 1 2 91. Unusually loud

0 1 2 92. Upset by new people or situations (describe): ______________________

0 1 2 93. Vomiting, throwing up (without medical cause)

0 1 2 94. Wakes up often at night

0 1 2 95. Wanders away

0 1 2 96. Wants a lot of attention

0 1 2 97. Whining

0 1 2 98. Withdrawn, doesn't get involved with others

0 1 2 99. Worries

0 1 2 100. Please write in any problems the child has that were not listed above.

0 1 2 ______________________

0 1 2 ______________________

0 1 2 ______________________

Please be sure you have answered all items. Underline any you are concerned about.

Does the child have any illness or disability (either physical or mental)? ☐ No ☐ **Yes—Please describe:**

What concerns you most about the child?

Please describe the best things about the child:

Language Development Survey for Ages 18-35 Months

For office use only
ID #

The Language Development Survey assesses children's word combinations and vocabulary. By carefully completing the Language Development Survey, you can help us obtain an accurate picture of the child's developing language. ***Please print your answers. Be sure to answer all items.***

I. Was the child born earlier than the usual 9 months after conception?

☐ No ☐ Yes—how many weeks early? ________weeks early

II. How much did the child weigh at birth? ________ pounds ________ounces; or ________ grams.

III. How many ear infections did the child have before age 24 months?

☐ 0-2 ☐ 3-5 ☐ 6-8 ☐ 9 or more

IV. Is any language beside English spoken in the child's home?

☐ No ☐ Yes—please list the languages: ____________ ____________ ____________ ____________

V. Has anyone in the child's family been slow in learning to talk?

☐ No ☐ Yes—please list their relationships to the child; for example, brother, father:

____

VI. Are you worried about the child's language development?

☐ No ☐ Yes—why? ____

____

VII. Does the child spontaneously say words in any language? (not just imitates or understands words)?

☐ No ☐ Yes—if yes, please complete item VIII and page 4.

VIII. Does the child combine 2 or more words into phrases? For example: "more cookie," "car bye-bye."

☐ No ☐ Yes—please print 5 of the child's longest and best phrases or sentences.

For each phrase that is not in English, print the name of the language.

1. ____
2. ____
3. ____
4. ____
5. ____

Be sure you answered all items. Then see other side.

Please circle each word that the child says SPONTANEOUSLY (not just imitates or understands). If your child says non-English versions of words on the list, circle the English word and write the first letter of the language (e.g., S for Spanish). Please include words even if they are not pronounced clearly or are in "baby talk" (for example: "baba" for bottle).

FOODS
1. apple
2. banana
3. bread
4. butter
5. cake
6. candy
7. cereal
8. cheese
9. coffee
10. cookie
11. crackers
12. drink
13. egg
14. food
15. grapes
16. gum
17. hamburger
18. hotdog
19. ice cream
20. juice
21. meat
22. milk
23. orange
24. pizza
25. pretzel
26. raisins
27. soda
28. soup
29. spaghetti
30. tea
31. toast
32. water

TOYS
33. ball
34. balloon
35. blocks
36. book
37. crayons
38. doll
39. picture
40. present
41. slide
42. swing
43. teddy bear

OUTDOORS
44. flower
45. house
46. moon
47. rain
48. sidewalk
49. sky
50. snow
51. star
52. street
53. sun
54. tree

ANIMALS
55. bear
56. bee
57. bird
58. bug
59. bunny
60. cat
61. chicken
62. cow
63. dog
64. duck
65. elephant
66. fish
67. frog
68. horse
69. monkey
70. pig
71. puppy
72. snake
73. tiger
74. turkey
75. turtle

BODY PARTS
76. arm
77. belly button
78. bottom
79. chin
80. ear
81. elbow
82. eye
83. face
84. finger
85. foot
86. hair
87. hand
88. knee
89. leg
90. mouth
91. neck
92. nose
93. teeth
94. thumb
95. toe
96. tummy

VEHICLES
97. bike
98. boat
99. bus
100. car
101. motorcycle
102. plane
103. stroller
104. train
105. trolley
106. truck

ACTIONS
107. bath
108. breakfast
109. bring
110. catch
111. clap
112. close
113. come
114. cough
115. cut
116. dance
117. dinner
118. doodoo
119. down
120. eat
121. feed
122. finish
123. fix
124. get
125. give
126. go
127. have
128. help
129. hit
130. hug
131. jump
132. kick
133. kiss
134. knock
135. look
136. love
137. lunch
138. make
139. nap
140. open
141. outside
142. pattycake
143. peekaboo
144. peepee
145. push
146. read
147. ride
148. run
149. see
150. show
151. shut
152. sing
153. sit
154. sleep
155. stop
156. take
157. throw
158. tickle
159. up
160. walk
161. want
162. wash

HOUSEHOLD
163. bathtub
164. bed
165. blanket
166. bottle
167. bowl
168. chair
169. clock
170. crib
171. cup
172. door
173. floor
174. fork
175. glass
176. knife
177. light
178. mirror
179. pillow
180. plate
181. potty
182. radio
183. room
184. sink
185. soap
186. spoon
187. stairs
188. table
189. telephone
190. towel
191. trash
192. T.V.
193. window

PERSONAL
194. brush
195. comb
196. glasses
197. key
198. money
199. paper
200. pen
201. pencil
202. penny
203. pocketbook
204. tissue
205. tooth brush
206. umbrella
207. watch

PLACES
208. church
209. home
210. hospital
211. library
212. park
213. school
214. store
215. zoo

MODIFIERS
216. all gone
217. all right
218. bad
219. big
220. black
221. blue
222. broken
223. clean
224. cold
225. dark
226. dirty
227. dry
228. good
229. happy
230. heavy
231. hot
232. hungry
233. little
234. mine
235. more
236. nice
237. pretty
238. red
239. stinky
240. that
241. this
242. tired
243. wet
244. white
245. yellow
246. yucky

CLOTHES
247. belt
248. boots
249. coat
250. diaper
251. dress
252. gloves
253. hat
254. jacket
255. mittens
256. pajamas
257. pants
258. shirt
259. shoes
260. slippers
261. sneakers
262. socks
263. sweater

OTHER
264. any letter
265. away
266. booboo
267. byebye
268. excuse me
269. here
270. hi, hello
271. in
272. me
273. meow
274. my
275. myself
276. nightnight
277. no
278. off
279. on
280. out
281. please
282. Sesame St
283. shut up
284. thank you
285. there
286. under
287. welcome
288. what
289. where
290. why
291. woofwoof
292. yes
293. you
294. yumyum
295. any number

PEOPLE
296. aunt
297. baby
298. boy
299. daddy
300. doctor
301. girl
302. grandma
303. grandpa
304. lady
305. man
306. mommy
307. own name
308. pet name
309. uncle
310. name of TV or story character

Other words your child says, including non-English words:

____

____

____

____

References

1. Ohayon, M. M., Caulet, M., & Lemoine, P. (1998). Comorbity of mental and insomnia disorders in the general population. *Comprehensive Psychiatry, 39*(4), 185–197.
2. Achenbach, T. M., & Rescorla, L. A. (2001). *Manual for the ASEBA School-Age Forms & Profiles*. Burlington, VT: University of Vermont.
3. Goodman, R., & Scott, S. (1999). Comparing the Strengths and Difficulties Questionnaire and the Child Behavior Checklist: is small beautiful? *Journal of Abnormal Child Psychology, 27*(1), 17–24.

Representative Studies Using Scale

Briggs-Gowan, M. J., & Carter, A. S. (2008). Social-emotional screening status in early childhood predicts elementary school outcomes. *Pediatrics, 121*(5), 957–962.

Ruiter, K. P., Dekker, M. C., Verhulst, F. C., & Koot, H. M. (2007). Developmental course of psychopathology in youths with and without intellectual disabilities. *Journal of Child Psychology and Psychiatry, 48*(5), 498–507.

20 Children's Morningness-Eveningness Scale

Purpose Recognizing that circadian rhythm shifts often occur during the transition between childhood and adolescence, the questionnaire developers designed an instrument to evaluate Morningness/Eveningness (M/E) preferences in these populations. Consisting of ten multiple-choice items, the survey examines sleep-schedule inclinations and subjective experiences of fatigue and alertness.

Population for Testing The scale was initially validated with populations of fourth, fifth, and sixth grade students, and most recently with a sample of Spanish adolescents aged 12–16 years [2].

Administration Requiring between 3 and 5 min for completion, the scale is a self-report, pencil-and-paper measure.

Reliability and Validity Developers' initial psychometric evaluation [1] found a significant correlation between M/E scale results and actual sleep and rise schedules. Similarly, Diaz-Morales and colleagues [2] found an internal consistency of $\alpha = .82$.

Obtaining a Copy A copy can be found in the original article published by developers [1].

Direct correspondence to:
Mary A. Carskadon
Phone: +1 401 421 9440
Email: mary_carskadon@brown.edu

Scoring Responses are scored using a Likert-type scale ranging from 1 to 5. For most items, a response of "a" receives a score of 1, and "e" receives 5. However, items marked with an asterisk are reversed in order to ensure that respondents attend carefully to questions. Higher scores indicate greater preferences toward morningness. Diaz-Morales and colleagues [2] suggest cutoffs at the 20th and 80th percentiles: Thus, scores of 10–20 would indicate eveningness, scores between 28 and 42 indicate morningness, and scores ranging from 21 to 27 are categorized as neither.

A. Shahid et al. (eds.), *STOP, THAT and One Hundred Other Sleep Scales*,
DOI 10.1007/978-1-4419-9893-4_20,

Children's Morningness-Eveningness Scale

*1. Imagine: School is cancelled! You can get up whenever you want to. When would you get out of bed? Between…
   a. 5:00 and 6:30 a.m.
   b. 6:30 and 7:45 a.m.
   c. 7:45 a.m. and 9:45 a.m.
   d. 11:00 a.m. and noon

*2. Is it easy for you to get up in the morning?
   a. No way!
   b. Sort of
   c. Pretty easy
   d. It's a cinch

*3. Gym class is set for 7:00 in the morning. How do you think you'll do?
   a. My best!
   b. Okay
   c. Worse than usual
   d. Awful

*4. The bad news: You have to take a two-hour test. The good news: You can take it when you think you'll do your best. What time is that?
   a. 8:00 to 10:00 a.m.
   b. 11:00 a.m. to 1:00 p.m.
   c. 3:00 to 5:00 p.m.
   d. 7:00 to 9:00 p.m.

*5. When do you have the most energy to do your favourite things?
   a. Morning! I'm tired in the evening
   b. Morning more than evening
   c. Evening more than morning
   d. Evening! I'm tired in the morning

*6. Guess what? Your parents have decided to let you set your own bedtime. What time would you pick? Between…
   a. 8:00 and 9:00 p.m.
   b. 9:00 and 10:15 p.m.
   c. 10:15 p.m. and 12:30 a.m.
   d. 12:30 and 1:45 a.m.
   e. 1:45 and 3:00 a.m.

*7. How alert are you in the first half hour you're up?
   a. Out of it
   b. A little dazed
   c. Okay
   d. Ready to take on the world

*8. When does your body start to tell you it's time for bed (even if you ignore it)?
Between...
   a. 8:00 and 9:00 p.m.
   b. 9:00 and 10:15 p.m.
   c. 10:15 p.m. and 12:30 a.m.
   d. 12:30 and 1:45 a.m.
   e. 1:45 and 3:00 a.m.

9. Say you had to get up at 6:00 a.m. every morning: What would it be like?
   a. Awful
   b. Not so great
   c. Okay (if I have to)
   d. Fine, no problem

*10. When you wake up in the morning how long does it take for you to be totally "with it?"
   a. 0 to 10 minutes
   b. 11 to 20 minutes
   c. 21 to 40 minutes
   d. More than 40 minutes

References

1. Carskadon, M. A., Viera, C., & Acebo, C. (1993). Association between puberty and delayed phase preference. *Sleep, 16*(3), 258–262.
2. Diaz-Morales, J. F., de León, M. C., & Sorroche, M. G. (2007). Validity of the morningness-eveningness scale for children among Spanish adolescents. *Chronobiology International, 24*(3), 435–447.

Representative Studies Using Scale

Goldstein, D., Hahn, C. S., Hasher, L., Wiprzycka, U. J., & Zelazo, P. D. (2007). Time of day, intellectual performance, and behavioral problems in morning versus evening type adolescents: is there a synchrony effect? *Personality and Individual Differences, 42*(3), 431–440.

21 Children's Sleep Habits Questionnaire (CSHQ)

Purpose A tool designed to screen for the most common sleep problems in children, the CSHQ consists of 33 items for scoring and several extra items intended to provide administrators with other potentially useful information about respondents. The instrument evaluates the child's sleep based on behavior within eight different subscales: bedtime resistance, sleep-onset delay, sleep duration, sleep anxiety, night wakings, parasomnias, sleep-disordered breathing, and daytime sleepiness.

Population for Testing The CSHQ has been validated with children aged 4–12.

Administration Parents should be able to complete the pencil-and-paper form within 10–15 min. A self-report version for children aged 7 and up is also available upon request from the developer's Web site: www.kidzzzsleep.org/

Reliability and Validity Developers evaluated several psychometric properties of the questionnaire [1]: Internal consistency ranged from .68 to .78, test-retest reliability fell between .62 and .79, sensitivity was .80, and specificity was .72.

Obtaining a Copy Questionnaires are available free from: www.kidzzzsleep.org/

Direct all correspondence to:
Judith Owens
Email: owensleep@aol.com

Scoring Parents are asked to indicate the frequency with which their child has engaged in certain sleep-related behaviors over the last typical week. A response of "Usually" indicates that the behavior has occurred from five to seven times; "Sometimes" means it has happened two to four times in the last week; and "Rarely" indicates that the behavior was observed once at the most. Scoring involves assigning values from 1 to 3 to responses. In most cases, "Usually" obtains a score of 3; however, some items are reversed in order to ensure that respondents are reading questions carefully and that responses are truthful. Though developers have not established norms for the scale, they determined that a total score of 41 points makes an effective cutoff for screening purposes as it correctly identified 80% of the clinical sample in their initial psychometric study.

A. Shahid et al. (eds.), *STOP, THAT and One Hundred Other Sleep Scales*,
DOI 10.1007/978-1-4419-9893-4_21, © Springer Science+Business Media, LLC 2012

Child's Sleep Habits
(Preschool and School-Aged)

____
Coding

The following statements are about your child's sleep habits and possible difficulties with sleep. Think about the past week in your child's life when answering the questions. If last week was unusual for a specific reason (such as your child had an ear infection and did not sleep well or the TV set was broken), choose the most recent typical week. Answer USUALLY if something occurs **5 or more times** in a week; answer SOMETIMES if it occurs **2-4 times** in a week; answer RARELY if something occurs **never or 1 time** during a week. Also, please indicate whether or not the sleep habit is a problem by circling "Yes," "No," or "Not applicable (N/A).

Bedtime

Write in child's bedtime: ________________

	3 Usually (5-7)	2 Sometimes (2-4)	1 Rarely (0-1)	Problem?
Child goes to bed at the same time at night	☐	☐	☐	Yes No N/A
Child falls asleep within 20 minutes after going to bed	☐	☐	☐	Yes No N/A
Child falls asleep alone in own bed	☐	☐	☐	Yes No N/A
Child falls asleep in parent's or sibling's bed	☐	☐	☐	Yes No N/A
Child falls asleep with rocking or rhythmic movements	☐	☐	☐	Yes No N/A
Child needs special object to fall asleep (doll, special blanket, etc.)	☐	☐	☐	Yes No N/A
Child needs parent in the room to fall asleep	☐	☐	☐	Yes No N/A
Child is ready to go to bed at bedtime	☐	☐	☐	Yes No N/A
Child resists going to bed at bedtime	☐	☐	☐	Yes No N/A
Child struggles at bedtime (cries, refuses to stay in bed, etc.)	☐	☐	☐	Yes No N/A
Child is afraid of sleeping in the dark	☐	☐	☐	Yes No N/A
Child is afraid of sleep alone	☐	☐	☐	Yes No N/A

Sleep Behavior

Child's usual amount of sleep each day: __________ hours and __________ minutes
(combining nighttime sleep and naps)

	3 Usually (5-7)	2 Sometimes (2-4)	1 Rarely (0-1)	Problem?
Child sleeps too little	☐	☐	☐	Yes No N/A
Child sleeps too much	☐	☐	☐	Yes No N/A
Child sleeps the right amount	☐	☐	☐	Yes No N/A
Child sleeps about the same amount each day	☐	☐	☐	Yes No N/A
Child wets the bed at night	☐	☐	☐	Yes No N/A
Child talks during sleep	☐	☐	☐	Yes No N/A
Child is restless and moves a lot during sleep	☐	☐	☐	Yes No N/A
Child sleepwalks during the night	☐	☐	☐	Yes No N/A
Child moves to someone else's bed during the night (parent, brother, sister, etc.)	☐	☐	☐	Yes No N/A

CSHQ- Rev 4/1/09

Coding

Sleep Behavior (continued)

	3 Usually (5-7)	2 Sometimes (2-4)	1 Rarely (0-1)	Problem?
Child reports body pains during sleep. If so, where? ______________	☐	☐	☐	Yes No N/A
Child grinds teeth during sleep (your dentist may have told you this)	☐	☐	☐	Yes No N/A
Child snores loudly	☐	☐	☐	Yes No N/A
Child seems to stop breathing during sleep	☐	☐	☐	Yes No N/A
Child snorts and/or gasps during sleep	☐	☐	☐	Yes No N/A
Child has trouble sleeping away from home (visiting relatives, vacation)	☐	☐	☐	Yes No N/A
Child complains about problems sleeping	☐	☐	☐	Yes No N/A
Child awakens during night screaming, sweating, and inconsolable	☐	☐	☐	Yes No N/A
Child awakens alarmed by a frightening dream	☐	☐	☐	Yes No N/A

Waking During the Night

	3 Usually (5-7)	2 Sometimes (2-4)	1 Rarely (0-1)	Problem?
Child awakes once during the night	☐	☐	☐	Yes No N/A
Child awakes more than once during the night	☐	☐	☐	Yes No N/A
Child returns to sleep without help after waking	☐	☐	☐	Yes No N/A

Write the number of minutes a night waking usually lasts: ______________

Morning Waking

Write in the time of day child usually wakes in the morning: ______________

	3 Usually (5-7)	2 Sometimes (2-4)	1 Rarely (0-1)	Problem?
Child wakes up by him/herself	☐	☐	☐	Yes No N/A
Child wakes up with alarm clock	☐	☐	☐	Yes No N/A
Child wakes up in negative mood	☐	☐	☐	Yes No N/A
Adults or siblings wake up child	☐	☐	☐	Yes No N/A
Child has difficulty getting out of bed in the morning	☐	☐	☐	Yes No N/A
Child takes a long time to become alert in the morning	☐	☐	☐	Yes No N/A
Child wakes up very early in the morning	☐	☐	☐	Yes No N/A
Child has a good appetite in the morning	☐	☐	☐	Yes No N/A

Coding

<u>Daytime Sleepiness</u>

	3 Usually (5-7)	2 Sometimes (2-4)	1 Rarely (0-1)	Problem?
Child naps during the day	☐	☐	☐	Yes No N/A
Child suddenly falls asleep in the middle of active behavior	☐	☐	☐	Yes No N/A
Child seems tired	☐	☐	☐	Yes No N/A

During the past week, your child has appeared very sleepy or fallen asleep during the following (check all that apply):

	1 Not Sleepy	2 Very Sleepy	3 Falls Asleep
Play alone	☐	☐	☐
Watching TV	☐	☐	☐
Riding in car	☐	☐	☐
Eating meals	☐	☐	☐

Reference

1. Owens, J. A., Spirito, A., McGuinn, M. (2000). The Children's Sleep Habits Questionnaire (CSHQ): psychometric properties of a survey instrument for school-aged children. *Sleep, 23*(8), 1043–1051.

Representative Studies Using Scale

Owens, J. A., Maxim, R., McGuinn, M., Nobile, C., Msall, M., & Alario, A. (1999). Television-viewing and sleep habits in school children. *Pediatrics, 104*(3), e27.

Liu, X., Liu, L., Owens, J. A., & Kaplan, D. L. (2005). Sleep patterns and sleep problems in schoolchildren in the United States and China. *Pediatrics, 115*(1), 241–249.

22 Circadian Type Inventory (CTI)

Purpose The CTI was initially developed to identify individuals capable of adapting to shift work. Thus, the scale assesses two factors that influence a person's ability to alter his or her sleeping rhythms: rigidity/flexibility of sleeping habits and ability/inability of overcome drowsiness [1]. Since its creation, the scale has undergone a number of revisions to improve its psychometric properties. An 18-item version was used as part of the larger Standard Shiftwork Index (SSI) in a study conducted by Barton and colleagues [2]. This shorter scale was then reduced and altered to make an 11 item scale by De Milia et al. [3].

Population for Testing The scale was initially validated with a population of 48 nightshift workers; it has since been analyzed in larger sample sizes using control participants as well.

Administration The CTI is a self-report, paper-and-pencil measure requiring between 5 and 10 min for completion.

Reliability and Validity The psychometric properties of the original 30-item CTI have been validated only minimally. A study by Smith and colleagues [4] found the scale to be satisfactory: Its two factors explained 27% of the variance in a population of students and its internal consistency was moderate, ranging from .58 to .74. The 18-item scale developed by Barton and colleagues [2] performed similarly, explaining 26% of the variance in the sample and demonstrating an internal reliability ranging from .73 to .79. The most recent 11-item version of the scale has proven to be the most psychometrically sound: The two factors of the scale explained 50% of the sample variance and the internal consistency ranged from .72 to .79 [5].

Obtaining a Copy An example of the scale can be found in the original article published by developers [1].

Direct correspondence to:
Simon Folkard
MRC Perceptual and Cognitive Unit,
Laboratory of Experimental Psychology
University of Sussex
Brighton, BN1 9QG, UK

Scoring Respondents use a 5-item, Likert-type scale to answer questions regarding their sleep habits and preferences. Scales range from 1 meaning "almost never," to 5 meaning "almost always." Higher scores on the rigidity subscale indicate a greater flexibility in circadian rhythm, while lower scores on the overcoming-drowsiness subscale indicate a greater ability to manage on less sleep.

A. Shahid et al. (eds.), *STOP, THAT and One Hundred Other Sleep Scales*,
DOI 10.1007/978-1-4419-9893-4_22, © Springer Science+Business Media, LLC 2012

Circadian Type Questionnaire

How easy do you find it to take short "cat naps" at odd times of day?

Very easy _______________________________________ Very difficult

If you have been out very late at a party, how easy do you find it to "sleep in" the following morning if there is nothing to prevent you doing so?

Very easy _______________________________________ Very difficult

After you've had several late-nights in a row, how easy do you find it to get to sleep if you go to bed early to try to "catch up"

Very easy _______________________________________ Very difficult

Do you have phases, *i.e.* several nights in a row, when you find it difficult to get to sleep?

Seldom _______________________________________ Frequently

How easy do you find it to sleep during the day if you have to?

Very easy _______________________________________ Very difficult

Do you go to bed at a regular time and get up at a regular time even if you don't have to?

Never _______________________________________ Always

To what extent do you prefer to have your meals at regular times?

No preference _______________________________________ Strong preference

When you are away on holiday, to what extent do you stick to your normal times of getting up and going to bed?

Very different _______________________________________ Exactly the same

If you have very little sleep one night, do you feel drowsy the following day?

Very much so _______________________________________ Hardly at all

To what extent are you better at working at certain times of day or night than at others?

Very much so _______________________________________ Hardly at all

Are you the sort of person who can easily miss out a night's sleep?

Definitely not _______________________________________ Definitely

If you are woken up at an unusual time can you "wake up" properly and do whatever it is you have to do?

Only with great difficulty ________________________________ Very easily

If you have something important to do but feel very drowsy can you overcome your drowsiness?

Only with great difficulty ________________________________ Very easily

Do you get a "second wind" if you stay up very late?

Always ________________________________ Never

How do you react to working at odd times of the day or night?

Enjoy it a lot ________________________________ Dislike it a lot

Are you the sort of person who feels far livelier during the day than early in the morning or late at night?

Definitely Not ________________________________ Definitely

If you don't have an alarm clock can you successfully "tell yourself" to wake up at a certain time?

Never ________________________________ Always

Do you find it easy to get up every early in the morning if, for example, you are setting off on holiday?

Very Difficult ________________________________ Very easy

When you have had to get up at a regular time for several days in a row do you start waking up just before your alarm clock goes off?

Never ________________________________ Frequently

Toward a predictive test of adjustment to shift work. Folkard and Monk [1], reprinted by permission of the publisher (Taylor & Francis Group).

References

1. Folkard, S. & Monk, T. H. (1979). Towards a predictive test of adjustment to shiftwork. *Ergonomics, 22*(1), 79–91.
2. Barton, J., Spelton, E. R., Totterdell, P. A., Smith, L. R., Folkard, S., & Costa, G. (1995). The standard shiftwork index: a battery of questionnaires for assessing shiftwork related problems. *Work and Stress, 9*, 4–30.
3. De Milia, L., Smith, P. A., & Folkard, S. (2004). Refining the psychometric properties of the circadian type inventory. *Personality and Individual Differences, 36*, 1953–1964.
4. Smith, P. A., Brown, D. F., Di Milia, L., & Wragg, C. (1993). The use of the circadian type inventory constructs of vigour and rigidity. *Ergonomics, 36*, 169–176.
5. Di Milia, L., Smith, P. A., & Folkard, S. (2005). A validation of the revised circadian type inventory in a working sample. *Personality and Individual Differences, 39*, 1293–1305.

Representative Studies Using Scale

Baehr, E. K., Revelle, W., & Eastman, C. I. (2000). Individual difference in the phase and amplitude of the human circadian temperature rhythm: with an emphasis on morningness-eveningness. *Journal of Sleep Research, 9*, 117–127.

Tucker, P., Smith, L., Macdonald, I., & Folkard, S. (2000). Effects of direction of rotation in continuous and discontinuous 8 hour shift systems. *Occupation and Environmental Medicine, 57*, 678–684.

23 Cleveland Adolescent Sleepiness Questionnaire (CASQ)

Purpose A 16-item, self-report questionnaire, the CASQ was designed to evaluate adolescent experiences of sleepiness and alertness in a variety of situations, including: in school, at home during the evening, and while in transit. Though similar scales have been developed in the past, the CASQ's creators suggest that these measures often contain items that are not applicable to children throughout the tested age range and that may not be particularly clear.

Population for Testing The scale has been validated with youth 11–17 years old.

Administration Requiring between 5 and 10 min, the scale is a self-report, pencil-and-paper measure.

Reliability and Validity In a psychometric analysis conducted by Spilsbury and colleagues [1], researchers demonstrated an internal consistency of .89. Total scores on the CASQ were negatively correlated with objective measures of sleep duration, while scores for youth in the obstructive sleep apnea group were significantly higher than those obtained by controls.

Obtaining a Copy A copy can be found in the original article published by developers [1].

Direct correspondence to:
James C. Spilsbury
Division of Clinical Epidemiology and Biostatistics
11400 Euclid Avenue
Cleveland, OH 44106-6083, USA
Email: jcs5@case.edu

Scoring Respondents use a 5-point, Likert-type scale to answer questions regarding their sleepiness in a variety of situations. Options range from "never," which receives a score of 1, to "almost always," which receives 5. Higher scores denote greater sleepiness.

A. Shahid et al. (eds.), *STOP, THAT and One Hundred Other Sleep Scales*,
DOI 10.1007/978-1-4419-9893-4_23, © Springer Science+Business Media, LLC 2012

Cleveland Adolescent Sleepiness Questionnaire

Today's Date: (fill in) __ __/__ __/__ __

What is your age? (fill in years) _____ **What is your sex? (check one)** 1. Female 2. Male

We would like to know about when you might feel sleepy during a usual week. For each statement, mark the circle under the response that best fits with how often it applies to you. It's important to answer them yourself – don't have people help you. There are no right or wrong answers. For example, if we asked "I sleep with a pillow," and the response that best fit how often you sleep with a pillow was "often," you would mark the item as follows:

EXAMPLE	**Never** (0 times per month)	**Rarely** (less than 3 times per month)	**Sometimes** (1-2 times per week)	**Often** (3-4 times per week)	**Almost every day** (5 or more times per week)
I sleep with a pillow	○	○	○	☒	○

Sleepiness Questions

	Never (0 times per month)	**Rarely** (less than 3 times per month)	**Sometimes** (1-2 times per week)	**Often** (3-4 times per week)	**Almost every day** (5 or more times per week)
1. I fall asleep during my morning classes	○	○	○	○	○
2. I go through the whole school day without feeling tired	○	○	○	○	○
3. I fall asleep during the last class of the day	○	○	○	○	○
4. I feel drowsy if I ride in a car for longer than five minutes	○	○	○	○	○
5. I feel wide-awake the whole day	○	○	○	○	○
6. I fall asleep at school in my afternoon classes	○	○	○	○	○

	Never (0 times per month)	Rarely (less than 3 times per month)	Sometimes (1-2 times per week)	Often (3-4 times per week)	Almost every day (5 or more times per week)
7. I feel alert during my classes	○	○	○	○	○
8. I feel sleepy in the evening after school	○	○	○	○	○
9. I feel sleepy when I ride in a bus to a school event like a field trip or sports game	○	○	○	○	○
10. In the morning when I am in school, I fall asleep	○	○	○	○	○
11. When I am in class, I feel wide-awake	○	○	○	○	○
12. I feel sleepy when I do my homework in the evening after school	○	○	○	○	○
13. I feel wide-awake the last class of the day	○	○	○	○	○
14. I fall asleep when I ride in a bus, car, or train	○	○	○	○	○
15. During the school day, there are times when I realize that I have just fallen asleep	○	○	○	○	○
16. I fall asleep when I do schoolwork at home in the evening	○	○	○	○	○

Reference

1. Spilsbury, J. C., Drotar, D., Rosen, C. L., Redline, S. (2007). The Cleveland adolescent sleepiness questionnaire: a new measure to assess excessive daytime sleepiness in adolescents. *Journal of Clinical Sleep Medicine, 3*(6), 603–612.

Representative Studies Using Scale

None

24 Columbia-Suicide Severity Rating Scale (C-SSRS)

Purpose The C-SSRS was designed to provide a prospective, standardized measure of suicidality. The scale allows clinicians and researchers alike to assess the severity and lethality of suicidal behaviors and ideations, and can be used to monitor treatment outcomes and establish suicide risk in a variety of research and clinical settings.

Population for Testing The scale has been used in a number of different populations, both adult and pediatric.

Administration Requiring approximately 5 min for completion, the C-SSRS is administered in the form of a clinical interview (though a self-report version is also available). Interviewers are not required to possess mental health training, allowing the scale to be used in any number of health care settings [1].

Reliability and Validity Though the scale itself has not been validated, it was created to be the prospective counterpart to the classification system called the Columbia Classification Algorithm for Suicide Assessment (C-CASA; [2]). The C-CASA was developed as a retrospective method for evaluating adverse events in clinical trials and was found to possess an overall reliability of .89.

Obtaining a Copy The scale is free for use in clinical settings. To obtain a copy, contact:
Kelly Posner
Center for Suicide Risk Assessment
Columbia University Department of Psychiatry
1051 Riverside Drive, Unit 74, New York, NY 10032, USA
Email: posnerk@childpsych.columbia.edu

Scoring In terms of suicidal behaviors, the scale is divided into several categories [3]: actual attempts, interrupted attempts, aborted attempts, and preparatory acts or behaviors. Interviewers establish the presence or absence of these behaviors and, where applicable, the number of attempts, both over the course of a lifetime and in the period of interest (the last week or month). Similarly, five aspects of suicidal ideation are queried: the wish to be dead, nonspecific active suicidal thoughts, active ideation without intent to act, active ideation with some intent to act, and active ideation with specific plan or intent. The presence and frequency of these different thoughts are evaluated.

A. Shahid et al. (eds.), *STOP, THAT and One Hundred Other Sleep Scales*,
DOI 10.1007/978-1-4419-9893-4_24, © Springer Science+Business Media, LLC 2012

COLUMBIA-SUICIDE SEVERITY RATING SCALE (C-SSRS)

Since Last Visit

Version 1/14/09

Posner, K.; Brent, D.; Lucas, C.; Gould, M.; Stanley, B.; Brown, G.; Fisher, P.; Zelazny, J.; Burke, A.; Oquendo, M.; Mann, J.

Disclaimer:

This scale is intended for use by trained clinicians. The questions contained in the Columbia-Suicide Severity Rating Scale are suggested probes. Ultimately, the determination of the presence of suicidality depends on clinical judgment.

Definitions of behavioral suicidal events in this scale are based on those used in **The Columbia Suicide History Form**, *developed by John Mann, MD and Maria Oquendo, MD, Conte Center for the Neuroscience of Mental Disorders (CCNMD), New York State Psychiatric Institute, 1051 Riverside Drive, New York, NY, 10032. (Oquendo M. A., Halberstam B. & Mann J. J., Risk factors for suicidal behavior: utility and limitations of research instruments. In M.B. First [Ed.]* Standardized Evaluation in Clinical Practice, *pp. 103 -130, 2003.)*

For reprints of the C-SSRS contact Kelly Posner, Ph.D., New York State Psychiatric Institute, 1051 Riverside Drive, New York, New York, 10032; inquiries and training requirements contact posnerk@childpsych.columbia.edu

SUICIDAL IDEATION	
Ask questions 1 and 2. If both are negative, proceed to "Suicidal Behavior" section. If the answer to question 2 is "yes," ask questions 3, 4 and 5. If the answer to question 1 and/or 2 is "yes", complete "Intensity of Ideation" section below.	Since Last Visit
1. Wish to be Dead Subject endorses thoughts about a wish to be dead or not alive anymore, or wish to fall asleep and not wake up. ***Have you wished you were dead or wished you could go to sleep and not wake up?*** If yes, describe:	**Yes** **No** ☐ ☐
2. Non-Specific Active Suicidal Thoughts General, non-specific thoughts of wanting to end one's life/commit suicide (e.g. *"I've thought about killing myself"*) without thoughts of ways to kill oneself/associated methods, intent, or plan during the assessment period. ***Have you actually had any thoughts of killing yourself?*** If yes, describe:	**Yes** **No** ☐ ☐
3. Active Suicidal Ideation with Any Methods (Not Plan) without Intent to Act Subject endorses thoughts of suicide and has thought of at least one method during the assessment period. This is different than a specific plan with time, place or method details worked out (e.g. thought of method to kill self but not a specific plan). Includes person who would say, *"I thought about taking an overdose but I never made a specific plan as to when, where or how I would actually do it.....and I would never go through with it".* ***Have you been thinking about how you might do this?*** If yes, describe:	**Yes** **No** ☐ ☐
4. Active Suicidal Ideation with Some Intent to Act, without Specific Plan Active suicidal thoughts of killing oneself and subject reports having some intent to act on such thoughts, as opposed to *"I have the thoughts but I definitely will not do anything about them".* ***Have you had these thoughts and had some intention of acting on them?*** If yes, describe:	**Yes** **No** ☐ ☐
5. Active Suicidal Ideation with Specific Plan and Intent Thoughts of killing oneself with details of plan fully or partially worked out and subject has some intent to carry it out. ***Have you started to work out or worked out the details of how to kill yourself? Do you intend to carry out this plan?*** If yes, describe:	**Yes** **No** ☐ ☐

INTENSITY OF IDEATION	
The following features should be rated with respect to the most severe type of ideation (i.e., 1-5 from above, with 1 being the least severe and 5 being the most severe). ***Most Severe Ideation:*** ____ ____________________ ***Type # (1-5)*** ***Description of Ideation***	Most Severe
Frequency ***How many times have you had these thoughts?*** (1) Less than once a week (2) Once a week (3) 2-5 times in week (4) Daily or almost daily (5) Many times each day	____
Duration ***When you have the thoughts, how long do they last?*** (1) Fleeting - few seconds or minutes (2) Less than 1 hour/some of the time (3) 1-4 hours/a lot of time (4) 4-8 hours/most of day (5) More than 8 hours/persistent or continuous	____
Controllability ***Could /can you stop thinking about killing yourself or wanting to die if you want to?*** (1) Easily able to control thoughts (2) Can control thoughts with little difficulty (3) Can control thoughts with some difficulty (4) Can control thoughts with a lot of difficulty (5) Unable to control thoughts (0) Does not attempt to control thoughts	____
Deterrents ***Are there things - anyone or anything (e.g. family, religion, pain of death) - that stopped you from wanting to die or acting on thoughts of committing suicide?*** (1) Deterrents definitely stopped you from attempting suicide (2) Deterrents probably stopped you (3) Uncertain that deterrents stopped you (4) Deterrents most likely did not stop you (5) Deterrents definitely did not stop you (0) Does not apply	____
Reasons for Ideation ***What sort of reasons did you have for thinking about wanting to die or killing yourself? Was it to end the pain or stop the way you were feeling (in other words you couldn't go on living with this pain or how you were feeling) or was it to get attention, revenge or a reaction from others? Or both?*** (1) Completely to get attention, revenge or a reaction from others. (2) Mostly to get attention, revenge or a reaction from others. (3) Equally to get attention, revenge or a reaction from others and to end/stop the pain. (4) Mostly to end or stop the pain (you couldn't go on living with the pain or how you were feeling). (5) Completely to end or stop the pain (you couldn't go on living with the pain or how you were feeling). (0) Does not apply	____

Version 1/14/09

SUICIDAL BEHAVIOR *(Check all that apply, so long as these are separate events; must ask about all types)*	Since Last Visit

Actual Attempt:
A potentially self-injurious act committed with at least some wish to die, *as a result of act.* Behavior was in part thought of as method to kill oneself. Intent does not have to be 100%. If there is ***any*** intent/desire to die associated with the act, then it can be considered an actual suicide attempt. ***There does not have to be any injury or harm,*** just the potential for injury or harm. If person pulls trigger while gun is in mouth but gun is broken so no injury results, this is considered an attempt.
Inferring Intent: Even if an individual denies intent/wish to die, it may be inferred clinically from the behavior or circumstances. For example, a highly lethal act that is clearly not an accident so no other intent but suicide can be inferred (e.g. gunshot to head, jumping from window of a high floor/story). Also, if someone denies intent to die, but they thought that what they did could be lethal, intent may be inferred.
Have you made a suicide attempt?
Have you done anything to harm yourself?
Have you done anything dangerous where you could have died?
    What did you do?
    Did you______ as a way to end your life?
    Did you want to die (even a little) when you_____?
    Were you trying to end your life when you _____?
    Or did you think it was possible you could have died from_____?
Or did you do it purely for other reasons / without ANY intention of killing yourself (like to relieve stress, feel better, get sympathy, or get something else to happen)? (Self-Injurious Behavior without suicidal intent)
If yes, describe:
 	
Has subject engaged in Non-Suicidal Self-Injurious Behavior?
	Yes **No**
	☐ ☐
	
	Total # of Attempts
	_____
	
	Yes **No**
	☐ ☐

Interrupted Attempt: When the person is interrupted (by an outside circumstance) from starting the potentially self-injurious act *(if not for that, actual attempt would have occurred).* Overdose: Person has pills in hand but is stopped from ingesting. Once they ingest any pills, this becomes an attempt rather than an interrupted attempt. Shooting: Person has gun pointed toward self, gun is taken away by someone else, or is somehow prevented from pulling trigger. Once they pull the trigger, even if the gun fails to fire, it is an attempt. Jumping: Person is poised to jump, is grabbed and taken down from ledge. Hanging: Person has noose around neck but has not yet started to hang - is stopped from doing so. ***Has there been a time when you started to do something to end your life but someone or something stopped you before you actually did anything?*** If yes, describe:	**Yes** **No** ☐ ☐ Total # of interrupted _____
Aborted Attempt: When person begins to take steps toward making a suicide attempt, but stops themselves before they actually have engaged in any self-destructive behavior. Examples are similar to interrupted attempts, except that the individual stops him/herself, instead of being stopped by something else. ***Has there been a time when you started to do something to try to end your life but you stopped yourself before you actually did anything?*** If yes, describe:	**Yes** **No** ☐ ☐ Total # of aborted _____
Preparatory Acts or Behavior: Acts or preparation towards imminently making a suicide attempt. This can include anything beyond a verbalization or thought, such as assembling a specific method (e.g. buying pills, purchasing a gun) or preparing for one's death by suicide (e.g. giving things away, writing a suicide note). ***Have you taken any steps towards making a suicide attempt or preparing to kill yourself (such as collecting pills, getting a gun, giving valuables away or writing a suicide note)?*** If yes, describe:	**Yes** **No** ☐ ☐
Suicidal Behavior: Suicidal behavior was present during the assessment period?	**Yes** **No** ☐ ☐
Completed Suicide:	**Yes** **No** ☐ ☐
Answer for Actual Attempts Only	Most Lethal Attempt Date:
Actual Lethality/Medical Damage: 0. No physical damage or very minor physical damage (e.g. surface scratches). 1. Minor physical damage (e.g. lethargic speech; first-degree burns; mild bleeding; sprains). 2. Moderate physical damage; medical attention needed (e.g. conscious but sleepy, somewhat responsive; second-degree burns; bleeding of major vessel). 3. Moderately severe physical damage; *medical* hospitalization and likely intensive care required (e.g. comatose with reflexes intact; third-degree burns less than 20% of body; extensive blood loss but can recover; major fractures). 4. Severe physical damage; *medical* hospitalization with intensive care required (e.g. comatose without reflexes; third-degree burns over 20% of body; extensive blood loss with unstable vital signs; major damage to a vital area). 5. Death	*Enter Code* _____
Potential Lethality: Only Answer if Actual Lethality=0 Likely lethality of actual attempt if no medical damage (the following examples, while having no actual medical damage, had potential for very serious lethality: put gun in mouth and pulled the trigger but gun fails to fire so no medical damage; laying on train tracks with oncoming train but pulled away before run over). 0 = Behavior not likely to result in injury 1 = Behavior likely to result in injury but not likely to cause death 2 = Behavior likely to result in death despite available medical care	*Enter Code* _____

References

1. Gangwisch, J. E., & Jacobson, C. M. (2009). New perspectives on assessment of suicide risk. *Current Treatment Opinions in Neurology, 11*(5), 371–376.
2. Posner, K. Oquendo, M. A., Gould, M., Stanley, B., & Davies, M. (2007). Columbia Classification Algorithm of Suicide Assessment (C-CASA): Classification of suicidal events in the FDA's pediatric suicidal risk analysis of antidepressants. *American Journal of Psychiatry, 164*(7), 1035–1043.
3. Posner, K. (2007). Suicidality issues in clinical trials: Columbia suicidal adverse event identification in PDA safety analysis [PowerPoint slides]. Retrieved from FDA website: http://www. fda.gov/ohrms/DOCKETS/ac/07/slides/2007-4306s1-01-CU-Posner.ppt#540,1,Slide 1

Representative Studies Using Scale

Faulconbridge, L. F., Wadden, T. A., Berkowitz, R. I., Sarwer, D. B., Womble, L. G., Hesson. L. A., Stunkard, A. J., & Fabricatore, A. N. (2009). Changes in symptoms of depression with weight loss. *Obesity, 17*(5), 1009–1016.

25 Composite Morningness Questionnaire

Purpose Finding the psychometric properties of alternative morningness questionnaires to be inadequate, developers culled items from two of these scales–the Horne Östberg Morningness-Eveningness Questionnaire [3] (Chap. 54)* and a diurnal type scale by Torsvall and Akerstedt [1] – to create the Composite Morningness Questionnaire. Through factor analysis, 13 items were selected from the two original questionnaires. Among these items, three factors were identified: morning activities, morning affect, and eveningness.

Population for Testing The scale has been validated in population of more than 500 undergraduate students.

Administration The scale is a self-report, paper-and-pencil measure requiring between 3 and 5 min for completion.

Reliability and Validity When developing the scale, Smith and colleagues [2] combined the two original questionnaires, analyzed out the three most reliable factors, and selected the items that best represented those factors. The resulting scale was found to have an internal consistency of .87.

Obtaining a Copy A copy can be found in the original article published by developers [2].

Direct correspondence to:
Carlla S. Smith, Department of Psychology
Bowling Green State University
Bowling Green, Ohio 43403, USA

Scoring For questions regarding preferred sleeping and waking times, respondents select the most suitable option from a list of time increments. Issues like ease of waking, alertness throughout the day, and exercise are also queried. Potential scores for the scale's items range from 1 to 4 or 5, with higher scores indicating a greater degree of morningness. Cutoffs for the scale were chosen using the upper and lower percentiles of the scale: A score of 22 or below indicates an evening type, a score above 44 indicates a morning type, and scores in between receive a classification of intermediate.

* Not included in this edition. Will be cited in the next version. In the interim, this and new emerging scales are listed and analysed in a similar way on our website www.sleepontario.com under "Scales".

A. Shahid et al. (eds.), *STOP, THAT and One Hundred Other Sleep Scales*,
DOI 10.1007/978-1-4419-9893-4_25, © Springer Science+Business Media, LLC 2012

Composite Morningness Questionnaire

Directions: Please *check* the response for *each* item that best describes *you*.

1. Considering only your own "feeling best" rhythm, at what time would you get up if you were entirely free to plan your day?

5:00-6:30 a.m.	_____ (5)
6:30-7:45 a.m.	_____ (4)
7:45-9:45 a.m.	_____ (3)
9:45-11:00 a.m.	_____ (2)
11:00 a.m. – 12:00 (noon)	_____ (1)

2. Considering your only "feeling best" rhythm, at what time would you go to bed if you were entirely free to plan your evening?

8:00-9:00 p.m.	_____ (5)
9:00-10:15 p.m.	_____ (4)
10:15 p.m. – 12:30 a.m.	_____ (3)
12:30–1:45 a.m.	_____ (2)
1:45-3:00 a.m.	_____ (1)

3. Assuming normal circumstance, how easy do you find getting up in the morning? (Check one.)

Not at all easy	_____ (1)
Slightly easy	_____ (2)
Fairly easy	_____ (3)
Very easy	_____ (4)

4. How alert do you feel during the first half hour after having awakened in the morning? (Check one.)

Not at all alert	_____ (1)
Slightly alert	_____ (2)
Fairly alert	_____ (3)
Very alert	_____ (4)

5. During the first half hour after having awakened in the morning, how tired do you feel? (Check one.)

Very tired	_____ (1)
Fairly tired	_____ (2)
Fairly refreshed	_____ (3)
Very refreshed	_____ (4)

6. You have decided to engage in some physical exercise. A friend suggests that you do this one hour twice a week and the best time for him is 7:00-8:00 a.m. Bearing in mind nothing else but your own "feeling best" rhythm, how do you think you would perform?

Would be in good form	_____ (4)
Would be in reasonable form	_____ (3)
Would find it difficult	_____ (2)
Would find it very difficult	_____ (1)

7. At what time in the evening do you feel tired and, as a result, in need of sleep?

8:00-9:00 p.m.	_____ (5)
9:00-10:15 p.m.	_____ (4)
10:15 p.m. – 12:30 a.m.	_____ (3)
12:30–1:45 a.m.	_____ (2)
1:45-3:00 a.m.	_____ (1)

8. You wish to be at your peak performance for a test which you know is going to be mentally exhausting and lasting for two hours. You are entirely free to plan your day, and considering only your own "feeling best" rhythm, which ONE of the four testing times would you choose?

8:00-10:00 a.m. _____ (4)
11:00 a.m. – 1:00 p.m. _____ (3)
3:00-5:00 p.m. _____ (2)
7:00-9:00 p.m. _____ (1)

9. One hears about "morning" and "evening" types of people. Which ONE of these types do you consider yourself to be?

Definitely a morning type _____ (4)
More a morning than an evening type _____ (3)
More an evening than a morning type _____ (2)
Definitely an evening type _____ (1)

10. When would you prefer to rise (provided you have a full day's work—8 hours) if you were totally free to arrange your time?

Before 6:30 a.m. _____ (4)
6:30-7:30 a.m. _____ (3)
7:30-8:30 a.m. _____ (2)
8:30 a.m. or later _____ (1)

11. If you always had to rise at 6:00 a.m., what do you think it would be like?

Very difficult and unpleasant _____ (1)
Rather difficult and unpleasant _____ (2)
A little unpleasant but no great problem _____ (3)
Easy and not unpleasant _____ (4)

12. How long a time does it usually take before you "recover your senses" in the morning after rising from a night's sleep?

0-10 minutes _____ (4)
11-20 minutes _____ (3)
21-40 minutes _____ (2)
More than 40 minutes _____ (1)

13. Please indicate to what extent you are a morning or evening *active* individual.

Pronounced morning active (morning alert and evening tired) _____ (4)
To some extent, morning active _____ (3)
To some extent, evening active _____ (2)
Pronounced evening active (morning tired and evening alert) _____ (1)

Note: Scoring is indicated in parentheses beside each score anchor.

References

1. Torsvall, L. & Akerstedt, T. (1980). A diurnal type scale. Construction, consistency and validation in shift work. *Scandinavian Journal of Work Environment Health, 6*, 283–290.
2. Smith, C. S., Reilly, C., & Midkiff, K. (1989). Evaluation of three circadian rhythm questionnaires with suggestions for an improved measure of morningness. *Journal of Applied Psychology, 74*(5), 728–738.
3. Home, J., & Ostberg, O. (1976). A self-assessment questionnaire to determine morningness-eveningness in human circadian rhythms. International Journal of Chronobiology,4, 97–110.

Representative Studies Using Scale

Mitchell, R. J. & Williamson, A. M. (2000). Evaluation an 8 hour versus a 12 hour shift roster on employees at a power station. *Applied Ergonomics, 31*(1), 83–93.

Waage, S., Moen, B. E., Pallesen, S., Eriksen, H. R., Ursin, H., Akerstedt, T., & Bjorvatn, B. (2009). Shift work disorder among oil rig workers in the North Sea. *Sleep, 32*(4), 558–565.

26 CPAP Use Questionnaire

Purpose The questionnaire consists of nine items designed to assess "cues to action" – signals from a variety of sources that can affect patients' perceptions of CPAP and can act as triggers for health-related behavior (e.g., compliance with CPAP therapy) [1]. The scale evaluates three separate factors: health cues (including concern about tiredness and potential health consequences), partner cues (those such as encouragement from the partner, and the partner's difficulty in sleeping due to snoring), and health professional cues (messages from a physician about the need for CPAP). Future studies using this scale are likely to focus on its utility in predicting CPAP compliance.

Population for Testing The scale was validated in a population of 63 patients diagnosed with obstructive sleep apnea following the first month of CPAP prescription [1].

Administration The questionnaire is a self-report, paper-and-pencil measure requiring between 2 and 5 min for completion.

Reliability and Validity In an initial evaluation, the scale was found to have an internal consistency of .63. Due to the novelty of such a scale, construct validity could not be fully assessed. Instead, scores on the three factor subscales were variables like relationship status (for the "partner cues" factor) and the Epworth Sleepiness Scale (for the "health cues" factor).

Obtaining a Copy A copy of the original scale can be found in the original article by the developers Olsen et al. [1]. The American Academy of Sleep Medicine must be contacted in order to reproduce or duplicate the scale.

Corresponding author:
Sara Olsen
University of Queensland, School of Psychology
St. Lucia, 4072, Queensland, Australia
Email: s.olsen2@uq.edu.au

Scoring Patients are asked to rate the importance of each cue on a 4-point Likert scale ranging from 0 ("not at all") to 3 ("extremely important"). Total scores are calculated by summing each item. A higher total score indicates greater overall importance attributed cues to start CPAP therapy.

A. Shahid et al. (eds.), *STOP, THAT and One Hundred Other Sleep Scales*,
DOI 10.1007/978-1-4419-9893-4_26, © Springer Science+Business Media, LLC 2012

Cues to CPAP Use Questionnaire (CCUQ)

In this section we would like you to indicate how important the following factors were in your decision to start using CPAP If a particular statement is not applicable for you, please indicate this by filling in the "⓪ not at all" response option. The scale is provided below:

⓪ Not At All ① A Little Important ② Moderately Important ③ Extremely Important

1. I started using CPAP because my sleep physician said that I should	⓪ ① ② ③
2. I started using CPAP because I was worried about my heart	⓪ ① ② ③
3. I started using CPAP because my partner couldn't sleep because of my snoring	⓪ ① ② ③
4. I started using CPAP because my sleep physician was worried about my sleep apnoea	⓪ ① ② ③
5. I started using CPAP following advice from a friend/acquaintance who does not have sleep apnoea	⓪ ① ② ③
6. My partner encouraged me to start using CPAP	⓪ ① ② ③
7. I started using CPAP because I was worried about the health consequences of my sleep problem	⓪ ① ② ③
8. I started using CPAP because I was so tired all of the time	⓪ ① ② ③
9. I started using CPAP because I was worried that I would have a car accident	⓪ ① ② ③

Reference

1. Olsen, S., Smith, S., Oei, T., & Douglas, J. (2010). Cues to starting CPAP in obstructive sleep apnea: development and validation of the cues to CPAP use questionnaire. *Journal of Clinical Sleep Medicine, 6*(3), 229–237.

Representative Studies Using Scale

None.

Depression and Somatic Symptoms Scale (DSSS)

27

Purpose The scale was developed as a simultaneous measure of depression and somatic symptoms – two issues that frequently co-occur [1]. Though many preexisting questionnaires for depression contain items relating to somatic complaints, the DSSS is specifically concerned with the relationship between the two. Consisting of 22 items, the DSSS includes 12 depression-related items and 10 somatic items – 5 of which query pain symptoms, forming a pain subscale. Two items of the depression subscale relate particularly to sleep, examining symptoms of insomnia and fatigue.

Population for Testing The scale was initially evaluated in a population of patients experiencing a major depressive episode (MDE) and in a group of non-MDE controls. Participants were aged 18–65 years.

Administration The scale is a self-report, pencil-and-paper measure requiring between 5 and 10 min for completion.

Reliability and Validity The scale's psychometric properties were first evaluated by developers Hung and colleagues [2]. They found an internal consistency ranging from .73 to .94 and a test-retest reliability of .88–.92. Additionally, scores on the DSSS were significantly correlated with those obtained on the Hamilton Rating Scale for Depression (Chap. 42), and results for both decreased significantly following treatment.

Obtaining a Copy A copy of the scale can be found in an article published by developers [2].

Direct correspondence to:
Chia-Yih Liu,
Department of Psychiatry
Chang Gung Memorial Hospital
5 Fu-Shing St, Kweishan
Taoyuan 333, Taiwan
Email: liucy752@cgmh.org.tw

Scoring Respondents are asked to indicate the degree to which they have experienced each symptom over the course of the previous week. The rating scale ranges from "absent" (0 points) to "severe" (3 points), and a total score is found by adding the results for all 22 items. Higher scores indicate more severe depressive and somatic issues.

A. Shahid et al. (eds.), *STOP, THAT and One Hundred Other Sleep Scales*,
DOI 10.1007/978-1-4419-9893-4_27, © Springer Science+Business Media, LLC 2012

Depression and somatic symptoms scale

Date: __/__/__

Please evaluate the severity of these symptoms you have experienced in the past week (7 days):

Absent: no symptoms.

Mild: symptoms caused **slight** discomfort or disturbance.

Moderate: symptoms caused **significant** discomfort or disturbance.

Severe: symptoms caused **very significant** discomfort or disturbance.

Please check one of absent, mild, moderate, or severe to indicate the severity of the following symptoms.

	Absent	Mild	Moderate	Severe
1. Headache				
2. Loss of interest in daily or leisure activities				
3. Tightness in the chest				
4. Insomnia				
5. Muscle tension				
6. Irritable mood				
7. Back pain				
8. Unable to feel happy or decreased ability to feel happy				
9. Dizziness				
10. Depressed mood or tearful				
11. Chest pain				
12. Feelings of self-reproach or guilt				
13. Neck or shoulder pain (or soreness)				
14. Loss of interest in sex				
15. Shortness of breath or difficulty breathing				
16. Anxious or nervous				
17. Soreness in more than half of the body's muscles				
18. Unable to concentrate				
19. Palpitations or increased heart rate				
20. Thoughts of death or suicidal ideas				
21. Fatigue or loss of energy				
22. Decreased appetite or loss of appetite				

References

1. Simon, G. E., VonKorff, M., Piccinelli, M., Fullerton, C., & Ormel, J. (1999). An international study of the relation between somatic symptoms and depression. *Journal of Medicine, 341*(18), 1329–1335.
2. Hung, C. I., Weng, L. J., Su, Y. J., & Liu, C. Y. (2006). Depression and somatic symptoms scale: a new scale with both depression and somatic symptoms emphasized. *Psychiatry and Clinical Neurosciences, 60*, 700–708.

Representative Studies Using Scale

Hung, C. I., Liu, C. Y., Cheng, Y. T., & Wang, S. J. (2009). Migraine: a missing link between somatic symptoms and major depressive disorder. *Journal of Affective Disorders, 117*(1), 108–115.

28 Dysfunctional Beliefs and Attitudes About Sleep Scale (DBAS)

Purpose Consisting of 28 items, the scale evaluates sleep-related beliefs, querying respondents' expectations and attitudes regarding the causes, consequences, and potential treatments of sleep issues. The scale may be particularly valuable in the formation of cognitive approaches to treatment. Identifying and targeting disordered cognitions about sleep may help to improve intervention outcomes.

Population for Testing The scale has been validated in an older population aged 55–88 years [1], as well as a younger patient population with a mean age of 49.8 years [2].

Administration The scale is a self-report, paper-and-pencil measure and it requires between 10 and 15 min for completion.

Reliability and Validity In an initial psychometric evaluation conducted by developers [1], the scale was shown to have an internal consistency ranging from .80 to .81. However, in a follow-up study by Espie and colleagues [2], only two of the scale's five domains were found to possess satisfactory internal consistencies, leading to the development of the DBAS-10 – a shorter, 10-item version of the original.

Obtaining a Copy A copy of the scale can be found in the original article published by developers [1].

Direct correspondence to:
Charles M. Morin
Virginia Commonwealth University
Medical College of Virginia, Department of Psychiatry
Box 268, Richmond, Virginia 23298-0268, USA

Scoring Each question consists of a 100-mm visual analogue scale which respondents use to indicate the degree to which they agree with statements related to sleep (with 0 indicating "strongly disagree" and 100 denoting "strongly agree"). Scores are calculated by measuring the distance, in millimeters, from the start of the line to the respondent's mark. A global score is found by averaging scores on all items, with higher scores indicating more dysfunctional beliefs and attitudes (item 23 is reverse-scored). While some researchers argue in favor of visual analogue scales and their sensitivity to subtle differences, others have found that certain items of the DBAS exhibit low mean and variance – evidence of a low sensitivity to individual differences [3].

A. Shahid et al. (eds.), *STOP, THAT and One Hundred Other Sleep Scales*,
DOI 10.1007/978-1-4419-9893-4_28, © Springer Science+Business Media, LLC 2012

Dysfunctional Beliefs and Attitudes about Sleep Scale (DBAS)

A number of statements reflecting people's beliefs and attitudes about sleep are provided below. Please indicate to what extent you personally agree or disagree with each statement. There is no right or wrong answer. For each statement, place a mark (/) somewhere along the line wherever your personal rating falls. Please consider the line to represent your own personal range. Try to use the whole scale rather than simply putting your marks at one end or the other of the line. Even if you do not have a sleep problem, please answer all questions.

1. I need 8 hours of sleep to feel refreshed and function well during the day.
2. When I don't get the proper amount of sleep on a given night, I need to catch up the next day by napping or the next night by sleeping longer.
3. Because I am getting older, I need less sleep.
4. I am worried that if I go for 1 or 2 nights without sleep, I may have a "nervous breakdown".
5. I am concerned that chronic insomnia may have serious consequences on my physical health.
6. By spending more time in bed, I usually get more sleep and feel better the next day.
7. When I have trouble falling asleep or getting back to sleep after nighttime awakening, I should stay in bed and try harder.
8. I am worried that I may lose control over my abilities to sleep.
9. Because I am getting older, I should go to bed earlier in the evening.
10. After a poor night's sleep, I know it will interfere with my activities the next day.
11. To be alert and function well during the day, I believe I would be better off taking a sleeping pill rather than having a poor night's sleep.
12. When I feel irritable, depressed, or anxious during the day, it is mostly because I did not sleep well the night before.
13. Because my bed partner falls asleep as soon as his or her head hits the pillow and stays asleep through the night, I should be able to do so too.
14. I feel insomnia is basically the result of aging and there isn't much that can be done about this problem.
15. I am sometimes afraid of dying in my sleep.
16. When I have a good night's sleep, I know that I will have to pay for it the next night.
17. When I sleep poorly one night, I know it will disturb my sleep schedule for the whole week.
18. Without an adequate night's sleep, I can hardly function the next day.
19. I can't ever predict whether I'll have a good or poor night's sleep.
20. I have little ability to manage the negative consequences of disturbed sleep.

21. When I feel tired, have no energy, or just seem not to function well during the day, it is generally because I did not sleep well the night before.
22. I get overwhelmed by my thoughts at night and often feel I have no control over this racing mind.
23. I can still lead a satisfactory life despite sleep difficulties.
24. I believe insomnia is essentially the result of a chemical imbalance.
25. I feel insomnia is ruining my ability to enjoy life and prevents me from doing what I want.
26. My sleep is getting worse all the time and I don't believe anyone can help.
27. A nightcap before bedtime is a good solution to sleep problems.
28. Medication is probably the only solution to sleeplessness.

Note: For each statement, the subject indicates his or her level of agreement or disagreement on a visual analog scale such as the following one.

Strongly Disagree ____ Strongly Agree

References

1. Morin. C. M., Stone, J. Trinkle, D., Mercer, J., & Remsberg, S. (1993). Dysfunctional beliefs and attitudes about sleep among older adults with and without insomnia complaints. *Psychology and Aging, 8*(3), 463–467.
2. Espie, C. A., Inglis, S. J., Harvey, L., & Tessier, S. (2000). Insomniacs' attributions: psychometric properties of the dysfunctional beliefs about sleep scale and the sleep disturbance questionnaire. *Journal of Psychosomatic Research, 48*, 141–148.
3. Morin, C. M., Vallières, A., & Ivers, H. (2007). Dysfunctional beliefs and attitudes about sleep (DBAS): validation of a brief version (DBAS-16). *Sleep, 30*(11), 1547–1554.

Representative Studies Using Scale

Edinger, J. D., Wohlgemuth, W. K., Radtke, R. A., March, G. R., & Quillian, R. E. (2001). Does cognitive-behavioral insomnia therapy alter dysfunctional beliefs about sleep? *Sleep, 24*(5), 591–599.

Morin, C. M., Blais, F., & Savard, J. (2002). Are changes in beliefs and attitudes about sleep related to sleep improvements in the treatment of insomnia? *Behaviour Research and Therapy, 40*(7), 741–752.

29 Epworth Sleepiness Scale (ESS)

Purpose Designed to evaluate overall daytime sleepiness, the questionnaire asks respondents to rate how likely they are to fall asleep in eight different situations. Each circumstance represents a moment of relative inactivity, from lying down for a nap in the afternoon to sitting in a car stopped in traffic. The scale may be indicated for use in research as well as for clinicians requiring an efficient screening devise for daytime sleepiness.

Population for Testing The scale has been validated with a population of adults with ages ranging from 18 to 78 years.

Administration A brief, pencil-and-paper self-report measure, the questionnaire should require approximately 2–5 min for completion.

Reliability and Validity The scale's psychometric properties were evaluated initially in a study by Johns [2]. When compared to the results of two other tests measuring daytime sleepiness [1], the ESS had a sensitivity of .94 and a specificity of 1.00.

Obtaining a Copy The scale is under copyright. The official website for this scale is www.epworthsleepinessscale.com.

Direct correspondence to:
Dr. Murray W. Johns,
Sleep Disorders Unit, Epworth Hospital
Melbourne, Victoria 3121
Australia

Scoring Using a scale of 0–3 (with 0 meaning "would *never* doze" and 3 meaning "*high* chance of dozing"), respondents rate their likelihood of falling asleep in a variety of situations. Total scores can range from 0 to 24. In terms of interpreting results, Johns and Hocking [3] have found a mean score of 4.6 ± 2.8 SD in normal participants. Thus, Johns [1] suggests a cutoff score 10 for identifying daytime sleepiness at a potentially clinical level.

A. Shahid et al. (eds.), *STOP, THAT and One Hundred Other Sleep Scales*,
DOI 10.1007/978-1-4419-9893-4_29, © Springer Science+Business Media, LLC 2012

Epworth Sleepiness Scale

Name: ____ Today's date: ______________

Your age (Yrs): ____________ Your sex (Male = M, Female = F): ______

How likely are you to doze off or fall asleep in the following situations, in contrast to feeling just tired?

This refers to your usual way of life in recent times.

Even if you haven't done some of these things recently try to work out how they would have affected you.

Use the following scale to choose the **most appropriate number** for each situation:

0 = would **never** doze
1 = **slight chance** of dozing
2 = **moderate chance** of dozing
3 = **high chance** of dozing

It is important that you answer each question as best you can.

Situation	**Chance of Dozing (0-3)**
Sitting and reading	___
Watching TV	___
Sitting, inactive in a public place (e.g. a theatre or a meeting)	___
As a passenger in a car for an hour without a break	___
Lying down to rest in the afternoon when circumstances permit	___
Sitting and talking to someone	___
Sitting quietly after a lunch without alcohol	___
In a car, while stopped for a few minutes in the traffic	

THANK YOU FOR YOUR COOPERATION

References

1. Johns, M. W. (2000). "Sensitivity and specificity of the multiple sleep latency test (MSLT), the maintenance of wakefulness test and the Epworth sleepiness scale: Failure of the MSLT as a gold standard." *Journal of Sleep Research, 9*, 5–11.
2. Johns, M. W. (1991). "A new method for measuring daytime sleepiness: the Epworth sleepiness scale." *Sleep, 14*(6), 540–545.
3. Johns, M. W. & Hocking, B. (1997). Daytime sleepiness and sleep habits of Australian workers. *Sleep, 20*, 844–849.

Representative Studies Using Scale

Choi, J. B., Nelesen, R., Loredo, J. S., Mills, P. J., Ancoli-Israel, S., Ziegler, M. G., & Dimsdale, J. E. (2006). Sleepiness in obstructive sleep apnea: a harbinger of impaired cardiac function? *Sleep, 29*(12), 1531–1536.

Arzt, M., Young, T., Finn, L., Skatrud, J. B., Clodagh, M. R., Newton, G. E., Mak, S., Parker, J. D., Floras, J. S., & Bradley, T. D. (2006). Sleepiness and sleep in patients with both systolic heart failure and obstructive sleep apnea. *Archives of Internal Medicine, 166*(16), 1716–1722.

Espie Sleep Disturbance Questionnaire (SDQ)

30

Purpose The SDQ is a 12-item scale designed to evaluate subjective experiences of insomnia. An analysis conducted by Espie and colleagues [1] revealed the four factors assessed by the scale: attributions regarding restlessness/agitation, attributions concerning mental overactivity, attributions concerning the consequences of insomnia, and attributions concerning lack of sleep readiness. While the questionnaire is similar to another scale created by developers – the Dysfunctional Beliefs and Attitudes about Sleep Scale (DBAS; (Chap. 28) – the SDQ is concerned specifically with beliefs about the sources of sleep issues, while the DBAS is more general in its focus.

Population for Testing The SDQ has been validated in a population of chronic insomnia patients with a mean age of 49.8 (SD 17.9).

Administration The scale is a self-administered, pencil-and-paper measure requiring between 3 and 5 min for completion.

Reliability and Validity According to a study conducted by Espie and colleagues [1], the scale possesses an internal consistency of .67. Though the scale was originally shown to possess three factors – mental activity, sleep pattern problem, and physical tension [2] – the current study elucidated a more suitable four-factor structure: attributions regarding restlessness/agitation, attributions concerning mental overactivity, attributions concerning the consequences of insomnia, and attributions concerning lack of sleep readiness.

Obtaining a Copy An example of the scale's items can be found in an article published by Espie and colleagues [1].

Direct correspondence to:
Colin A. Espie Telephone: 0141-211-3903
Email: c.espie@clinmed.gla.ac.uk

Scoring Respondents use a five-point, Likert-type scale to indicate how often certain statements about insomnia are representative of their experience – 1 means "never true," while 5 means "very often true." Higher scores are indicative of more dysfunctional beliefs about the causes and correlates of insomnia.

References

1. Espie, C. A., Inglis, S. J., Harvey, L., & Tessier, S. (2000). Insomniacs' attributions: psychometric properties of the dysfunctional beliefs and attitudes about sleep scale and the sleep disturbance scale. *Journal of Psychosomatic Research, 48*(2), 141–148.
2. Espie, C. A., Brooks, D. N., & Lindsay, W. R. (1989). An evaluation of tailored psychological treatment of insomnia. *Journal of Behavior Therapy and Experimental Psychology, 20*, 143–153.

A. Shahid et al. (eds.), *STOP, THAT and One Hundred Other Sleep Scales*,
DOI 10.1007/978-1-4419-9893-4_30, © Springer Science+Business Media, LLC 2012

Representative Studies Using Scale

Harvey, A. G., Schmidt, D. A., Scarnà, A., Semler, C. N., & Goodwin, G. M. (2005). Sleep-related functioning in euthymic patients with bipolar disorder, patients with insomnia, and subjects without sleep problems. *American Journal of Psychiatry, 162*(1), 50–59.

Watts, F. N., Coyle, K., & East, M. P. (1994). The contribution of worry to insomnia. *British Journal of Clinical Psychology, 33*(2), 211–220.

31 FACES (Fatigue, Anergy, Consciousness, Energy, Sleepiness)

Purpose The original purpose of this adjectival checklist was to distinguish between tiredness, sleepiness, and fatigue. With such a wide spectrum of adjectives available to describe fatigue and its associated energy states, scale developers hoped to create a measure that would be sensitive to a variety of experiences related to these states of energy deficiency. The checklist consists of 50 adjectives found to cluster into five subscales prompted by the acronym FACES: Fatigue (adjectives like "exhausted," "drained," and "weary"), Anergy ("indolent," "languid"), Consciousness ("comatose," "unconscious"), Energy ("vigorous," "lively"), and Sleepiness ("sleepy," "drowsy"). Unlike the Fatigue Assessment Scale (FAS; Chap. 33), the FACES is a multidimensional approach to the construct of fatigue.

Population for Testing The scale has been validated with a population of insomnia patients with a mean age of 43.5 ± 13.9 years.

Administration Requiring between 5 and 10 min for completion, the scale is a self-report, paper-and-pencil measure.

Reliability and Validity Developers Shapiro and colleagues [1] evaluated the psychometric properties of the scale and found an internal consistency ranging from .78 to .97. The checklist also possessed good convergent validity, with the sleepiness and consciousness subscales correlating highly with scores on the Epworth Sleepiness Scale.

Obtaining a Copy A copy of the scale's items can be found in an article published by developers [1].

Direct correspondence to:
Colin M. Shapiro
Telephone: +1-416-603-5273
Email: suzanne.alves@uhn.on.ca

Scoring Respondents use a scale ranging from 0 ("not at all") to 3 ("strongly") to indicate the degree to which they have experienced each feeling or energy state over the course of the previous week. Higher scores indicate more acute states of tiredness or fatigue, except for those items belonging to the energy subscale.

A. Shahid et al. (eds.), *STOP, THAT and One Hundred Other Sleep Scales*,
DOI 10.1007/978-1-4419-9893-4_31,

FACES ADJECTIVE CHECKLIST

Below is a list of words that describe feelings people have. Please read each one carefully. Then circle the ONE number corresponding to the adjective phrase that best describes **HOW YOU HAVE BEEN FEELING DURING THE PAST WEEK INCLUDING TODAY**. If you are unfamiliar with any of the words, please circle the question mark (?) to the right of the rating scale. The numbers refer to the following descriptive phrases:

1. Fatigued	0	1	2	3	4	?		26. Comatose	0	1	2	3	4	?
2. Worn-out	0	1	2	3	4	?		27. Unconscious	0	1	2	3	4	?
3. Exhausted	0	1	2	3	4	?		28. Dormant	0	1	2	3	4	?
4. Wacked-out	0	1	2	3	4	?		29. Bombed	0	1	2	3	4	?
5. Drained	0	1	2	3	4	?		30. Blurry-eyed	0	1	2	3	4	?
6. Pooped	0	1	2	3	4	?		31. Vigorous	0	1	2	3	4	?
7. Overtired	0	1	2	3	4	?		32. Full of pep	0	1	2	3	4	?
8. Weary	0	1	2	3	4	?		33. Lively	0	1	2	3	4	?
9. Tired	0	1	2	3	4	?		34. Charged-up	0	1	2	3	4	?
10. Spent	0	1	2	3	4	?		35. Wide-eyed	0	1	2	3	4	?
11. Bushed	0	1	2	3	4	?		36. Energetic	0	1	2	3	4	?
12. Out of Steam	0	1	2	3	4	?		37. Carefree	0	1	2	3	4	?
13. Frazzled	0	1	2	3	4	?		38. Active	0	1	2	3	4	?
14. Limited Endurance	0	1	2	3	4	?		39. Cheerful	0	1	2	3	4	?
15. Achy Muscles	0	1	2	3	4	?		40. Alert	0	1	2	3	4	?
16. Indolent	0	1	2	3	4	?		41. Snoozy	0	1	2	3	4	?
17. Languid	0	1	2	3	4	?		42. Sleepy	0	1	2	3	4	?
18. Soporific	0	1	2	3	4	?		43. Drowsy	0	1	2	3	4	?
19. Lassitude	0	1	2	3	4	?		44. Slumber	0	1	2	3	4	?
20. Supine	0	1	2	3	4	?		45. Heavy-eyed	0	1	2	3	4	?
21. Accidie	0	1	2	3	4	?		46. Half-Awake	0	1	2	3	4	?
22. Phlegmatic	0	1	2	3	4	?		47. Sluggish	0	1	2	3	4	?
23. Line of Least Resistance	0	1	2	3	4	?		48. Yawning	0	1	2	3	4	?
24. Jaded	0	1	2	3	4	?		49. Dozy	0	1	2	3	4	?
25. Apathetic	0	1	2	3	4	?		50. Somnambulant	0	1	2	3	4	?

Reference

1. Shapiro, C. M., Flanigan, M., Fleming, J. A. E., Morehouse, R., Moscovitch, A., Plamondon, J., Reinish, L., & Devins, G. M. (2002). Development of an adjective checklist to measure five FACES of fatigue and sleepiness: data from a national survey of insomniacs. Journal of Psychosomatic Research, 52, 467–473.

Representative Studies Using Scale

Shen, J., Hossain, N., Streiner, D. L., Ravindran, A. V., Wang, X., Deb, P., Huang, X., Sun, F., & Shapiro, C. M. (2011). Excessive daytime sleepiness and fatique in depression patients and therapeutic response of a sedating antidepression. *Journal of Affective Disorder*, 134, 421–426.

Shahid, A., Shen, J., & Shapiro, C. M. (2010) Measurements of sleepiness and fatigue. *Journal of Pshchosomatic Research*, 69, 81–89.

32 Fatigue Assessment Inventory (FAI)

Purpose The 29-item scale is designed to evaluate four domains of fatigue: its severity, pervasiveness, associated consequences, and response to sleep. It may be valuable for screening individuals in clinical practice, and may also be useful for research endeavours.

Population for Testing The scale has been validated with patients experiencing symptoms of fatigue as well as with healthy controls. No age range for the scale has been provided.

Administration The scale is a self-report, pencil-and-paper measure requiring between 5 and 10 min for administration.

Reliability and Validity In a validation study conducted by developers [1], the scale was found to have an internal consistency from .70 to .92 and a test–retest reliability of .50–.70. In the patient group, 81.3% scored more than 4 on the FAI, and in the control group 89.2% scored less than 4. Scores on the scale also correlated highly with two other measures of fatigue and energy level.

Obtaining a Copy A copy of the scale can be found in the original article published by developers [1].

Direct correspondence to:
Lauren B. Krupp
Department of Neurology
Stony Brook, NY 11794-8121, USA

Scoring Respondents use a scale ranging from 1 ("completely disagree") to 7 ("completely agree") to indicate how accurately certain statements about fatigue represent their experiences over the previous 2 weeks. Higher scores are indicative of greater problems with fatigue. The scale provides a global severity score that can be used both for screening and research purposes.

A. Shahid et al. (eds.), *STOP, THAT and One Hundred Other Sleep Scales*,
DOI 10.1007/978-1-4419-9893-4_32, © Springer Science+Business Media, LLC 2012

Fatigue Assessment Inventory

Instructions:

Below are a series of statements regarding your Fatigue. By Fatigue we mean a sense of tiredness, lack of energy or total body give-out. Please read each statement and choose a number from 1 to 7, where #1 indicates you completely disagree with the statement and #7 indicates you completely agree. Please answer these questions as they apply to the past TWO WEEKS.

Circle the appropriate number on the answer sheet!

Questions:

	Completely Disagree						Completely agree
1. I feel drowsy when I am fatigued.	1	2	3	4	5	6	7
2. When I am fatigued, I lose my patience.	1	2	3	4	5	6	7
3. My motivation is lower when I am fatigued.	1	2	3	4	5	6	7
4. When I am fatigued, I have difficulty concentrating.	1	2	3	4	5	6	7
5. Exercise brings on my fatigue.	1	2	3	4	5	6	7
6. Heat brings on my fatigue.	1	2	3	4	5	6	7
7. Long periods of inactivity bring on my fatigue	1	2	3	4	5	6	7
8. Stress brings on my fatigue.	1	2	3	4	5	6	7
9. Depression brings on my fatigue.	1	2	3	4	5	6	7
10. Work brings on fatigue.	1	2	3	4	5	6	7
11. My fatigue is worse in the afternoon.	1	2	3	4	5	6	7
12. My fatigue is worse in the morning.	1	2	3	4	5	6	7
13. Performance of routine daily activities increases my fatigue.	1	2	3	4	5	6	7
14. Resting lessens my fatigue.	1	2	3	4	5	6	7
15. Sleeping lessens my fatigue.	1	2	3	4	5	6	7
16. Cool temperatures lessen my fatigue.	1	2	3	4	5	6	7
17. Positive experiences lessen my fatigue.	1	2	3	4	5	6	7
18. I am easily fatigued.	1	2	3	4	5	6	7
19. Fatigue interferes with my physical functioning.	1	2	3	4	5	6	7
20. Fatigue causes frequent problems for me.	1	2	3	4	5	6	7
21. My fatigue prevents sustained physical functioning.	1	2	3	4	5	6	7
22. Fatigue interferes with carrying out certain duties and responsibilities.	1	2	3	4	5	6	7
23. Fatigue predated other symptoms of my condition.	1	2	3	4	5	6	7
24. Fatigue is my most disabling symptom	1	2	3	4	5	6	7
25. Fatigue is among my 3 most disabling symptoms.	1	2	3	4	5	6	7
26. Fatigue interferes with my work, family or social life.	1	2	3	4	5	6	7
27. Fatigue makes other symptoms worse.	1	2	3	4	5	6	7
28. Fatigue that I now experience is different in quality or severity than the fatigue I experienced before I developed this condition	1	2	3	4	5	6	7
29. I experienced prolonged fatigue after exercise.	1	2	3	4	5	6	7

Reference

1. Schwartz, J. E., Jandorf, L., & Krupp, L. B. (1993). The measurement of fatigue: a new instrument. *Journal of Psychosomatic Research, 37*(7), 753–762.

Representative Studies Using Scale

O'Dell, M. W., Meighen, M., & Riggs, R. V. (1996). Correlates of fatigue in HIV infection prior to AIDS: a pilot study. *Disability and Rehabilitation, 18*(5), 249–254.

McAndrews, M. P., Farcnik, K., Carlen, P., Damyanovich, A., Mrkonjic, M., Jones, S., & Heathcote, E. J. (2005). Prevalence and significance of neurocognitive dysfunction in hepatitis C in the absence of correlated risk factors. *Hepatology, 41*(4), 801–808.

Note: The Fatigue Severity Scale (Chap. 35) by the same author is a short form (9 item) using similar descriptions.

33 Fatigue Assessment Scale (FAS)

Purpose The FAS is a 10-item scale evaluating symptoms of chronic fatigue. In contrast to other similar measures (e.g., the Multidimensional Fatigue Inventory Chap. 57), the FAS treats fatigue as a unidimensional construct and does not separate its measurement into different factors. However, in order to ensure that the scale would evaluate all aspects of fatigue, developers chose items to represent both physical and mental symptoms.

Population for Testing The scale has been validated in a population of both male and female respondents with mean ages of 45 ± 8.4 years and 43 ± 9.5 years, respectively.

Administration The FAS is a self-report, paper-and-pencil measure requiring approximately 2 min for administration.

Reliability and Validity Developers Michielsen and colleagues [1] analyzed the scale's psychometric properties and found an internal consistency of .90. Results on the scale also correlated highly with the fatigue-related subscales of other measures like the Checklist Individual Strength. In subsequent analyses, four of the scale's ten items were shown to possess a gender bias – women tended to score significantly higher than men [2]. However, when adjusted scores were calculated, researchers found that this bias had only a negligible effect on each individual's total score, indicating that the scale's original simplified scoring method is still appropriate.

Obtaining a Copy A copy of the scale can be found in the original article published by developers [1].

Direct correspondence to:
Helen J. Michielsen
Telephone: +31-13-466-2299
Email: h.j.michielsen@kub.nl

Scoring Each item of the FAS is answered using a five-point, Likert-type scale ranging from 1 ("never") to 5 ("always"). Items 4 and 10 are reverse-scored. Total scores can range from 10, indicating the lowest level of fatigue, to 50, denoting the highest.

A. Shahid et al. (eds.), *STOP, THAT and One Hundred Other Sleep Scales*,
DOI 10.1007/978-1-4419-9893-4_33, © Springer Science+Business Media, LLC 2012

Fatigue Assessment Scale (FAS)

The following 10 statements refer to how you usually feel. For each statement you can choose one out of five answer categories, varying from *never* to *always*. 1 = *never*; 2 = *sometimes;* 3 = *regularly*; 4 = *often*; 5 = *always*.

	Never	Sometimes	Regularly	Often	Always
1. I am bothered by fatigue (WHOQOL)	1	2	3	4	5
2. I get tired very quickly (CIS)	1	2	3	4	5
3. I don't do much during the day (CIS)	1	2	3	4	5
4. I have enough energy for everyday life (WHOQOL)	1	2	3	4	5
5. Physically, I feel exhausted (CIS)	1	2	3	4	5
6. I have problems starting things (FS)	1	2	3	4	5
7. I have problems thinking clearly (FS)	1	2	3	4	5
8. I feel no desire to do anything (CIS)	1	2	3	4	5
9. Mentally, I feel exhausted	1	2	3	4	5
10. When I am doing something, I can concentrate quite well (CIS)	1	2	3	4	5

Note: The abbreviations after the items indicate the scale from which the items has been abstracted. The following are the scales:

CIS - Checklist Individual Strength

WHOQOL - World Health Organization Quality of Life assessment instrument

FS - Fatigue Scale

References

1. Michielsen, H. J., De Vries, J., & Van Heck, G. L. (2003). Psychometric qualities of a brief self-rated fatigue measure the fatigue assessment scale. Journal of Psychosomatic Research, 54, 345–352.
2. De Vries, J., Michielsen, H. J., Van Heck, G. L., & Drent, M. (2004). Measuring fatigue in sarcoidosis: the fatigue assessment scale (FAS). *British Journal of Health Psychology, 9*(3), 279–291.

Representative Studies Using Scale

Michielsen, H. J., Drent, M., Peros-Golubicic, T., & De Vries, J. (2006). Fatigue is associated with quality of life in sarcoidosis patients. Chest, 130(4), 989–994.

Smith, O. R. F., Michielsen, H. J., Pelle, A. J., Schiffer, A. A., Winter, J. B., & Denollet, J. (2007). Symptoms of chronic fatigue in chronic heart failure patients: clinical and psychological predictors. European Journal of Heart Failure, 9(9), 922–927.

34 Fatigue Impact Scale (FIS)

Purpose The FIS was developed to assess the symptom of fatigue as part of an underlying chronic disease or condition. Consisting of 40 items, the instrument evaluates the effect of fatigue on three domains of daily life: cognitive functioning, physical functioning, and psychosocial functioning [1]. In addition to the original version, a shorter 21-item measure called the Modified Fatigue Impact Scale (MFIS) has been developed and validated for use in those situations where a longer instrument might be fatiguing [2]. Similarly, Fisk and Doble used Rasch analyses to reduce the original to a mere eight items that could be used for monitoring daily changes in fatigue, creating the Daily Fatigue Impact Scale (D-FIS; [3]).

Population for Testing The scale was initially validated in a population of adult patients presenting at a clinic for the treatment of infectious diseases. The FIS and its variants have been used to assess symptoms of fatigue associated with a variety of conditions, including multiple sclerosis [4] and hepatitis C [5].

Administration The FIS is a self-report, paper-and-pencil measure requiring between 5 and 10 min for completion.

Reliability and Validity The original FIS was validated initially by developers [1], who found an internal consistency of >than .87 for all three subscales. The FIS also accurately distinguished between the patient group with multiple sclerosis and the group with chronic fatigue. More recently, Mathiowetz [6] found a test–retest reliability ranging from .68 to .85 in patients with multiple sclerosis. Additionally, scores on the FIS were moderately correlated with those obtained on the SF-36 (Chap. 76) – though this support for the scale's convergent validity was undermined by a low correlation between results on the FIS and the Fatigue Severity Scale (Chap. 35). The MFIS has been shown to possess an internal consistency ranging from .65 to .92 [2] and the D-FIS has an internal consistency of .92 [7].

Obtaining a Copy A copy of the original FIS cannot be found in the article published by developers [1]; however, examples of the items in the scale can be found in this article. The MFIS can be found in an article by Kos and colleagues [2] and the D-FIS is available in an article by Fisk and Doble [3]. The original FIS can be obtained through MAPI Research Trust at their website www.mapi-trust.org/test/123-fis

Direct correspondence to:
John D. Fisk
Department of Psychiatry
Dalhousie University
QEII Health Sciences Centre
Halifax, Nova Scotia B3H 2E2

A. Shahid et al. (eds.), *STOP, THAT and One Hundred Other Sleep Scales*,
DOI 10.1007/978-1-4419-9893-4_34, © Springer Science+Business Media, LLC 2012

Scoring Respondents are asked to rate the extent to which fatigue has interfered with certain aspects of their day-to-day functioning using a scale that ranges from 0 ("no problem") to 4 ("extreme problem"). Scores are then tallied to produce an overall score with a potential maximum of 160. Subscale scores can also be calculated to give a more nuanced impression of fatigue.

Daily Fatigue Impact Scale

Fatigue is a feeling of physical tiredness and lack of energy that many people experience from time to time. In certain medical conditions, feelings of fatigue can be more frequent and more of a problem than usual. The following questionnaire has been designed to help us understand how you experience fatigue and how it has affected your life. Below is a list of statements that describe how fatigue may cause problems in people's lives. Please read each statement carefully and place an 'X' in the box that indicates best HOW MUCH OF A PROBLEM FATIGUE HAS BEEN FOR YOU TODAY. Please check ONE box for each statement and do not skip any items.

	No problem 0	Small problem 1	Moderate problem 2	Big problem 3	Extreme problem 4
1. Because of fatigue, I feel less alert.					
2. Because of fatigue, I have to reduce my workload or responsibilities.					
3. Because of fatigue, I am less motivated to do anything that requires physical effort.					
4. Because of fatigue, I have trouble maintaining physical effort for long periods.					
5. Because of fatigue, I find it difficult to make decisions					
6. Because of fatigue, I am less able to finish tasks that require thinking.					
7. Because of fatigue, I feel slowed down in my thinking.					
8. Because of fatigue, I have to limit my physical activities.					

References

1. Fisk, J. D., Ritvo, P. G., Ross, L., Haase, D. A., Marrie, T. J., & Schlech, W. F. (1994a). Measuring the functional impact of fatigue: initial validation of the fatigue impact scale. *Clinical Infectious Diseases, 18*, S79–83.
2. Kos, D., Kerckhofs, E., Carrea, I., Verza, R., Ramos, M., & Jansa, J. (2005). Evaluation of the modified fatigue impact scale in four different European countries. *Multiple Sclerosis, 11*, 76–80.
3. Fisk, J. D., & Doble, S. E. (2002). Construction and validation of a fatigue impact scale for daily administration. *Quality of Life Research, 11*, 263–272.
4. Fisk, J. D., Pontefract, A., Ritvo, P. G., Archibald, C. J., & Murray, T. J. (1994b). The impact of fatigue on patients with multiple sclerosis. *Canadian Journal of Neurological Sciences, 21*(1), 9–14.
5. Hassoun, Z., Willems, B., Deslauriers, J., Nguyen, B. N., & Huet, P. M. (2002). Assessment of fatigue in patients with chronic hepatitis C using the fatigue impact scale. *Digestive Diseases and Sciences, 47*(12), 2674–2681.
6. Mathiowetz, V. (2003). Test-retest reliability and convergent validity of the fatigue impact scale for persons with multiple sclerosis. *The American Journal of Occupational Therapy, 57*(4), 389–395.
7. Martinez-Martin, P., Catalan, M. J., Benito-Leon, J., Moreno, A. O., Zamarbide, I., Cubo, E., van Blercon, N., Arillo, V. C., Pondal, M., Linazasoro, G., Alonso, F., Ruiz, P. G., & Frades, B. (2006). Impact of fatigue in Parkinson's disease: the fatigue impact scale for daily use (D-FIS). *Quality of Life Research, 15*, 597–606.

Fatigue Impact Scale

Vanage, S. M., Gilbertson, K. K., & Mathiowetz, V. (2003). Effects of an energy conservation course on fatigue impact for persons with progressive multiple sclerosis. *The American Journal of Occupational Therapy, 57*(3), 315–323.

Modified Fatigue Impact Scale

Chwastiak, L., Gibbons, L., Ehde, E., Sullivan, M., Bowen, J., Bombardier, C., & Kraft, G. (2005). Fatigue and psychiatric illness in a large community sample of persons with multiple sclerosis. *Journal of Psychosomatic Research, 59*(5), 291–298.

35 Fatigue Severity Scale (FSS)

Purpose The FSS is a nine-item instrument designed to assess fatigue as a symptom of a variety of different chronic conditions and disorders. The scale addresses fatigue's effects on daily functioning, querying its relationship to motivation, physical activity, work, family, and social life, and asking respondents to rate the ease with which they are fatigued and the degree to which the symptom poses a problem for them.

Population for Testing The scale was initially validated in a population of patients with multiple sclerosis and systemic lupus erythematosus. Participants had a mean age of 35.6 ± 8.9 years. The scale has also been used to assess patients with chronic hepatitis C [1], Parkinson's disease [2], and chronic renal failure [3].

Administration The scale is a self-report, paper-and-pencil measure requiring 2–3 min for completion.

Reliability and Validity Developers Krupp and colleagues [4] conducted an initial psychometric evaluation of the FSS and found an internal consistency of.88 and a test–retest reliability of .84. Scores on the FSS were significantly higher for individuals with multiple sclerosis and systemic lupus erythematosus than they were for healthy control participants; additionally, results on the FSS were found to be significantly correlated with scores obtained using a previously established measure of fatigue.

Obtaining a Copy A copy of the scale's items can be found in the original article published by developers [4].

Direct correspondence to:
Lauren R. Krupp
Department of Neurology, School of Medicine
Health Sciences Center, State University of New York at Stony Brook
Stony Brook, NY 11794-8121, USA

Scoring Respondents use a scale ranging from 1 ("completely disagree") to 7 ("completely agree") to indicate their agreement with nine statements about fatigue. A visual analogue scale is also included with the scale; respondents are asked to denote the severity of their fatigue over the past 2 weeks by placing a mark on a line extending from "no fatigue" to "fatigue as bad as could be." Higher scores on the scale are indicative of more severe fatigue.

A. Shahid et al. (eds.), *STOP, THAT and One Hundred Other Sleep Scales*,
DOI 10.1007/978-1-4419-9893-4_35, © Springer Science+Business Media, LLC 2012

FATIGUE SEVERITY SCALE

During the past week, I have found that:	Strongly Disagree			Neither Agree Nor Disagree			Strongly Agree
1. My motivation is lower when I am fatigued.	1	2	3	4	5	6	7
2. Exercise brings on my fatigue.	1	2	3	4	5	6	7
3. I am easily fatigued.	1	2	3	4	5	6	7
4. Fatigue interferes with my physical functioning.	1	2	3	4	5	6	7
5. Fatigue causes frequent problems for me.	1	2	3	4	5	6	7
6. My fatigue prevents sustained physical functioning.	1	2	3	4	5	6	7
7. Fatigue interferes with carrying out certain duties and responsibilities.	1	2	3	4	5	6	7
8. Fatigue is among my three most disabling symptoms.	1	2	3	4	5	6	7
8. Fatigue interferes with my work, family, or social life.	1	2	3	4	5	6	7

References

1. Kleinman, L., Zodet, M. W., Hakim, Z., Aledort, J., Barker, C., Chan, K., Krupp, L., & Revicki, D. (2000). Psychometric evaluation of the fatigue severity scale for use in chronic hepatitis C. *Quality of Life Research, 9*, 499–508.
2. Herlofson, L., & Larsen, J. P. (2002). Measuring fatigue in patients with Parkinson's disease – the fatigue severity scale. *European Journal of Neurology, 9*, 595–600.
3. Schneider, R. A. (2004). Chronic renal failure: assessing the fatigue severity scale for use among caregivers. *Journal of Clinical Nursing, 13*(2), 219–225.
4. Krupp, L. B., LaRocca, N. G., Muir-Nash, J., & Steinberg, A. D. (1989). The fatigue severity scale: application to patients with multiple sclerosis and systemic lupus erythematosus. *Archives of Neurology, 46*, 1121–1123.

Representative Studies Using Scale

Téllez, N., Río, J., Tintoré, M., Nos, C., Galán, I., & Montalban, X. (2006). Fatigue in multiple sclerosis persists over time. *Journal of Neurology, 253*(11), 1466–1470.

Naess, H., Waje-Andreassen, U., Thomassen, L., Nyland, H., & Myhr, K. M. (2006). Health-related quality of life among young adults with ischemic stroke on long-term follow-up. *Stroke, 37*, 1232–1236.

Fatigue Symptom Inventory (FSI)

36

Purpose The scale is composed of 14 items (one of which is not scored) and is designed to evaluate multiple aspects of fatigue, including its perceived severity, frequency, and interference with daily functioning. Though multiple measures of fatigue have been created for use with a variety of clinical and research populations, many of these focus on specific aspects of fatigue – intensity or duration, for example – and the developers hoped to design an instrument for examining a wide range of fatigue-related issues. The scale has been primarily validated in patients with cancer, though it has been tested minimally in a variety of other groups as well.

Population for Testing The scale has been validated with both female and male cancer patients with an age range of 18–24 [1]. An initial study also suggests that the FSI possesses some reliability and validity with healthy controls as well [2].

Administration A brief self-report, pencil-and-paper measure, the scale should require between 5 and 10 min for completion.

Reliability and Validity The largest study examining the scale's psychometric properties found an internal consistency of .94 [1]. Results on the instrument were also significantly correlated with an established measure of fatigue.

Obtaining a Copy An example of the items used in the questionnaire can be found in the original article published by developers [2].

Direct correspondence to:
D.M. Hann
Behavioral Research Center, American Cancer Society
1599 Clifton Road NE
Atlanta, GA 30329, USA

Scoring Items use an 11-point, Likert-type scale that ranges from one fatigue-related extreme to another (lower points on the scale denote less acute problems with fatigue). A global score can be obtained for items 1–13. Question 14 is meant to provide qualitative data only. Additionally, a Disruption Index score can be calculated by adding scores obtained on items 5–11.

A. Shahid et al. (eds.), *STOP, THAT and One Hundred Other Sleep Scales*,
DOI 10.1007/978-1-4419-9893-4_36, © Springer Science+Business Media, LLC 2012

Fatigue Symptom Inventory (FSI)

For each of the following, circle the one number that best indicates how that item applies to you.

1. Rate your level of fatigue on the day you felt most fatigued during the past week.

0 1 2 3 4 5 6 7 8 9 10

Not at all Fatigued — As fatigued as I could be

2. Rate your level of fatigue on the day you felt least fatigued during the past week.

0 1 2 3 4 5 6 7 8 9 10

Not at all fatigued — As fatigued as I could be

3. Rate your level of fatigue on the average in the last week.

0 1 2 3 4 5 6 7 8 9 10

Not at all fatigued — As fatigued as I could be

4. Rate your level of fatigue right now.

0 1 2 3 4 5 6 7 8 9 10

Not at all fatigued — As fatigued as I could be

5. Rate how much, in the past week, fatigue interfered with your general level of activity.

0 1 2 3 4 5 6 7 8 9 10

No interference — Extreme interference

6. Rate how much, in the past week, fatigue interfered with your ability to bathe and dress yourself.

0 1 2 3 4 5 6 7 8 9 10

No interference — Extreme interference

7. Rate how much, in the past week, fatigue interfered with your normal work activity (includes both work outside the home and housework).

0 1 2 3 4 5 6 7 8 9 10

No Interference — Extreme Interference

8. Rate how much, in the past week, fatigue interfered with your ability to concentrate.

0 1 2 3 4 5 6 7 8 9 10

No Interference — Extreme Interference

9. Rate how much, in the past week, fatigue interfered with your relations with other people.

0 1 2 3 4 5 6 7 8 9 10

No Interference — Extreme Interference

10. Rate how much, in the past week, fatigue interfered with your enjoyment of life.

0 1 2 3 4 5 6 7 8 9 10

No Interference — Extreme Interference

11. Rate how much, in the past week, fatigue interfered with your mood:

0 1 2 3 4 5 6 7 8 9 10

No Interference — Extreme Interference

12. Indicate how many days, in the past week, you felt fatigued for any part of the day.

0 1 2 3 4 5 6 7

Days — Days

13. Rate how much of the day, on average you felt fatigued in the past week.

0 1 2 3 4 5 6 7 8 9 10

None of the day — The entire day

References

1. Hann, D. M., Denniston, M. M., & Baker, F. (2000). Measurement of fatigue in cancer patients: further validation of the fatigue symptom inventory. *Quality of Life Research, 9*(7), 847–854.
2. Hann, D. M., Jacobsen, P. B., Azzarello, L. M., Martin, S. C., Curran, S. L., Fields, et al. (1998). Measurement of fatigue in cancer patients: development and validation of the fatigue symptom inventory. *Quality of Life Research, 7*, 301–310.

Representative Studies Using the Scale

Jacobsen, P. B., Donovan, K. A., Small, B. J., Jim, H. S., Munster, P. N., & Andrykowski, M. A. (2007). Fatigue after treatment for early stage breast cancer: a controlled comparison. *Cancer, 110*(8), 1851–1859.

Luciani, A., Jacobsen, P. B., Extermann, M., Foa, P., Marussi, D., Overcash, J. A., & Balducci, L. (2008). Fatigue and functional dependences in older cancer patients. *American Journal of Clinical Oncology – Cancer Clinical Trials, 31*(5), 424–430.

37 FibroFatigue Scale

Purpose The instrument is an observer rating scale, designed to measure the severity of symptoms in fibromyalgia and chronic fatigue syndrome patients. Consisting of 12 items, the scale evaluates pain, muscular tension, fatigue, concentration difficulties, failing memory, irritability, sadness, sleep disturbances, autonomic disturbances, irritable bowel, headache, and subjective experience of infection. Scale developers were specifically interested in creating a tool that could be used to monitor treatment outcomes. However, the scale requires a trained administrator, making it potentially unsuitable for large-scale research studies.

Population for Testing The majority of the scale's properties were assessed in a population of 100 female patients between the ages of 20 and 66 years. However, a group of 13 men were added to the sample when examining interrater reliability in order to rule out the effects of gender.

Administration The FibroFatigue Scale is an observer-rated instrument to be administered by a trained individual. It requires between 10 and 15 min for completion.

Reliability and Validity During an initial psychometric evaluation, developers Zachrisson and colleagues [1] found an interrater reliability of .98 for the total scale. Items for the FibroFatigue Scale were chosen from the Comprehensive Psychopathological Rating Scale (CPRS) if they had a baseline incidence rate of at least 70% within a population of chronic fatigue syndrome and fibromyalgia patients.

Obtaining a Copy A copy of the scale can be found in an article published by developers (Zachrisson, 2002).

Direct correspondence to:
Olof Zachrisson
Psychiatry Section, Institute of Clinical Neuroscience
Sahlgrenska University Hospital/Mölndal
SE 431 80 Mölndal, Sweden
Email: olof.zachrisson@neuro.gu.se

Scoring Over the course of a clinical interview, administrators rate each symptom on a scale from 0 (absence of the symptom) to 6 (maximal degree of the symptom). In order to provide interviewers with a point of reference for evaluating severity, symptom descriptions are included for scores of 0, 2, 4, and 6. However, the points between these anchoring scores may also be used and can help to increase the instrument's sensitivity. Total scores can be calculated and compared longitudinally with scores from the same individual or they can be used as one-time measures of severity.

A. Shahid et al. (eds.), *STOP, THAT and One Hundred Other Sleep Scales*,
DOI 10.1007/978-1-4419-9893-4_37, © Springer Science+Business Media, LLC 2012

FibroFatigue Scale

Item list

1. Aches and pain	7. Sadness
2. Muscular tension	8. Sleep disturbances
3. Fatigue	9. Autonomic disturbances
4. Concentration difficulties	10. Irritable bowel
5. Failing memory	11. Headache
6. Irritability	12. Subjective experience

of infection

1. Aches and pain
Representing reports of bodily discomfort, aches and pain. Rate according to intensity, frequency, duration, and requests for relief. Disregard any statement about the cause being organic.

0	Absent or transient aches
1	
2	Occasional definite aches and pain
3	
4	Prolonged and inconvenient aches and pain; requests for effective analgesics
5	
6	Severely interfering or crippling pains

2. Muscular tension
Representing the description of increased tension in the muscles and difficulty in relaxing physically.

0	No increase in muscular tension
1	
2	Some occasional increase in muscular tension, more evident in demanding situations
3	
4	Considerable difficulty in finding a comfortable position when sitting or lying; disturbing muscular tension
5	
6	Painful muscular tension; completely incapable of relaxing physically

3. Fatigue
Representing the experience of debilitating fatigue and lack of energy and the experience of tiring more easily than usual.

0	Ordinary staying power; not easily fatigued
1	
2	Tires easily but does not have to take a break more often than usual
3	
4	Considerable fatigue and lack of energy; easily wearied; frequently forced to pause or rest
5	
6	Exhaustion interrupts almost all activities or even makes them impossible

4. Concentration difficulties
Representing difficulties in collecting one's thoughts mounting to incapacitating lack of concentration.
Rate according to intensity, frequency, and degree of incapacity.

0	No difficulties in concentrating
1	
2	Occasional difficulties in collecting thoughts
3	
4	Difficulties in concentrating and sustaining thought which interfere with reading or conversation
5	
6	Incapacitating lack of concentration

5. Failing memory
Representing subjective disturbances of recall compared with previous ability.

0	Memory as usual
1	
2	Occasional increased lapses of memory
3	
4	Reports of socially inconvenient or disturbing loss of memory
5	
6	Complaints of complete inability to remember

6. Irritability
Representing the subjective experience of irritable mood (dysphoria), anger, and having a short fuse, regardless of whether the feelings are acted out or not. Rate according to intensity, frequency, and the amount of provocation tolerated.

0	Not easily irritated
1	
2	Easily irritated or angered; reports irritability, which is easily dissipated
3	
4	Pervasive feelings of irritability or anger; outbursts may occur
5	
6	Persistent irritability or anger which is difficult or impossible to control

7. Sadness
Representing subjectively experienced mood, regardless of whether it is reflected in appearance or not; includes depressed mood, low spirits, despondency, and the feeling of being beyond help and without hope.
Rate according to intensity, duration, and the extent to which the mood is influenced by events.

0	Occasional sadness may occur in the circumstances
1	
2	Predominant feelings of sadness, but brighter moments occur
3	
4	Pervasive feelings of sadness or gloominess; the mood is hardly influenced by external circumstances
5	
6	Continuous experience of misery or extreme despondency

8. Sleep disturbances
Representing a subjective experience of disturbed sleep compared to the subject's own normal pattern when well.

0	Sleeps as usual
1	
2	Slight difficulty dropping off to sleep, reduced duration of sleep, light or fitful sleep, or sleeps deeper or longer than usual
3	
4	Frequent or intense sleep disturbances; sleep reduced or broken by at least 2 hours, or several hours extra sleep
5	
6	Severe sleep disturbances; less than 2 or 3 hours sleep, or spends a great part of the day asleep in spite of normal or increased sleep at night

9. Autonomic disturbances
Representing descriptions of palpitations, breathing difficulties, dizziness, increased sweating, cold hands and feet, dry mouth, and frequent micturition. Rate according to intensity and frequency and duration of one or many symptoms.

0	No autonomic disturbances
1	
2	Occasional autonomic symptoms which occur under emotional stress
3	
4	Frequent or intense autonomic disturbances (two or more of above-mentioned symptoms) which are experienced as discomforting or socially inconvenient
5	
6	Very frequent autonomic disturbances, which interrupt other activities or are incapacitating

10. Irritable bowel
Representing a subjective experience of abdominal discomfort or pain along with descriptions of altered stool frequency or diarrhoea/obstipation, bloating or feeling of distension. Rate according to intensity, frequency, and degree of inconvenience produced.

0	No irritable bowel
1	
2	Occasional irritable bowel symptoms which may occur under emotional stress
3	
4	Frequent or intense irritable bowel, which is experienced as discomforting or socially inconvenient
5	
6	Very frequent irritable bowel, which interrupts other activities or are incapacitating

11. Headache
Representing reports of discomfort, aches, and pain at the head. Rate according to intensity, frequency, duration, and requests for relief. Disregard any statement about the cause being organic.

0	Absent or transient headache
1	
2	Occasional definite headache
3	
4	Prolonged and inconvenient headache; requests for effective analgesics
5	
6	Severe interfering or crippling headache

12. Subjective experience of infection
Representing descriptions of symptoms (e.g., mild fever or chills, sore throat, lymph node pain) and reports of infection (e.g., infection in upper/lower respiratory tract, urinary tract, gyn, derma). Rate according to intensity, frequency, and duration and also requests for treatment.

0	No symptoms of infection
1	
2	Occasional definite symptoms of infection
3	
4	Frequent or intense symptoms of infection; requests for treatment
5	
6	Severe interfering or crippling symptoms of infection

Reference

1. Zachrisson, O., Regland, B., Jahreskog, M., Kron, M., & Gottfries, C. G. (2002). A rating scale for fibromyalgia and chronic fatigue syndrome (the FibroFatigue scale). *Journal of Psychosomatic Research, 52*, 501–509.

Representative Studies Using Scale

Gottfries, C. G., Hager, O., Regland, B., & Zachrisson, O. (2006). Long-term treatment with a staphylococcus toxoid vaccine in patients with fibromyalgia and chronic fatigue syndrome. *Journal of Chronic Fatigue Syndrome, 13*(4), 29–40.

Maes, M., Mihaylova, I., & De Ruyter, M. (2006). Lower serum zinc in Chronic Fatigue Syndrome (CFS): Relationships to immune dysfunctions and relevance for the oxidative stress status in CFS. *Journal of Affective Disorders, 90*(2–3), 141–147.

Frontal Lobe Epilepsy and Parasomnias (FLEP) Scale

38

Purpose Created by Derry and colleagues [1], the 11-item FLEP scale is designed to aid clinicians in distinguishing frontal lobe seizures from parasomnias. While polysomnography is considered the gold standard approach for differentiating the two conditions, scale developers cite the need for an efficient, cost-effective alternative for those who, for whatever reason, do not have access to sleep clinic facilities. In order to distinguish nocturnal events caused by epilepsy from those related to parasomnias, the scale queries several factors, including: age of onset and event duration, frequency, timing, symptoms, stereotypy, and recall.

Population for Testing The scale was initially validated in a population of patients referred to a sleep clinic experiencing nocturnal events of uncertain cause. Participant ages depended significantly on which condition group they belonged to: nocturnal frontal lobe epilepsy patients had a mean age of 27.9, the NREM arousal parasomnia group had a mean age of 13.2 years, and the REM behavior disorder group had a mean age of 69.1 years.

Administration The FLEP scale consists of a semi-structured interview to be conducted by a trained administrator. It requires approximately 10 min for completion.

Reliability and Validity In a psychometric evaluation of the scale, Derry and colleagues [1] found that the FLEP possessed an interrater reliability of .97, a sensitivity of 1.00, a specificity ranging from .90 to .93, a positive predictive value ranging from .91 to .94, and a negative predictive value of 1.00. A follow-up evaluation found slightly less promising results [2], indicating a sensitivity of .71, a specificity of 1.00, a positive predictive value of 1.00, and a negative predictive value of .91. In nocturnal frontal lobe epilepsy patients, the scale gave an incorrect diagnosis 28.5% of the time.

Obtaining a Copy An example of the scale's items can be found in the original article published by developers [1].

Direct correspondence to:
Dr. Reisberg
Aging and Dementia Research and Treatment Center
New York University School of Medicine
550 First Ave., New York, NY 10016, USA
Email: barry.reisberg@med.nyu.edu

Scoring Most questions require only a "yes" or "no" answer, though a few ask specifically for estimates of duration or frequency. For each item, responses are classified as either indicating epilepsy (these receive either +1 or +2), indicating parasomnia (these receive either −1 or −2), or neutral (a score of 0). Total scores are then calculated. Developers suggest that individuals with scores greater than +3 are very likely to have epilepsy, while those with scores of 0 or less are very unlikely to have epilepsy. However, these boundaries have been called into question by other research suggesting that they provide misleading results [2].

A. Shahid et al. (eds.), *STOP, THAT and One Hundred Other Sleep Scales*,
DOI 10.1007/978-1-4419-9893-4_38, © Springer Science+Business Media, LLC 2012

The Frontal Lobe Epilepsy and Parasomnias (FLEP) Scale

Clinical Feature		Score
Age at onset		
At what age did the patient have their first clinical event?	<55 y	0
	≥55 y	−1
Duration		
What is the duration of a typical event?	<2 min	+1
	2-10 min	0
	>10 min	−2
Clustering		
What is the typical number of events to occur in a single night?	1 or 2	0
	3-5	+1
	>5	+2
Timing		
At what time of night do the events most commonly occur?	Within 30 min of sleep onset	+1
	Other times (including if no clear pattern identified)	0
Symptoms		
Are the events associated with a definite aura?	Yes	+2
	No	0
Does the patient ever wander outside the bedroom during the events?	Yes	-2
	No (or uncertain)	0
Does the patient perform complex, directed behaviors (eg, picking up objects, dressing) during events?	Yes	−2
	No (or uncertain)	0
Is there a clear history of prominent dystonic posturing, tonic limb extension, or cramping during events?	Yes	+1
	No (or uncertain)	0
Stereotypy		
Are the events highly stereotyped or variable in nature?	Highly stereotyped	+1
	Some variability/uncertain	0
	Highly variable	−1
Recall		
Does the patient recall the events?	Yes, lucid recall	+1
	No or vague recollection only	0
Vocalization		
Does the patient speak during the events and, if so, is there subsequent recollection of this speech?	No	0
	Yes, sounds only or single words	0
	Yes, coherent speech with incomplete or no recall	−2
	Yes, coherent speech with recall	+2
Total score		

References

1. Derry, C. P., Davey, M., Johns, M., Kron, K., Glencross, D., Marini, C., Scheffer, I. E., & Berkovic, S. F. (2006). Distinguishing sleep disorders from seizures: diagnosing bumps in the night. *Archives of Neurology, 63*(5), 705–709.
2. Manni, R., Terzaghi, M., & Repetto, A. (2008). The FLEP scale in diagnosing nocturnal frontal lobe epilepsy, NREM and REM parasomnias: data from a tertiary sleep and epilepsy unit. *Epilepsia, 49*(9), 1581–1585.

Representative Studies Using Scale

None.

39 Functional Outcomes of Sleep Questionnaire (FOSQ)

Purpose Consisting of 30 questions related to the effects of fatigue on daily activities, the instrument was designed to evaluate the respondent's quality of life as it relates to disorders of excessive sleepiness. Five domains of day-to-day life are examined: activity levels, vigilance, intimacy and sexual relationships, productivity, and social outcomes. The questionnaire is indicated for both research and clinical purposes (screening, assessing treatment outcomes, etc.). Recently, Chasens and colleagues [1] created a shorter, 10-item version of the scale in order to allow for rapid and efficient administration.

Population for Testing With approximately a fifth-grade reading level, the questionnaire is designed for adults suffering from disorders of excessive sleepiness.

Administration Requiring between 10 and 15 min for completion, the instrument is designed for self-report using pencil and paper.

Reliability and Validity Developers Weaver and colleagues [2] conducted a psychometric study of the instrument and demonstrated an internal reliability of $\alpha = .95$ and a test–retest reliability ranging from .81 to .90. In a validation study of the 10-item version, Chasens and colleagues [1] found an internal consistency of .87. Results on the shorter scale were also highly correlated with the original FOSQ.

Obtaining a Copy A copy can be found in the developers' original published article [2].

Direct correspondence to:
Terri Weaver
University of Pennsylvania School of Nursing
Room 348 NEB
420 Guardian Drive, Philadelphia
Pennsylvania 19104-6096, USA

Scoring For each of the five domains examined, respondents indicate the degree of difficulty they experience when attempting certain activities because they are sleepy or tired. Lower scores designate more acute issues with sleepiness: 4 means "no difficulty," 3 is "yes, a little difficulty," 2 is "yes, moderate difficulty," and 1 means "yes, extreme difficulty."

A. Shahid et al. (eds.), *STOP, THAT and One Hundred Other Sleep Scales*,
DOI 10.1007/978-1-4419-9893-4_39, © Springer Science+Business Media, LLC 2012

Functional Outcomes of Sleep Questionnaire (FOSQ)

Here are some sample questions from the scale: (Approval for full scale is not received)

Item	1 yes, extreme difficulty	2 yes, moderate difficulty	3 yes, a little difficulty	4 no difficulty
Difficulty keeping pace with others your own age	1	2	3	4
Rating of general level of activity	1	2	3	4
Relationship with family/friends been affected	1	2	3	4
Difficulty watching television	1	2	3	4
Difficulty operating motor vehicle for long distances	1	2	3	4
Difficulty participating in meetings of a group	1	2	3	4
Ability to become sexually aroused affected	1	2	3	4
Desire for intimacy or sex affected	1	2	3	4
Difficulty concentrating on things	1	2	3	4
Difficulty getting things done because too sleepy to drive	1	2	3	4
Difficulty performing employed or volunteer work	1	2	3	4
Difficulty visiting with family/friends in their house	1	2	3	4

References

1. Chasens, E. R., Ratcliffe, S. J., & Weaver, T. E. (2009). Development of the FOSQ-10: a short version of the functional outcomes of sleep questionnaire. *Sleep, 32*(7), 915–919.
2. Weaver, T. E., Laizner, A. M., Evans, L. K., Maislin, G., Chugh, D. K, Lyon, K., et al. (1997). An instrument to measure functional status outcomes for disorders of excessive sleepiness. *Sleep, 20*(10), 835–843.

Representative Studies Using Scale

Weaver, T. E., & Cueller, N. (2006). A randomized trial evaluating the effectiveness of sodium oxybate therapy on quality of life in narcolepsy. *Sleep, 29*, 1189–1194.

Shaheen, N. J., Madanick, R. D., Alattar, M., Morgan, D. R., Davis, P. H., Galanko, J. A., Spacek, M. B., & Vaughn, B. V. (2008). Gastroesophageal reflux disease as an etiology of sleep disturbance in subjects with insomnia and minimal reflux symptoms: a pilot study of prevalence and response to therapy. *Digestive Diseases and Sciences, 53*(6), 1493–1499.

40 General Sleep Disturbance Scale (GSDS)

Purpose The GSDS is a 21-item scale initially designed to evaluate the incidence and nature of sleep disturbances in employed women. Questions pertain to a variety of general sleep issues, including: problems initiating sleep, waking up during sleep, waking too early from sleep, quality of sleep, quantity of sleep, fatigue and alertness at work, and the use of substances to induce sleep.

Population for Testing The scale was initially used to evaluate sleep in a population of registered nurses with a mean age of 40.6±9.9 years. It has since been validated in a sample of both males and females with a mean age of 33.4±4.6, and a Chinese version has been developed [1]. Additionally, it has been employed in studies examining diverse patient populations, including those with Parkinson's disease [2] and cancer [3].

Administratin The GSDS is a self-report, paper-and-pencil measure requiring 5 to 10 min for completion.

Reliability and Validity In an initial psychometric evaluation of the scale, developer Lee [4] found an internal consistency of .88 for the whole scale. More recently, researchers Gay and colleagues [5] found an internal consistency ranging from .77 to .85.

Obtaining a Copy

Direct correspondence to:
Kathryn A. Lee
N411Y, Box 0606
School of Nursing, University of California
San Francisco, California 94193-0606, USA

Scoring The GSDS queries respondents regarding the frequency with which they've experienced certain sleep difficulties within the previous week. Respondents use an eight-point, Likert-type scale ranging from 0 (meaning "never") to 7 ("every day") to respond to each item. As guidelines set forth in the Diagnostic and Statistical Manual of Mental Disorders require symptoms to occur at least three times a week in order to establish a diagnosis of insomnia, researchers have suggested that individuals with an average score of three on the GSDS should be considered at risk for sleep disturbance [1].

A. Shahid et al. (eds.), *STOP, THAT and One Hundred Other Sleep Scales*,
DOI 10.1007/978-1-4419-9893-4_40, © Springer Science+Business Media, LLC 2012

GENERAL SLEEP DISTURBANCE SCALE

How often in the past week did you:	NO DAYS							EVERY DAY
1. have difficulty getting to sleep	0	1	2	3	4	5	6	7
2. wake up during your sleep period	0	1	2	3	4	5	6	7
3. wake up too early at the end of a sleep period	0	1	2	3	4	5	6	7
4. feel rested upon awakening at the end of a sleep period	0	1	2	3	4	5	6	7
5. sleep poorly	0	1	2	3	4	5	6	7
6. feel sleepy during the day	0	1	2	3	4	5	6	7
7. struggle to stay awake during the day	0	1	2	3	4	5	6	7
8. feel irritable during the day	0	1	2	3	4	5	6	7
9. feel tired or fatigued during the day	0	1	2	3	4	5	6	7
10. feel satisfied with the quality of your sleep	0	1	2	3	4	5	6	7
11. feel alert and energetic during the day	0	1	2	3	4	5	6	7
12. get too much sleep	0	1	2	3	4	5	6	7
13. get too little sleep	0	1	2	3	4	5	6	7
14. take a nap at a scheduled time	0	1	2	3	4	5	6	7
15. fall asleep at an unscheduled time	0	1	2	3	4	5	6	7
16. drink an alcoholic beverage to help you get to sleep	0	1	2	3	4	5	6	7
17. use tobacco to help you get to sleep	0	1	2	3	4	5	6	7
18. use herbal product to help you get to sleep	0	1	2	3	4	5	6	7
19. use an over-the-counter sleeping pill to help you get to sleep	0	1	2	3	4	5	6	7
20. use a prescription sleeping pill to help you get to sleep	0	1	2	3	4	5	6	7
21. use aspirin or other pain medication to help you get to sleep	0	1	2	3	4	5	6	7

References

1. Lee, S. Y. (2007). Validating the general sleep disturbance scale among Chinese American parents with hospitalized infants. *Journal of Transcultural Nursing, 18*(2), 111–117.
2. Dowling, G., Mastick, J., Colling, E., Carter, J., Singer, C., & Aminoff, M. (2005). Melatonin for sleep disturbances in Parkinson's disease. *Sleep Medicine, 6*(5), 459–466.
3. Lee, K., Cho, M., Miaskowski, C., & Dodd, M. (2004). Impaired sleep and rhythms in persons with cancer. *Sleep Medicine Reviews, 8*(3), 199–212.
4. Lee, K. A. (1992). Self-reported sleep disturbances in employed women. *Sleep, 15*, 493–498.
5. Gay, C. L., Lee, K. A., & Lee, S. Y. (2004). Sleep patterns and fatigue in new mothers and fathers. *Biological Research for Nursing, 5*, 311–318.

Representative Studies Using Scale

Lee, K. A., Zaffke, M. E., Baratte-Beebee, K. (2004). Restless legs syndrome and sleep disturbance during pregnancy: the role of folate and iron. *Journal of Women's Health and Gender-Based Medicine, 10*(4), 335–341.

Gay, C. L., Lee, K. A., & Lee, S. Y. (2004). Sleep patterns and fatigue in new mothers and fathers. *Biological Research for Nursing, 5*(4), 311–318.

41 Glasgow Content of Thoughts Inventory (GCTI)

Purpose This 25-item questionnaire was developed to evaluate the content, character, and intrusiveness of cognitions in adults in the moments prior to sleep onset. The tool is specifically intended for assessing the cognitive processes of individuals with insomnia, particularly when those processes may affect the creation of treatment plans and the interpretation of treatment outcomes.

Population for Testing The questionnaire has been validated with a sample of insomniac participants between the ages of 16 and 65.

Administration Completed by self-report using pencil and paper, the scale requires between 5 and 10 min for administration.

Reliability and Validity Developed by Harvey and Espie [1], the GCTI has been validated on a variety of psychometric measures: an initial study found a construct validity of $r = .88$, a concurrent validity ranging from .48 to .82, a test–retest reliability of .88, and an internal consistency of $\alpha = .87$.

Obtaining a Copy A copy can be found in the developers' original published article [1].

Direct correspondence to:
Colin Espie
Department of Psychological Medicine,
University of Glasgow,
Academic Centre Gartnaval Royal Hospital
1055 Great Western Road, Glasgow G12 0XH
Scotland, UK

Scoring Respondents are asked to indicate how frequently in the last week they have been kept awake by certain thoughts. Individuals rate each of the questionnaire's 25 statements on a scale from 1 ("never") to 4 ("always"). Higher scores indicate more intrusive cognitions that may lead to increased sleep-onset latency. Developers suggest a cutoff score of 42, which yields a sensitivity of 100% and a specificity of 83%.

A. Shahid et al. (eds.), *STOP, THAT and One Hundred Other Sleep Scales*,
DOI 10.1007/978-1-4419-9893-4_41, © Springer Science+Business Media, LLC 2012

Glasgow Content of Thoughts Inventory (GCTI)

Here are some thoughts that people have when they can't sleep. Please indicate by placing a tick in the appropriate box how often over the past 7 nights the following thoughts have kept you awake.

		Never	Sometimes	Often	Always
1.	Things in the future				
2.	How tired/sleepy you feel				
3.	Things that happened during the day				
4.	How nervous/anxious you feel				
5.	How mentally awake you feel				
6.	Checking the time				
7.	Trivial things				
8.	How you can't stop your mind from racing				
9.	How long you've been awake				
10.	Your health				
11.	Ways you can get to sleep				
12.	Things you have to do tomorrow				
13.	How hot/cold you feel				
14.	Your work/responsibilities				
15.	How frustrated/annoyed you feel				
16.	How light/dark the room is				
17.	Noises you hear				
18.	Being awake all night				
19.	Pictures of things in your mind				
20.	The effects of not sleeping well				
21.	Your personal life				
22.	How thinking too much is the problem				
23.	Things in your past				
24.	How bad you are at sleeping				
25.	Things to do to help you sleep				

Reference

1. Harvey, K. J., & Espie, C. A. (2004). Development and preliminary investigation of the Glasgow Content of Thoughts Inventory (GCTI): a new measure for the assessment of pre-sleep cognitive activity. *British Journal of Clinical Psychology, 43*, 409–420.

Representative Studies Using Scale

None.

Hamilton Rating Scale for Depression (HAM-D)

42

Purpose One of the most frequently used instruments for evaluating depression in adults, the questionnaire allows clinicians to assess the nature and severity of mood disorders in patient populations. The scale is comprised of 21 items for inquiry, though only the first 17 are used in scoring. Each question examines a different symptom or aspect of depression, including: mood, guilty feelings, suicidal ideation, insomnia, agitation, and somatic symptoms. The scale is suitable for use in a variety of research and clinical settings, and can be applied as both a single-use instrument for measuring depression severity and as a tool for monitoring changes in depressive symptoms over the course of treatment. Items 4, 5, and 6 refer specifically to sleep, inquiring about insomnia prior to sleep onset, disturbed sleep in the middle of the night, and trouble falling back sleep in the early morning, respectively. Other items may be peripherally involved with sleep difficulties as they refer to fatigue, retardation, and somatic symptoms in general. It should be noted that there have been different iterations with longer, shorter, and one version with specific modifications for seasonal affective disorder [10].

Population for Testing The scale has been validated across a variety of studies, primarily in adult populations possessing major depressive disorder.

Administration The scale is administered through an interview conducted by a trained clinician. Its administration time will vary depending on the specific needs of the patient and the interviewer's preferred approach. On average, it should require approximately 10–15 min. Some have expressed concern regarding the interpretive nature of the instrument. The scale requires a trained clinician capable of distilling information regarding both frequency and intensity of symptoms into a single score, potentially making it inefficient for use in large research projects. To address this, a number of researchers (including Potts and colleagues [1]) have designed structured-interview versions of the HAM-D which can be administered in a variety of settings by interviewers without backgrounds in psychiatry. For even greater ease of use, a self-report, paper-and-pencil version is also available – the Hamilton Depression Inventory developed by Reynolds and Kobak [2]. Additional alternative versions include tests with fewer items and questionnaires with modified rating scales.

Reliability and Validity The psychometric properties of the HAM-D have been examined in a wide array of studies since its creation by Hamilton in 1960 [3]. One of the most recent reviews conducted by Bagby and colleagues [4] evaluated psychometric properties reported in 70 different articles, finding an internal reliability ranging from .46 to .97, an inter-rater reliability of .82 to .98, and a test–retest reliability of .81 to .98. Though scores for the scale as a whole appear to be quite high, studies examining inter-rater reliabilities and

A. Shahid et al. (eds.), *STOP, THAT and One Hundred Other Sleep Scales*,
DOI 10.1007/978-1-4419-9893-4_42, © Springer Science+Business Media, LLC 2012

test–retest coefficients at the level of individual items have found values that are much lower. Others have criticized the scale as outdated in terms of the DSM-IV definition of depression and have claimed that its scoring is unclear. Overall, the HAM-D's tremendous staying power has made it the subject of studies both laudatory and critical in nature [5, 6]. Decisions regarding its psychometric suitability should be undertaken carefully and on a case-by-case basis. For one of Hamilton's final writings on the subject of depression and the selection of depression scales, turn to a review written by Hamilton and Shapiro in *Measuring Human Problems: A Practical Guide* [7].

Obtaining a Copy A copy of the original scale can be found in Hamilton [3]. A large number of modified versions are available from their respective designers.

Scoring Though all 21 items may be valuable for both research and clinical purposes, only the first 17 are used for scoring. During the interview, clinicians solicit patient reports on a variety of depressive symptoms and use their clinical expertise to assign each a score for severity. For the majority of questions, scores range from 0 to 4, with 4 representing more acute signs of depression. Several questions have ranges that extend only as high as 2 or 3. A total score is tallied and can then be compared with previous scores or can be contrasted with a pre-defined cutoff score. Over the decades, a number of values have been suggested as potential cutoffs – total scores to be used as indicators of remission. Though the cutoff of 7 suggested by Frank and colleagues [8] has become a consensus for determining remission, others suggest that it should be as low as 2 [9].

Hamilton Depression Rating Scale (HDRS)

PLEASE COMPLETE THE SCALE BASED ON A STRUCTURED INTERVIEW

Instructions: for each item select the one "cue" which best characterizes the patient. Be sure to record the answers in the appropriate spaces (positions 0 through 4).

1 DEPRESSED MOOD *(sadness, hopeless, helpless, worthless)*

0 |__| Absent.
1 |__| These feeling states indicated only on questioning.
2 |__| These feeling states spontaneously reported verbally.
3 |__| Communicates feeling states non-verbally, i.e. through facial expression, posture, voice and tendency to weep.
4 |__| Patient reports virtually only these feeling states in his/her spontaneous verbal and non-verbal communication.

2 FEELINGS OF GUILT

0 |__| Absent.
1 |__| Self reproach, feels he/she has let people down.
2 |__| Ideas of guilt or rumination over past errors or sinful deeds.
3 |__| Present illness is a punishment. Delusions of guilt.
4 |__| Hears accusatory or denunciatory voices and/or experiences threatening visual hallucinations.

3 SUICIDE

0 |__| Absent.
1 |__| Feels life is not worth living.
2 |__| Wishes he/she were dead or any thoughts of possible death to self.
3 |__| Ideas or gestures of suicide.
4 |__| Attempts at suicide (any serious attempt rate 4).

4 INSOMNIA: EARLY IN THE NIGHT

0 |__| No difficulty falling asleep.
1 |__| Complains of occasional difficulty falling asleep, i.e. more than ½ hour.
2 |__| Complains of nightly difficulty falling asleep.

5 INSOMNIA: MIDDLE OF THE NIGHT

0 |__| No difficulty.
1 |__| Patient complains of being restless and disturbed during the night.
2 |__| Waking during the night – any getting out of bed rates 2 (except for purposes of voiding).

11 ANXIETY SOMATIC (physiological concomitants of anxiety) such as:

gastro-intestinal – dry mouth, wind, indigestion, diarrhea, cramps, belching
cardio-vascular – palpitations, headaches
respiratory – hyperventilation, sighing
urinary frequency
sweating

0 |__| Absent.
1 |__| Mild.
2 |__| Moderate.
3 |__| Severe.
4 |__| Incapacitating.

12 SOMATIC SYMPTOMS GASTRO-INTESTINAL

0 |__| None.
1 |__| Loss of appetite but eating without staff encouragement. Heavy feelings in abdomen.
2 |__| Difficulty eating without staff urging. Requests or requires laxatives or medication for bowels or medication for gastro-intestinal symptoms.

6 INSOMNIA: EARLY HOURS OF THE MORNING
0 |__| No difficulty.
1 |__| Waking in early hours of the morning but goes back to sleep.
2 |__| Unable to fall asleep again if he/she gets out of bed.

7 WORK AND ACTIVITIES
0 |__| No difficulty.
1 |__| Thoughts and feelings of incapacity, fatigue or weakness related to activities, work or hobbies.
2 |__| Loss of interest in activity, hobbies or work – either directly reported by the patient or indirect in listlessness, indecision and vacillation (feels he/she has to push self to work or activities).
3 |__| Decrease in actual time spent in activities or decrease in productivity. Rate 3 if the patient does not spend at least three hours a day in activities (job or hobbies) excluding routine chores.
4 |__| Stopped working because of present illness. Rate 4 if patient engages in no activities except routine chores, or if patient fails to perform routine chores unassisted.

8 RETARDATION (slowness of thought and speech, impaired ability to concentrate, decreased motor activity)
0 |__| Normal speech and thought.
1 |__| Slight retardation during the interview.
2 |__| Obvious retardation during the interview.
3 |__| Interview difficult.
4 |__| Complete stupor.

9 AGITATION
0 |__| None.
1 |__| Fidgetiness.
2 |__| Playing with hands, hair, etc.
3 |__| Moving about, can't sit still.
4 |__| Hand wringing, nail biting, hair-pulling, biting of lips.

10 ANXIETY PSYCHIC
0 |__| No difficulty.
1 |__| Subjective tension and irritability.
2 |__| Worrying about minor matters.
3 |__| Apprehensive attitude apparent in face or speech.
4 |__| Fears expressed without questioning.

13 GENERAL SOMATIC SYMPTOMS
0 |__| None.
1 |__| Heaviness in limbs, back or head. Backaches, headaches, muscle aches. Loss of energy and fatigability.
2 |__| Any clear-cut symptom rates 2.

14 GENITAL SYMPTOMS (symptoms such as loss of libido, menstrual disturbances)
0 |__| Absent.
1 |__| Mild.
2 |__| Severe.

15 HYPOCHONDRIASIS
0 |__| Not present.
1 |__| Self-absorption (bodily).
2 |__| Preoccupation with health.
3 |__| Frequent complaints, requests for help, etc.
4 |__| Hypochondriacal delusions.

16 LOSS OF WEIGHT ***(RATE EITHER a OR b)***

a) According to the patient:	b) According to weekly measurements:
0 |__| No weight loss.	0 |__| Less than 1 lb weight loss in week.
1 |__| Probable weight loss associated with present illness.	1 |__| Greater than 1 lb weight loss in week.
2 |__| Definite (according to patient) weight loss.	2 |__| Greater than 2 lb weight loss in week.
3 |__| Not assessed.	3 |__| Not assessed.

17 INSIGHT
0 |__| Acknowledges being depressed and ill.
1 |__| Acknowledges illness but attributes cause to bad food, climate, overwork, virus, need for rest, etc.
2 |__| Denies being ill at all.

Total score: |__|__|

References

1. Potts, M. K., Daniels, M., Burnam, M. A., & Wells, K. B. (1991). A structured interview version of the Hamilton Depression Rating Scale: evidence of reliability and versatility of administration.
2. Reynolds, W. M., & Kobak, K. A. (1995). *Hamilton Depression Inventory*. Odessa, FL: Psychological Assessment Resources.
3. Hamilton, M. (1960). A rating scale for depression. *Journal of Neurology, Neurosurgery, and Psychiatry, 23*, 56–62.
4. Bagby, R. M., Ryder, A. G., Schuller, D. R., & Marshall, M. B. (2004) The Hamilton Depression Rating Scale: has the gold standard become a lead weight? *American Journal of Psychiatry, 161*(12), 2163–2177.
5. Hedlund, J. L., & Vieweg, B. W. (1979). The Hamilton Rating Scale for Depression: a comprehensive review. *Journal of Operational Psychiatry, 10*, 149–165.
6. Knesevich, J. W., Biggs, J. T., Clayton, P. J., & Ziegler, V. E. (1977). Validity of the Hamilton Rating Scale for Depression. *The British Journal of Psychiatry, 131*, 49–52.
7. Hamilton, M., & Shaprio, C. M. (1990). Depression. In D. F. Peck & C. M. Shapiro (Eds.), *Measuring Human Problems* (25–65). Great Britain: John Wiley & Sons.
8. Frank, E., Prien, R. F., Jarrett, R. B., Keller, M. B., Kupfer, D. J., Lavori, P. W., Rush, A. J., & Weissman, M. M. (1991). Conceptualization and rationale for consensus definitions of terms in major depressive disorder: remission, recovery, relapse, and recurrence. *Archives of General Psychiatry, 48*(9), 851–855.

9. Zimmerman, M., Posternak, M. A., & Chelminski, I. (2005). Is the cutoff to define remission on the Hamilton Rating Scale for Depression too high? *The Journal of Nervous and Mental Disease, 193*(3), 170–175.
10. Williams, J. B. W., Link, M. J., Rosenthal, N. E., Terman, M. (1998). Structured Interview Guide for the Hamilton Depression Rating Scale, Seasonal Affective Disorders Version (SIGHSAD). New York Psychiatric Institute, New York.

Representative Studies Using Scale

Reynolds, C. F., Dew, M. A., Pollock, B. G., Mulsant, B. H., Frank, E., Miller, M. D., Houck, P. R., Mazumdar, S., Butters, M. A., Stack, J. A., Schlernitzauer, M. A., Whyte, E. M., Gildengers, A., Karp, J., Lenze, E., Szanto, K., Bensasi, S., & Kupfer, D. J. (2006). Maintenance treatment of major depression in old age. *New England Journal of Medicine, 354*(11), 1130–1138.

Brecht, S., Kajdasz, D., Ball, S., & Thase, M. E. (2008). Clinical impact of duloxetine treatment on sleep in patients with major depressive disorder. *International Clinical Psychopharmacology, 23*(6), 317–324.

Levitan, R., Shen, J., Jindal, J., Driver, H. S., Kennedy, S. H., & Shapiro, C. M. (2000). A preliminary randomized double-blind placebo controlled trial of tryptophan combined with fluoxetine in the treatment of major depression: anti-depressant and hypnotic effects. *Journal of Psychiatry & Neuroscience, 25*, 337–346.

Insomnia Severity Index (ISI)

43

Purpose Designed as a brief screening tool for insomnia, the seven-item questionnaire asks respondents to rate the nature and symptoms of their sleep problems using a Likert-type scale. Questions relate to subjective qualities of the respondent's sleep, including the severity of symptoms, the respondent's satisfaction with his or her sleep patterns, the degree to which insomnia interferes with daily functioning, how noticeable the respondent feels his or her insomnia is to others, and the overall level of distress created by the sleep problem.

Population for Testing The scale has been validated on two separate insomnia patient populations with ages ranging from 17 to 84.

Administration Requiring only about 5 min for completion, the brief scale is a self-report measure administered with pencil and paper.

Reliability and Validity Developers Bastien and colleagues [1] performed an initial psychometric study and demonstrated an internal consistency of $\alpha = .74$ and found item-total correlations that were quite variable, ranging from .36 to .54.

Obtaining a Copy A copy can be found in the developers' original published article [1].

Direct correspondence to:
C.M. Morin
École de Psychologie and Centre d'Étude des Troubles du Sommeil
Université Laval
St. Foy, Quebec G1K 7P4
Canada

Scoring Respondents rate each element of the questionnaire using Likert-type scales. Responses can range from 0 to 4, where higher scores indicate more acute symptoms of insomnia. Scores are tallied and can be compared both to scores obtained at a different phase of treatment and to the scores of other individuals. Though developers point out that their chosen cutoff scores have not been validated, they offer a few guidelines for interpreting scale results: a total score of 0–7 indicates "no clinically significant insomnia," 8–14 means "subthreshold insomnia," 15–21 is "clinical insomnia (moderate severity)," and 22–28 means "clinical insomnia (severe)."

A. Shahid et al. (eds.), *STOP, THAT and One Hundred Other Sleep Scales*,
DOI 10.1007/978-1-4419-9893-4_43,

Insomnia Severity Index (ISI)

Name: ______________________ **Date:** ____________________

1. Please rate the current (i.e., last 2 weeks) **SEVERITY** of your insomnia problem(s).

	None	Mild	Moderate	Severe	Very
Difficulty falling asleep:	0	1	2	3	4
Difficulty staying asleep:	0	1	2	3	4
Problem waking up too early:	0	1	2	3	4

2. How **SATISFIED**/dissatisfied are you with your current sleep pattern?

Very Satisfied				Very Dissatisfied
0	1	2	3	4

3. To what extent do you consider your sleep problem to **INTERFERE** with your daily functioning (e.g. daytime fatigue, ability to function at work/daily chores, concentration, memory, mood, etc.).

Not at all Interfering	A Little	Somewhat	Much	Very Much Interfering
0	1	2	3	4

4. How **NOTICEABLE** to others do you think your sleeping problem is in terms of impairing the quality of your life?

Not at all Noticeable	Barely	Somewhat	Much	Very Much Noticeable
0	1	2	3	4

5. How **WORRIED**/distressed are you about your current sleep problem?

Not at all	A Little	Somewhat	Much	Very Much
0	1	2	3	4

Guidelines for Scoring/Interpretation:

Add scores for all seven items (1a+1b+1c+ 2+3+4+5) = _____
Total score ranges from 0-28
0-7 = No clinically significant insomnia
8-14 = Subthreshold insomnia
15-21 = Clinical insomnia (moderate severity)
22-28 = Clinical insomnia (severe)

Reference

1. Bastien, C. H., Vallières, A., & Morin, C. M. (2001). Validation of the insomnia severity index as an outcome measure for insomnia research. *Sleep Medicine, 2*, 297–307.

Representative Studies Using Scale

Manber, R., Edinger, J. D., Gress, J. L., San Pedro-Salcedo, M. G., Kuo, T. F., & Kalista, T. (2008). Cognitive behavioral therapy for insomnia enhances depression outcome in patients with comorbid major depressive disorder and insomnia. *Sleep, 31*(4), 489–495.

LeBlanc, M., Beaulieu-Bonneau, S., Merette, C., Savard, J., Ivers, H., & Morin, C. M. (2007). Psychological and health-related quality of life factors associated with insomnia in a population-based sample. *Journal of Psychosomatic Research, 63*(2), 157–166.

International Restless Legs Syndrome Study Group Rating Scale

44

Purpose Developed as a tool for assessing the severity Restless Legs Syndrome (RLS), the 10-item questionnaire asks respondents to use Likert-type ratings to indicate how acutely the disorder has affected them over the course of the past week. Questions can be divided into one of two categories: disorder symptoms (nature, intensity, and frequency) and their impact (sleep issues, disturbances in daily functioning, and resultant changes in mood).

Population for Testing The instrument has been validated with a sample of RLS patients aged 22–91.

Administration A self-report, pencil-and paper instrument, the scale requires approximately 5–10 min for completion.

Reliability and Validity A large psychometric study conducted by Walters and colleagues [1] found an internal consistency ranging from .93 to .95, an inter-rater reliability of .93 to .97, a test–retest reliability of .87, a concurrent validity of .78 to .84, and a correlation of about .73 with the diagnostic judgments of a clinician.

Obtaining a Copy An example can be found in the developers' original published article [1]. However, the scale is under copyright.

Direct correspondence and reprint requests to:
Caroline Anfray
Information Resources Centre, MAPI Research Institute
27 rue de la Villette
69003 Lyon, France
Phone: +33(0) 472 13 66 67
FAX: +33 (0) 472 13 66 82
Email: canfray@mapi.fr or instdoc@mapi.fr

Scoring Each of the ten questions requires respondents to rate their experiences with RLS on a scale from 0 to 4, with 4 representing the most severe and frequent symptoms and 0 representing the least. Total scores can range from 0 to 40. As a brief scale with excellent psychometric qualities, the instrument may be suitable for a variety of research and clinical purposes, including screening and assessment of treatment outcomes.

A. Shahid et al. (eds.), *STOP, THAT and One Hundred Other Sleep Scales*,
DOI 10.1007/978-1-4419-9893-4_44, © Springer Science+Business Media, LLC 2012

International Restless Legs Syndrome Study Group Rating Scale (IRLS)

(Investigator Version 2.2)

Have the patient rate his/her symptoms for the following ten questions. The patient and not the examiner should make the ratings, but the examiner should be available to clarify any misunderstandings the patient may have about the questions. The examiner should mark the patient's answers on the form.

In the past week…

(1) Overall, how would you rate the RLS discomfort in your legs or arms?

- 4☐ Very severe
- 3☐ Severe
- 2☐ Moderate
- 1☐ Mild
- 0☐ None

In the past week…

(2) Overall, how would you rate the need to move around because of your RLS symptoms?

- 4☐ Very severe
- 3☐ Severe
- 2☐ Moderate
- 1☐ Mild
- 0☐ None

In the past week…

(3) Overall, how much relief of your RLS arm or leg discomfort did you get from moving around?

- 4☐ No relief
- 3☐ Mild relief
- 2☐ Moderate relief
- 1☐ Either complete or almost complete relief
- 0☐ No RLS symptoms to be relieved

In the past week…

(4) How severe was your sleep disturbance due to your RLS symptoms?

4☐ Very severe
3☐ Severe
2☐ Moderate
1☐ Mild
0☐ None

In the past week…

(5) How severe was your tiredness or sleepiness during the day due to your RLS symptoms?

4☐ Very severe
3☐ Severe
2☐ Moderate
1☐ Mild
0☐ None

In the past week…

(6) How severe was your RLS as a whole?

4☐ Very severe
3☐ Severe
2☐ Moderate
1☐ Mild
0☐ None

In the past week…

(7) How often did you get RLS symptoms?

4☐ Very often (This means 6 to 7 days a week)
3☐ Often (This means 4 to 5 days a week)
2☐ Sometimes (This means 2 to 3 days a week)
1☐ Occasionally (This means 1 day a week)
0☐ Never

In the past week…

(8) When you had RLS symptoms, how severe were they on average?

- 4☐ Very severe (This means 8 hours or more per 24 hour day)
- 3☐ Severe (This means 3 to 8 hours per 24 hour day)
- 2☐ Moderate (This means 1 to 3 hours per 24 hour day)
- 1☐ Mild (This means less than 1 hour per 24 hour day)
- 0☐ None

In the past week…

(9) Overall, how severe was the impact of your RLS symptoms on your ability to carry out your daily affairs, for example carrying out a satisfactory family, home, social, school or work life?

- 4☐ Very severe
- 3☐ Severe
- 2☐ Moderate
- 1☐ Mild
- 0☐ None

In the past week…

(10) How severe was your mood disturbance due to your RLS symptoms - for example angry, depressed, sad, anxious or irritable?

- 4☐ Very severe
- 3☐ Severe
- 2☐ Moderate
- 1☐ Mild
- 0☐ None

The sum of the item scores serves as the global score for the scale.
Higher scores indicate more impairment /higher severity

INVESTIGATOR VERSION 2.2 February 2004

SCALING AND SCORING OF THE

'International Restless Legs Syndrome Study Group Rating Scale' (IRLS)

Mapi Research Trust
27 rue de la Villette
69003 Lyon
France
Phone: +33 (0) 4 72 13 65 75
Fax: +33 (0) 4 72 13 66 82

Contact:
Marie-Pierre Emery
E-mail : mpemery@mapigroup.com

The International Restless Legs Syndrome Study Group (IRLSSG)

Represented by
Dr Arthur Walters
E-mail: ArtUMDNJ@aol.com

Dr Richard Allen
E-mail: RichardJHU@aol.com

MAPI RESEARCH TRUST Education Information Dissemination

International Restless Legs Syndrome Study Group Rating Scale (IRLS)

The IRLS is composed of 10 items.
It gives a global score for all 10 items that is most commonly used as an overall severity score.
9 of the 10 items investigate two dimensions of the RLS severity.

DESCRIPTION OF THE QUESTIONNAIRE:

Dimensions	Number of Items	Cluster of Items	Item Reversion	Direction of Dimensions
Symptoms	6	1, 2, 4, 6, 7 and 8	No	Higher score = Higher severity
Symptoms impact	3	5, 9 and 10	No	Higher score = Higher impact

Item 3 is part of the diagnostic criteria and does not belong to any of the two dimensions. It is used for the total score for overall RLS severity.

SCORING OF DIMENSIONS:

Item scaling	5-point Likert scale from 0 "None" to 4 "very severe"
Weighting of Items	No
Extension of the Scoring Scale	Symptom severity subscale: 0-24 Impact on daily living subscale: 0-12 Global score: 0-40
Scoring Procedure	The score of each subscale is calculated by summing the scores of all items of the subscale The global score is obtained by summing all the 10 items scores
Interpretation and Analysis of missing data*	All 10 items should be completed to calculate the global score For the symptoms subscale, all six items should be completed to calculate the subscale score For the symptoms impact subscale, all three items should be completed to calculate the subscale score
Interpretation and Analysis of 'non-concerned' answers	Not applicable for this questionnaire. Subjects should not be administered the scale unless they meet the 4 IRLSSG criteria for Restless Legs Syndrome

* This scale should be read to the patient by a trained staff member with the patient looking at the questions and providing a verbal answer. The staff member and not the patient records the patient's answer. In this situation there should be no missing items. If missing items occur the staff member failed to properly administer the scale and the results should probably not be accepted. Pro-rating for missing answers should not be needed for this scale.

REFERENCE(S):

The International Restless Legs Syndrome Study Group. Validation of the International Restless Legs Syndrome Study Group rating scale for restless legs syndrome. Sleep medicine. 2003;4:121-132

Allen RP, Kushida CA, Atkinson MJ and RLS QoL Consortium. Factor analysis of the International Restless Legs Syndrome Study Group's scale for restless legs severity. Sleep Medicine. 2003; 4:133-135

Abetz L, Arbuckle R, Allen RP, Garcia-Borreguero D, Hening W, Walters AS, Mavraki E, Kirsch JM. The reliability, validity and responsiveness of the International Restless Legs Syndrome Study Group rating scale and subscales in a clinical-trial setting. Sleep Med. 2006 Jun;7(4):340-9. Epub 2006 May 19

Reference

1. Walters, A. S., LeBrocq, C., Dhar, A., Hening, W., Rosen, R., Allen, R. P., Trenkwalder, C., & International Restless Legs Syndrome Study Group. (2003). Validation of the International Restless Legs Syndrome Study Group rating scale for restless legs syndrome. *Sleep Medicine, 4*(2), 121–132.

Representative Studies Using Scale

Bjorvatn, B., Leissner, L., Ulfberg, J., Gyring, J., Karlsborg, M., Regeur, L., Skeidsvoll, H., Nordhus, I. H., & Pallesen, S. (2005). Prevalence, severity and risk factors of restless legs syndrome in the general adult population in two Scandinavian countries. *Sleep Medicine, 6*(4), 307–312.

Hornyak, M., Hundemer, H., Quail, D., Riemann, D., Voderholzer, U., Trenkwalder, C. (2007). Relationship of periodic leg movements and severity of restless legs syndrome: A study in unmedicated and medicated patients. *Clinical Neurophysiology, 118*(7), 1532–1537.

Jenkins Sleep Scale

45

Purpose Designed as an efficient and brief instrument for use in research, the four-item question evaluates the frequency and intensity of certain sleep difficulties in respondents. Questions address difficulty falling asleep, frequent awakenings during the night, trouble remaining asleep, and subjective feelings of fatigue and sleepiness despite receiving a typical night's rest. Though the questionnaire is short, developers suggest that its four items have been shown to possess good predictive value in previous studies [1]. However, with only four items, it cannot begin to address the entire spectrum of sleep disorders and should only be considered for use as a preliminary screening device.

Population for Testing The scale has been validated with two different testing populations, ages 25–69 years.

Administration Requiring between 2 and 5 min for completion, the instrument can be administered through an interview or in a self-report, pencil-and-paper format.

Reliability and Validity In an initial psychometric analysis conducted by the developers [1], the scale possessed an internal consistency ranging from .63 to .79.

Obtaining a Copy A copy of the questionnaire is published in the original article published by Jenkins and colleagues [1].

Direct correspondence to:
C.D. Jenkins
Department of Preventive Medicine
and Community Health
University of Texas Medical Branch
Galveston, TX 77550, USA

Scoring Respondents use a Likert-type scale to answer questions regarding the frequency with which they have experienced certain sleep difficulties over the past month: 0 means "not at all," while 5 means "22–31 days." Higher scores indicate more acute sleep difficulties.

A. Shahid et al. (eds.), *STOP, THAT and One Hundred Other Sleep Scales*,
DOI 10.1007/978-1-4419-9893-4_45, © Springer Science+Business Media, LLC 2012

Jenkins Sleep Scale

How often in the past month did you:	(0) Not at all	(1) 1-3 days	(2) 4-7 days	(3) 8-14 days	(4) 15-21 days	(5) 22-31 days
1. Have trouble falling asleep?	0	1	2	3	4	5
2. Wake up several times per night?	0	1	2	3	4	5
3. Have trouble staying asleep (including waking far too early)?	0	1	2	3	4	5
4. Wake up after your usual amount of sleep feeling tired and worn out?	0	1	2	3	4	5

Reference

1. Jenkins, C. D., Stanton, B. A., Niemcryk, S. J., & Rose, R. M. (1988). A scale for the estimation of sleep problems in clinical research. *Journal of Clinical Epidemiology, 41*(4), 313–321.

Representative Studies Using Scale

Jerlock, M., Gaston-Johansson, F., Kjellgren, K., & Welin, C. (2006). Coping strategies, stress, physical activity and sleep in patients with unexplained chest pain. *BMC Nursing, 5*(7).

46 Johns Hopkins Restless Legs Severity Scale (JHRLSS)

Purpose Using this single-item scale, trained clinicians assign individuals a Restless Legs Syndrome (RLS) severity score based on the time of day at which symptoms begin to appear. This score acts as a subjective measure of RLS which can be used as a quick screening device and also as a longitudinal instrument for evaluating treatment outcomes.

Population for Testing The scale has been validated with patients aged 29–81 years, though it should presumably be indicated for use with younger adult RLS patients as well.

Administration Rating is conducted by a trained clinician and does not necessarily even require face-to-face interview – raters in a study conducted by Allen and Earley [1] used patient charts to assign scores. Administration time will depend on the individual rater and the situation in which the patient is being evaluated. However, 5–10 min should be sufficient.

Reliability and Validity Developers Allen and Earley [1] evaluated the psychometric properties of the scale against the results of overnight polysomnography. They demonstrated an inter-rater reliability of .91, and results of the scale correlated highly with sleep efficiency ($r=.60$) and periodic leg movements per hour of sleep ($r=.45$) as measured by the polysomnogram.

Obtaining a Copy The developers' original article explains the scoring of the scale [1].

Direct correspondence to:
Richard P. Allen
Department of Neurology,
John Hopkins University
Bayview Medical Center,
Neurology and Sleep Disorders
A Building 6-C, Room 689
4940 Eastern Avenue
Baltimore, MD 21224, USA

Scoring Clinicians assign patients ratings based on the following criterion: a score of 0 means that symptoms are never experienced, 1 (mild) means symptoms begin within an hour of bedtime, 2 (moderate) designates symptoms that begin in the evening (sometime after 6:00), and 3 (severe) means that symptoms begin during the day (before 6:00).

A. Shahid et al. (eds.), *STOP, THAT and One Hundred Other Sleep Scales*,
DOI 10.1007/978-1-4419-9893-4_46, © Springer Science+Business Media, LLC 2012

Johns Hopkins Restless Legs Severity Scale (JHRLSS)

Score	Usual time of day when RLS symptoms start (after 12 noon)
0 (NEVER)	No Symptoms
0.5 infrequent	Symptoms less than daily or almost daily
1 (Mild)	AT BEDTIME and/or during the sleep period. (Symptoms may occur within 60 minutes before the usual bed or simply at the time of going to bed or during the night after in bed.)
2 (Moderate)	IN THE EVENING (6 P.M. or later). Symptoms may start at anytime between 6 P.M. and the usual bedtime. (The definition of evening may need to be adjusted for patients who routinely have much later bedtimes, such as those who have an afternoon siesta.)
3 (Severe)	AFTERNOON (Before 6 P.M.). Symptoms start in the afternoon and persist into the evening and night
4 (Very Severe)	MORNING (Before noon). Symptoms may start in the morning or they may be present virtually all day. There is usually a "protected period" in the mid-morning (8-10 a.m.) with few if any symptoms. Even the protected period may have symptoms for the most severe RLS, often occurring with significant RLS augmentation.

(Note, since RLS symptoms once started tend to persist until morning, the number of hours in the day with RLS will be about 1-6 for mild, 7-12 for moderate and 13 or more for severe RLS on this scale).

Sample Standard Questions:

1. How many days in a week or month do you have RLS symptoms ____________ per week ___________ per month

2. On a usual day what is the earliest time after 12 noon that these sensations or movements likely to occur if you were to sit down or rest? _____ P.M. _____A.M.

Reference

1. Allen R. P., & Earley, C. J. (2001). Validation of the Johns Hopkins restless legs severity scale. *Sleep Medicine, 2*(3), 239–242.

Representative Studies Using Scale

Earley, C. J., Barker, P. B., Horska, K., & Allen, R. P. (2006). MRI-determined regional brain iron concentrations in early-and late-onset restless legs syndrome. *Sleep Medicine, 7*(5), 458–461.

Pearson, V. E., Allen, R. P., Dean, T., Gamaldo, C. E., Lesage, S. R., & Earley, C. J. (2006). Cognitive deficits associated with restless legs syndrome (RLS). *Sleep Medicine, 7*(1), 25–30.

47 Karolinska Sleepiness Scale (KSS)

Purpose This scale [1] measures the subjective level of sleepiness at a particular time during the day. On this scale subjects indicate which level best reflects the psycho-physical sate experienced in the last 10 min. The KSS is a measure of situational sleepiness. It is sensitive to fluctuations.

Population for Testing It has been used in studies of shift work, jetlag, for driving abilities [2], attention and performance, and in clinical settings. It is used for both males and females.

It is helpful in assessing the changes in response to environmental factors, circadian rhythm, and effects of drugs. Because the KSS is not a measure of 'Trait' sleepiness, it has not been widely used for clinical purposes.

Administration This is self-report measure. It takes 5 min to complete.

Reliability and Validity In a study conducted by Kaida et al. [3], the authors investigated the validity of the KSS and found that it was highly correlated to EEG and behavioral variables. The results show that KSS has a high validity. However, because the scores of the KSS vary according to earlier sleep, time of day, and other parameters, it is difficult to deduce its test–retest reliability.

Scoring This is a 9-point scale (1 = extremely alert, 3 = alert, 5 = neither alert nor sleepy, 7 = sleepy – but no difficulty remaining awake, and 9 = extremely sleepy – fighting sleep). There is a modified KSS that contains one other item: 10 = extremely sleepy, falls asleep all the time. Scores on the KSS increase with longer periods of wakefulness and it strongly correlate with the time of the day.

Obtaining a Copy A copy can be obtained from the authors.

Direct correspondence:
Torbjörn Åkerstedt
IPM & Karolinska Institutet
Box 230
17177 Stockholm, Sweden
Email: Torbjorn.Akerstedt@ki.se

A. Shahid et al. (eds.), *STOP, THAT and One Hundred Other Sleep Scales*,
DOI 10.1007/978-1-4419-9893-4_47, © Springer Science+Business Media, LLC 2012

Karolinska Sleepiness Scale (KSS)

Extremely alert	1
Very alert	2
Alert	3
Rather alert	4
Neither alert nor sleepy	5
Some signs of sleepiness	6
Sleepy, but no effort to keep awake	7
Sleepy, but some effort to keep awake	8
Very sleepy, great effort to keep awake, fighting sleep	9
Extremely sleepy, can't keep awake	10

References

1. Akerstedt T, Gillberg M. (1990). Subjective and objective sleepiness in the active individual. International Journal of Neuroscience, 52, 29–37.
2. Kecklund G, Akerstedt T. (1993). Sleepiness in long distance truck driving: an ambulatory EEG study of night driving. Ergonomics, 36, 1007–17.
3. Kaida M, Takahashi T, Åkerstedt A, Nakata Y, Otsuka T, Haratani K, et al. (2006). Validation of the Karolinska sleepiness scale against performance and EEG variables. Clinical Neurophysiology, 117, 1574–81.

Representative Studies Using Scale

Gillberg M, Kecklund G, Akerstedt T. (1994). Relations between performance and subjective ratings of sleepiness during a night awake. Sleep, 17, 236–241.

Kaida, K., Åkerstedt, T., Kecklund, G., Nilsson, J.P., Axelsson, J. (2007). Use of subjective and physiological indicators of sleepiness to predict performance during a vigilance task. Industrial Health, 45, 520–526.

Maimberg, B., Kecklund, G., Karlson, B., Persson, R., Flisberg, P., Ørbaek, P. (2010). Sleep and recovery in physicians on night call: a longitudinal field study. BMC Health Services Research, 10, 239.

Sallinen, M., Harma, M., Akila, R., Holm, A., Luukkonen, R., Mikola, H., et al. (2004). The effects of sleep debt and monotonous work on sleepiness and performance during a 12-h dayshift. *Journal of Sleep Research*, 13, 285–94.

Leeds Sleep Evaluation Questionnaire (LSEQ)

48

Purpose A 10-item, subjective, self-report measure, the LSEQ was designed to assess changes in sleep quality over the course of a psychopharmacological treatment intervention. The scale evaluates four domains: ease of initiating sleep, quality of sleep, ease of waking, and behavior following wakefulness.

Population for Testing Developers initially validated the LSEQ with individuals aged 18–49 years [1]. The scale is available in a wide range of languages.

Administration The scale is a self-report, paper-and-pencil measure requiring between 5 and 10 min for completion.

Reliability and Validity A psychometric evaluation conducted by Parrott and Hindmarch [1] revealed the four-factor structure of the scale. The "initiating sleep" and the "quality of sleep" factors were correlated with one another, while the "awakening from sleep" and the "behavior following wakefulness" factors were also correlated.

Obtaining a Copy A copy of the questionnaire can be found in the original article published by developers [1].

Direct correspondence to:
A.C. Parrott
Department of Psychology,
University of Leeds
Leeds LS2 9JT, UK

Scoring A visual analogue scale, the LSEQ requires respondents to place marks on a group of 10-cm lines representing the changes they have experienced in a variety of symptoms since beginning treatment. Lines extend between extremes like "more difficult than usual" and "easier than usual" (item 6, querying ease of waking). Responses are measured using a 100-mm scale and are then averaged to provide a score for each domain. These can then be used to evaluate the efficacy and sleep-related side effects of a drug treatment.

A. Shahid et al. (eds.), *STOP, THAT and One Hundred Other Sleep Scales*,
DOI 10.1007/978-1-4419-9893-4_48,

Leeds Sleep Evaluation Questionnaire

How would you describe the way you currently fall asleep in comparison to usual?

1. More difficult than usual	________________	Easier than usual	
2. Slower than usual	________________	More quickly than usual	GTS – getting to sleep
3. I feel less sleepy than usual	________________	More sleepy than usual	

How would you describe the quality of your sleep compared to normal sleep?

4. More restless than usual	________________	Calmer than usual	QOS – quality of sleep
5. With more wakeful periods than usual	________________	With less wakeful periods than usual	

How would you describe your awakenings in comparison to usual?

6. More difficult than usual	________________	Easier than usual	AFS – Awake following sleep
7. Requires a period of time longer than usual	________________	Shorter than usual	

How do you feel when you wake up?

8. Tired	________________	Alert	BFW - Behaviour Following Wakening

How do you feel now?

9. Tired	________________	Alert	

How would you describe your balance and co-ordination upon awakening?

10. More disrupted than usual	________________	Less disrupted than than usual	

Reference

1. Parrott, A. C., & Hindmarch, I. (1978). Factor analysis of a sleep evaluation questionnaire. *Psychological Medicine, 8*(2), 325–329.

Representative Studies Using Scale

Luthringer, R., Staner, L., Noel, N., Muze, M., Gassmann-Mayer, C., Talluri, K., Cleton, A., Eerdekens, M., Battisti, W. P., & Palumbo, J. M. (2007). A double-blind, placebo-controlled, randomized study evaluating the effect of paliperidone extended-release tablets on sleep architecture in patients with schizophrenia. *International Clinical Psychopharmacology, 22*(5), 299–308.

Lemoine, P., Nir, T., Laudon, M., & Zisapel, N. (2007). Prolonged release melatonin improves sleep quality and morning alertness in insomnia patients aged 55 years and older and has no withdrawal effects. *Journal of Sleep Research, 16*(4), 372–380.

Maastricht Vital Exhaustion Questionnaire (MQ)

49

Purpose Having observed that patients who experience myocardial infarction often present with unexplained tiredness for some time prior, developers of the questionnaire hoped to create a tool that could be used to assess these feelings of "vital exhaustion" [1]. The scale consisting of 21 items honed from an original pool of 58 and chosen for their capacity to predict future coronary events. There is also a 37 item version shown on the following page. The asterisked items are all included in the 21 item scale as are a further six items which are listed on the following page. Sleep physicians may be particularly interested in incorporating the scale into their practice due to the strong association between sleep disordered breathing and cardiac problems [2].

Population for Testing The MQ was initially developed through a survey that was answered by 3,877 male civil servants [1]. Its predictive capability has since been assessed in women as well [3].

Administration The Maastricht Questionnaire is a short, paper-and-pencil measure requiring between 5 and 10 min for completion.

Reliability and Validity In an initial validation, the questionnaire was found to possess an internal consistency of .89. Further assessment of the scale confirmed that "vital exhaustion" is significantly associated with future angina and future myocardial infarction [4].

Obtaining a Copy A copy of the scale can be found in the original article by the developers [1].

Direct Correspondence:
Ad Appels
Department of Medical Psychology
Maastricht University, Box 616, 62000 MD
Maastricht, the Netherlands
Email: ad.appels@mp.unimaas.nl

Scoring Patients are asked a number of questions which they can answer with "yes," "no," or "?" (e.g., "Do you often feel tired?"). Responses of "yes" are scored as 2, "?" is given 1 point, and "no" receives 0. For items 9 and 14, this scoring system is reversed. A total score can then be calculated by summing each item. Developers defined "vital exhaustion" as scores that fell above the median of the MQ.

A. Shahid et al. (eds.), *STOP, THAT and One Hundred Other Sleep Scales*,
DOI 10.1007/978-1-4419-9893-4_49, © Springer Science+Business Media, LLC 2012

Maastricht Vital Exhaustion Questionnaire

*1. Do you often feel tired?
*2. Do you often have difficulty falling asleep?
*3. Do you wake up repeatedly during the night?
4. Have you felt less confident lately?
5. Do you sometimes have a feeling that you have got problems you cannot work out, in recent months?
*6. Do you feel weak all over?
7. Have you been unable to stand loud noises lately?
*8. Do you have a feeling that you haven't been accomplishing much lately?
*9. Do you have the feeling that you can't cope with everyday problems as well as you used to?
10. Do you have a feeling that the future is becoming less and less certain?
11. Have you though about deceased acquaintances or relatives more often lately?
*12. Do you believe that you have come to a "dead end"?
13. Are you continuously worrying about your health?
14. Have demands been made on you lately that you could not cope with?
15. Do minor hassles easily irritate you in recent months?
*16. Do you feel more listless recently than before?
17. Do you feel as if you are losing your self-control?
18. Do you have a feeling that nobody can help you with those problems deep down inside?
19. Have demands been made on you lately that you could only meet by making extra efforts?
*20. I enjoy sex as much as ever. (no)
*21. Have you experienced a feeling of hopelessness recently?
22. Do you often worry about your health?
23. Do you sometimes wonder whether you will still be alive tomorrow?
24. Does the feeling that you are a failure ever come upon you?
*25. Do little things irritate you more lately than they used to do?
*26. Do you feel you want to give up trying?
27. Are you becoming less satisfied with yourself?
28. Have you lately had a feeling, like "I do not achieve enough, I could achieve more if only I were healthier, not so weak, not so limp"?
29. Do you feel downcast?
*30. Do you sometimes feel that your body is like a battery that is losing its power?
31. Do you sometimes have a feeling that you don't know exactly where you stand?
32. Do you feel less capable of doing something useful nowadays.
33. Do you have a feeling that you family doesn't understand you too well?
*34. Would you want to be dead at times?
35. Have you felt strange bodily sensation lately?
*36. Do you have the feeling that you don't have what it takes anymore these days?
37. Can you bring yourself less and less to leave the house and go somewhere for a visit?

Further items making up the 21 item Maastricht scale are:

(a) Does it take more time to grasp a difficult problem than it did a year ago?

(b) I feel fine

(c) Do you feel dejected?

(d) Do you feel like crying sometimes?

(e) Do you ever wake up with a feeling of exhaustion and fatigue?

(f) Do you have increasing difficulty on concentrating on a single subject for long?

References

1. Appels, A., Höppener, P., Mulder, P. (1987). A questionnaire to assess premonitory symptoms of myocardial infarction. *International Journal of Cardiology, 17*, 15–24
2. Ancoli-Israel, S., DuHamel, E., Stepnowsky, C., Engler, R., Cohen-Zion, M., & Marler, M. (2003). The relationship between congestive heart failure, sleep apnea, and mortality in older men. *Chest, 124*(4), 1400–1405.
3. Appels, A., Falger, P., & Schouten, E. (1993). Vital exhaustion as a risk indicator for myocardial infarction in women. *Journal of Psychosomatic Research, 37*(8), 881–890.
4. Appels, A. & Mulder, P. (1989). Fatigue and heart disease. The association between "vital exhaustion" and past, present and future coronary heart disease. *Journal of Psychosomatic Research, 33*(6), 727–738.

Representative Studies Using Scale

Hayakawa, T., Fujita, O., Ishida, K., Usami, T., Sugiura, S. Kayukawa, Y., Terashima, M., Ohta, T., & Okada, T. (2002). Evaluating mental fatigue in patients with obstructive sleep apnea syndrome by the Maastricht Questionnaire. *Psychiatry and Clinical Neurosciences, 56*(3), 313–314.

Van Diest, R., & Appels, W. (1994). Sleep characteristics of exhausted men. *Psychosomatic Medicine, 56*(1), 28–35.

Medical Outcomes Study Sleep Scale (MOS-SS) 50

Purpose The MOS-SS was created as part of a larger initiative to evaluate health status in a population of more than 10,000 patient participants. Consisting of 12 items, the sleep scale is only a small part of the complete Patient Assessment Questionnaire (PAQ), a 20-page instrument querying a broad range of health-related issues including physical functioning, psychological well-being, health distress, and pain. The sleep scale examines six factors: sleep initiation, maintenance, respiratory problems, quantity, perceived adequacy, and somnolence. The MOS-SS can be administered separately, or it can be used as part of a complete battery of testing to provide a more general picture of health.

Population for Testing The questionnaire was initially validated in a baseline sample of more than 3,000 individuals. Participants ranged in age from 18 to 98 years, with a mean age of 54.

Administration The scale itself is quite short, requiring approximately 5 min for administration. However, the complete PAQ is much longer and more time-consuming. Both are self-report, pencil-and-paper measures.

Reliability and Validity In a baseline psychometric evaluation of the scale [1], MOS developers found an internal consistency ranging from .75 to .86. Measures of sleep disturbance, quantity, and optimal sleep were found to be highly related to perceptions of adequacy.

Obtaining a Copy A copy of the scale can be found in a chapter regarding sleep measures written by Hays and Stewart [1]. The complete PAQ can be found in the book's Appendix [2].

Scoring The scale uses predominantly Likert-type questions to evaluate sleep. Scales range from 1 (meaning "all of the time") to 6 ("none of the time"), and require respondents to indicate how frequently during the previous 4 weeks they have experienced certain sleep-related issues. Several of these items are reverse scored. Another Likert-type item queries sleep latency (1 = "0–15 min" and 5 = "more than 60 min"). Finally, a fill-in-the-blank question asks participants to estimate the average number of hours they have slept each night in the past month – a response of 8 h or greater receives a 1, while answers below 8 h receive 0.

A. Shahid et al. (eds.), *STOP, THAT and One Hundred Other Sleep Scales*,
DOI 10.1007/978-1-4419-9893-4_50, © Springer Science+Business Media, LLC 2012

Sleep Scale from the Medical Outcomes Study

1. How long did it usually take for you to fall asleep during the past 4 weeks?

(Circle One)

0-15 minutes................1

16-30 minutes................2

31-45 minutes................3

46-60 minutes................4

More than 60 minutes 5

---

2. On the average, how many hours did you sleep each night during the past 4 weeks?

Write in number
of hours per night: ☐☐

How often during the <u>past 4 weeks</u> did you…

(Circle One Number On Each Line)

	All of the Time ▼	Most of the Time ▼	A Good Bit of the Time ▼	Some of the Time ▼	A Little of the Time ▼	None of the Time ▼
3. feel that your sleep was not quiet (moving restlessly, feeling tense, speaking, etc., while sleeping)?	1	2	3	4	5	6
4. get enough sleep to feel rested upon waking in the morning?	1	2	3	4	5	6
5. awaken short of breath or with a headache?	1	2	3	4	5	6
6. feel drowsy or sleepy during the day?	1	2	3	4	5	6
7. have trouble falling asleep?	1	2	3	4	5	6
8. awaken during your sleep time and have trouble falling asleep again?	1	2	3	4	5	6
9. have trouble staying awake during the day?	1	2	3	4	5	6
10. snore during your sleep?	1	2	3	4	5	6
11. take naps (5 minutes or longer) during the day?	1	2	3	4	5	6
12. get the amount of sleep you needed?	1	2	3	4	5	6

References

1. Hays, R. D., & Stewart, A. L. (1992). Sleep measures. In A. L. Stewart & J. E. Ware (Eds.), *Measuring functioning and well-being* (235–259). Durham: Duke University Press.
2. Stewart, A. L., & Ware, J. E. (1992). *Measuring functioning and well-being*. Durham: Duke University Press.

Representative Studies Using Scale

Haut, S. R., Katz, M., Masur, J., & Lipton, R. B. (2009). Seizures in the elderly: impact on mental status, mood, and sleep. *Epilepsy and Behavior, 14*(3), 540–544.

Zelman, D. C., Brandenburg, N. A., & Gore, M. (2006). Sleep impairments in patients with painful diabetic peripheral neuropathy. *The Clinical Journal of Pain, 22*(8), 681–685.

Katz, D. A., & McHorney, C. A. (1998). Clinical correlates of insomnia in patients with chronic illness. *Archives of Internal Medicine, 158*(10), 1099–1107.

Mini-Mental State Examination (MMSE)

51

Purpose A simplified version of a much more extensive instrument for assessing cognitive mental status, the MMSE was designed to accommodate patients who cannot maintain attention for long periods, particularly elderly individuals with delirium or dementia. The instrument is divided into two parts, both of which are administered by a clinician or nurse: The first concerns the respondent's memory, attention span, and orientation in location and time, while the second asks the respondent to name certain objects, repeat phrases, follow verbal directions, and to copy both a sentence and a figure using pencil and paper. The questionnaire can be used as a measure of the severity of cognitive impairment at a single moment, or it can be employed across different times and treatments to reflect an individual's changing cognitive abilities. As disturbed sleep is quite prevalent in elderly individuals – particularly those with dementia [1] – a cognitive status exam like the MMSE may be especially useful for sleep specialists attempting to address the diagnosis and treatment of this patient population.

Population for Testing Though the test was designed with elderly individuals in mind, it has been validated on a variety of adult patient populations, including those presenting with depressed and manic affective disorders, schizophrenia, and drug abuse issues.

Administration Requiring between 10 and 15 min for completion, the test is administered both verbally and using pencil and paper by trained third party. To purchase the scale from its publishers, individuals are required to complete a "PAR Customer Qualification Form for Medical and Allied Health Professionals," proving that they are trained in the administration, scoring, and interpretation of psychometric measures, or that they possess equivalent experience in the field.

Reliability and Validity An initial psychometric study performed by Folstein and colleagues [2] found a test-retest reliability of .89 for the same tester and a reliability of .83 when two different examiners were used. More recently, the instrument has also been validated for use with cancer patients [3], and individuals with acquired brain injury [4].

Obtaining a Copy An example of the original questionnaire is available from Folstein and colleagues [2]. The test is under copyright and recent versions can be purchased from publishers *Psychological Assessment Resources* online at www.minimental.com.

Scoring The instrument's 11 items are scored using Likert-type scales that range from two to six options in length. Higher scores indicate better cognitive function, with a maximum score of 30. Though developers initially suggested a cutoff score of 24, more recent normative data and cutoff scores are available for a variety of different age groups and education levels in a clinical guidebook published by the developers.

A. Shahid et al. (eds.), *STOP, THAT and One Hundred Other Sleep Scales*,
DOI 10.1007/978-1-4419-9893-4_51, © Springer Science+Business Media, LLC 2012

Additionally, scoring software can be purchased that generates detailed reports based on respondent results.

References

1. Ancoli-Israel, S., Poceta, J. S., Stepnowsky, C., Martin, J., & Gehrman, P. (1997). Identification and treatment of sleep problems in the elderly. *Sleep Medicine Reviews, 1*(1), 3–17.
2. Folstein, M. F., Folstein, S. E., & McHugh, P. R. (1975). "Mini-mental state:" a practical method for grading the cognitive state of patients for the clinician. *Journal of Psychiatric Research, 12*(3), 189–198.
3. Mystakidou, K., Tsilika, E., Parpa, E., Galanos, A., Vlahos, L. (2007). Brief cognitive assessment of cancer patients: evaluation of the mini-mental state examination (MMSE) psychometric properties. *Psycho-Oncology, 16*(4), 352–357.
4. Elhan, A. H., Kutley, S., Kucukdeveci, A. A., Cotuk, C., Ozturk, G., Tesio, L., & Tennant, A. (2005). Psychometric properties of the mini-mental state examination in patients with acquired brain injury in Turkey. *Journal of Rehabilitation Medicine, 37*(5), 306–311.

Representative Studies Using Scale

Slavin, M. J., Sandstrom, C. K., Tran, T. T., Doraiswamy, P. M., & Petrella, J. R. (2007). Hippocampal volume and the mini-mental state examination in the diagnosis of amnestic mild cognitive impairment. *American Journal of Roentgenology, 188*(5), 1404–1410.

Sinforiani, E., Zangaglia, R., Manni, R., Cristina, S., Marchion, E., Nappi, G., Mancini, F., & Pacchetti, C. (2006). REM sleep behavior disorder, hallucinations, and cognitive impairment in Parkinson's disease. *Movement Disorders, 21*(4), 462–466.

Modified Checklist for Autism in Toddlers (M-CHAT)

52

Purpose As the original Checklist for Autism in Toddlers (CHAT) requires a home health visitor to observe the child in the family environment, the M-CHAT was designed to accommodate health-care systems in which home visits are not covered. Both questionnaires assess the risk for autism spectrum disorders (ASD) – the M-CHAT is designed to do so using only the behavioral reports of parents. Consisting of 23 "yes or no" questions, the instrument can be quickly administered by a family doctor at the time of the child's 18-month checkup, or can be used by specialists and other professionals for screening, research, or educational purposes. Though researchers have only recently begun to explore the manifestation of sleep disorders in children with autism and other Pervasive Developmental Disorders, one review of the literature conducted by Johnson [1] suggests that between 34% and 80% of these children have a sleep problem. Thus, these children may be particularly overrepresented in a sleep clinic setting: The ability to properly screen for developmental disorders should be considered an asset for sleep specialists of all kinds.

Population for Testing Studies validating the instrument have used sample of toddlers between 16 and 30 months of age.

Administration The questionnaire can be administered through interview or can be completed by parents with pencil and paper. About 5–10 min should be enough time for completion.

Reliability and Validity Robins and colleagues [2] found the test possessed an internal reliability of $\alpha = .85$, a sensitivity of .87, specificity of .99, a positive predictive power of .80, and a negative predictive power of .99.

Obtaining a Copy The questionnaire is free for download and can be found, along with scoring materials, at: www.firstsigns.org

Direct correspondence to:
Diana Robins, Department of Psychology,
University of Connecticut, 406 Babbidge Road,
U-1020,
Storrs, Connecticut 06269-1020, USA

Scoring Each "yes or no" answer is assigned a value of "pass" or "fail" using the scoring sheet provided at www.firstsigns.org. Those behaviors that are considered indicative of either autism or another pervasive developmental disorder count as "fails" – a total of three failed items may be cause for concern and the child should be referred for evaluation by a specialist. Developers also identified 6 of the 23 items as highly discriminating factors in evaluating autism. Questions 7, 14, 2, 9, 15, and 13 ask parents to assess their child's response to his or her name, ability to use and understand pointing gestures, interest in other children, showing behavior, and ability to imitate. A "fail" on only two of these items would also represent a fail on the checklist.

A. Shahid et al. (eds.), *STOP, THAT and One Hundred Other Sleep Scales*,
DOI 10.1007/978-1-4419-9893-4_52, © Springer Science+Business Media, LLC 2012

Instructions and Permissions for Use of the M-CHAT

The Modified Checklist for Autism in Toddlers (M-CHAT; Robins, Fein, & Barton, 1999) is available for free download for clinical, research, and educational purposes. There are two authorized websites: the M-CHAT and supplemental materials can be downloaded from **www.firstsigns.org** or from Dr. Robins' website, at **http://www2.gsu.edu/~wwwpsy/faculty/robins.htm**

Users should be aware that the M-CHAT continues to be studied, and may be revised in the future. Any revisions will be posted to the two websites noted above.

Furthermore, the M-CHAT is a copyrighted instrument, and use of the M-CHAT must follow these guidelines:

(1) Reprints/reproductions of the M-CHAT must include the copyright at the bottom (© 1999 Robins, Fein, & Barton). No modifications can be made to items or instructions without permission from the authors.

(2) The M-CHAT must be used in its entirety. There is no evidence that using a subset of items will be valid.

(3) Parties interested in reproducing the M-CHAT in print (e.g., a book or journal article) or electronically (e.g., as part of digital medical records or software packages) must contact Diana Robins to request permission (drobins@gsu.edu).

Instructions for Use

The M-CHAT is validated for screening toddlers between 16 and 30 months of age, to assess risk for autism spectrum disorders (ASD). The M-CHAT can be administered and scored as part of a well-child check-up, and also can be used by specialists or other professionals to assess risk for ASD. The primary goal of the M-CHAT was to maximize sensitivity, meaning to detect as many cases of ASD as possible. Therefore, there is a high false positive rate, meaning that not all children who score at risk for ASD will be diagnosed with ASD. To address this, we have developed a structured follow-up interview for use in conjunction with the M-CHAT; it is available at the two websites listed above. Users should be aware that even with the follow-up questions, a significant number of the children who fail the M-CHAT will not be diagnosed with an ASD; however, these children are at risk for other developmental disorders or delays, and therefore, evaluation is warranted for any child who fails the screening.

The M-CHAT can be scored in less than two minutes. Scoring instructions can be downloaded from **http://www2.gsu.edu/~wwwpsy/faculty/robins.htm or www.firstsigns.org**. We also have developed a scoring template, which is available on these websites; when printed on an overhead transparency and laid over the completed M-CHAT, it facilitates scoring. Please note that minor differences in printers may cause your scoring template not to line up exactly with the printed M-CHAT.

Children who fail more than 3 items total or 2 critical items (particularly if these scores remain elevated after the follow-up interview) should be referred for diagnostic evaluation by a specialist trained to evaluate ASD in very young children. In addition, children for whom there are physician, parent, or other professional's concerns about ASD should be referred for evaluation, given that it is unlikely for any screening instrument to have 100% sensitivity.

M-CHAT

Please fill out the following about how your child usually is. Please try to answer every question. If the behavior is rare (e.g., you've seen it once or twice), please answer as if the child does not do it.

1. Does your child enjoy being swung, bounced on your knee, etc.?	Yes No
2. Does your child take an interest in other children?	Yes No
3. Does your child like climbing on things, such as up stairs?	Yes No
4. Does your child enjoy playing peek-a-boo/hide-and-seek?	Yes No
5. Does your child ever pretend, for example, to talk on the phone or take care of a doll or pretend other things?	Yes No
6. Does your child ever use his/her index finger to point, to ask for something?	Yes No
7. Does your child ever use his/her index finger to point, to indicate interest in something?	Yes No
8. Can your child play properly with small toys (e.g. cars or blocks) without just mouthing, fiddling, or dropping them?	Yes No
9. Does your child ever bring objects over to you (parent) to show you something?	Yes No
10. Does your child look you in the eye for more than a second or two?	Yes No
11. Does your child ever seem oversensitive to noise? (e.g., plugging ears)	Yes No
12. Does your child smile in response to your face or your smile?	Yes No
13. Does your child imitate you? (e.g., you make a face-will your child imitate it?)	Yes No
14. Does your child respond to his/her name when you call?	Yes No
15. If you point at a toy across the room, does your child look at it?	Yes No
16. Does your child walk?	Yes No
17. Does your child look at things you are looking at?	Yes No
18. Does your child make unusual finger movements near his/her face?	Yes No
19. Does your child try to attract your attention to his/her own activity?	Yes No
20. Have you ever wondered if your child is deaf?	Yes No
21. Does your child understand what people say?	Yes No
22. Does your child sometimes stare at nothing or wander with no purpose?	Yes No
23. Does your child look at your face to check your reaction when faced with something unfamiliar?	Yes No

References

1. Johnson, C. R. (1996). Sleep problems in children with mental retardation and autism. *Child and Adolescent Psychiatric Clinics of North America, 5*, 673–683.
2. Robins, D. L., Fein, D., Barton, M. L., & Green, J. A. (2001). The modified checklist for autism in toddlers: an initial study investigating the early detection of autism and pervasive developmental disorders. *Journal of Autism and Developmental Disorders, 31*(2), 131–144.

Representative Studies Using Scale

Limperopoulos, C., Bassan, H., Sullivan, N. R., Soul, J. S., Robertson, R. L., Moore, M., Ringer, S. A., Volpe, J. J., & du Plessis, A. J. (2008). Positive screening for autism in ex-preterm infants: prevalence and risk factors. *Pediatrics, 121*(4), 758–765.

53 Mood Disorder Questionnaire (MDQ)

Purpose The MDQ is a 13-item questionnaire designed to screen for bipolar spectrum disorders using DSM-IV criteria [1]. Items refer to a variety of manifestations of mania, including hyperactivity, irritability, sleeping behavior, concentration, activity levels, and risky behavior.

Population for Testing The scale was initially validated in a population of psychiatric clinic outpatients aged 18–80 years, and has since been employed in a sample of the general population as well.

Administration The scale is a self-report, paper-and-pencil measure requiring 3–5 min for completion.

Reliability and Validity In an initial psychometric evaluation of the scale, Hirschfeld and colleagues [1] administered both a diagnostic interview and the MDQ by telephone and found an internal consistency of .90. Researchers chose a cutoff score of 7, which provided a sensitivity of .73 and a specificity of .90. In a follow-up study, the scale was evaluated as a measure for screening within the general population. Hirschfeld and colleagues [2] found an internal consistency of .84, a sensitivity of .28, and a specificity of .97.

Obtaining a Copy A copy of the scale can be found in the original article published by developers [1].

Scoring Each item describes a symptom or behavior characteristic of mania (e.g., racing thoughts, increased energy) and asks respondents to indicate whether there has been a period in their life when they have experienced these issues. A response of "yes" is scored as a positive indication of a bipolar spectrum disorder. Hirschfeld and colleagues [1] recommend a cutoff score of seven for screening purposes.

A. Shahid et al. (eds.), *STOP, THAT and One Hundred Other Sleep Scales*,
DOI 10.1007/978-1-4419-9893-4_53, © Springer Science+Business Media, LLC 2012

1.	Has there ever been a period of time when you were not your usual self and...	YES	NO
	...you felt so good or so hyper that other people thought you were not your normal self or you were so hyper that you got into trouble?		
	...you were so irritable that you shouted at people or started fights or arguments?		
	...you felt much more self-confident than usual?		
	...you got much less sleep than usual and found you didn't really miss it?		
	...you were much more talkative or spoke faster than usual?		
	...thoughts raced through your head or you couldn't slow your mind down?		
	...you were so easily distracted by things around you that you had trouble concentrating or staying on track?		
	...you had much more energy than usual?		
	...you were much more active or did many more things than usual?		
	...you were much more social or outgoing than usual, for example, you telephoned friends in the middle of the night?		
	...you were much more interested in sex than usual?		
	...you did things that were unusual for you or that other people might have thought were excessive, foolish, or risky?		
	...spending money got you or your family into trouble?		
2.	If you checked YES to more than one of the above, have several of these ever happened during the same period of time? *Please circle one response only.* **YES** **NO**		
3.	How much of a problem did any of these cause you—like being unable to work; having family, money, or legal troubles; getting into arguments or fights? *Please circle one response only.* **No problem** **Minor problem** **Moderate problem** **Serious problem**		

References

1. Hirschfeld, R. M., Williams, J. B., Spitzer, R. L., Calabrese, J. R., Flynn, L., Keck, P. E., Lewis, L., McElroy, S. L., Post, R. M., Rapport, D. J., Russell, J. M., Sachs, G. S., & Zajecka, J. (2000). Development and validation of a screening instrument for bipolar spectrum disorder: the mood disorder questionnaire. *American Journal of Psychiatry, 157*, 1873–1875.
2. Hirschfeld, R. M., Holzer, C., Calabrese, J. R., Weissman, M., Reed, M., Davies, M., Frye, M. A., Keck, P., McElroy, S., Lewis, L., Tierce, J., Wagner, K. D., & Hazard, E. (2003). Validity of the mood disorder questionnaire: a general population study. *American Journal of Psychiatry, 160*(1), 178–180.

Representative Studies Using Scale

Kripke, D. F., Rex, K. M., Ancoli-Israel, S., Nievergelt, C. M., Klimecki, W., & Kelsoe, J. R. (2008). Delayed sleep phase cases and controls. *Journal of Circadian Rhythms, 6*(6), 6–6.

54 Morningness-Eveningness Questionnaire

Purpose Consisting of 19 items, the scale was developed to assess individual differences in morningness and eveningness – the degree to which respondents are active and alert at certain times of day. Scale items query preferences in sleep and waking times, and subjective "peak" times at which respondents feel their best.

Population for Testing The questionnaire was first validated with individuals aged 18–32 years.

Administration A self-report, paper-and-pencil measure, the scale requires between 10 and 15 min for completion.

Reliability and Validity Horne and Östberg [1] conducted an evaluation of the scale's psychometric properties and found that individuals placed within each of the scale's five diagnostic categories possessed significantly different waking oral temperatures. More recently, research has indicated that the scale's inter-item correlations are merely moderate, ranging from – .02 to + .61, suggesting that the scale is actually composed of two factors [2]. Still, the full scale internal consistency remained sufficient at .82, supporting the use of a global score.

Obtaining a Copy A copy can be found in the original article published by developers [1].

Scoring The scale is composed of both Likert-type and time-scale questions. The Likert-type items present four options with the lowest values indicating definite eveningness. Similarly, the time-scale items are divided into periods of 15 min spanning a time frame of 7 h. Each section of the scale is assigned a value of 1 through 5. To obtain a global score, each item is totaled and the sum is converted to a 5-point scale: definitely morning type (70–86), moderately morning type (59–69), neither type (42–58), moderately evening type (31–41), and definitely evening type (16–30). However, finding that these cutoffs under-identified morningness types in a population of Austrian students, researcher Neubauer [3] suggested that the scale may need to be adapted to the specific region in which it is being used to accommodate variations in circadian rhythms.

A. Shahid et al. (eds.), *STOP, THAT and One Hundred Other Sleep Scales*,
DOI 10.1007/978-1-4419-9893-4_54, © Springer Science+Business Media, LLC 2012

Morningness-Eveningess Questionnaire

Instructions:

1. Please read each question very carefully before answering.
2. Answer ALL questions
3. Answer questions in numerical order.
4. Each question should be answered independently of others. Do NOT go back and check your answers.
5. All questions have a selection of answers. For each question place a cross alongside ONE answer only. Some questions have a scale instead of a selection of answers. Place a cross at the appropriate point along the scale.
6. Please answer each question as honestly as possible. Both your answers and the results will be kept, in strict confidence.
7. Please feel free to make any comments in the section provided below each question.

The Questionnaire with scores for each choice

1. Considering only your own "feeling best" rhythm, at what time would you get up if you were entirely free to plan your day?

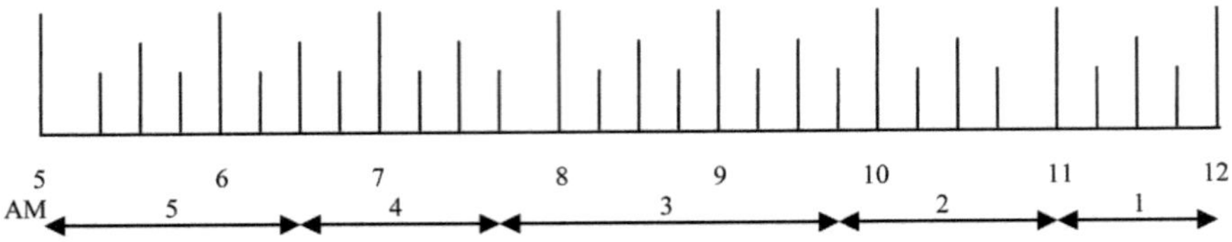

2. Considering only your own "feeling best" rhythm, at what time would you go to bed if you were entirely free to plan your evening?

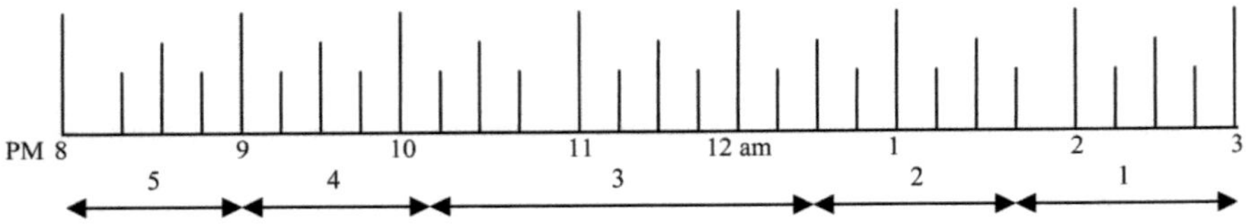

3. If there is a specific time at which you have to get up in the morning, to what extent are you dependent on being woken up by an alarm clock?

Not at all dependent ☐ 4
Slightly dependent ☐ 3
Fairly dependent ☐ 2
Very dependent ☐ 1

4. Assuming adequate environmental conditions, how easy do you find getting up in the mornings?

Not at all easy ☐ 1
Not very easy ☐ 2
Fairly easy ☐ 3
Very easy ☐ 4

5. How alert do you feel during the first half hour after having woken in the mornings?

Not at all alert ☐ 1
Slightly alert ☐ 2
Fairly alert ☐ 3
Very alert ☐ 4

6. How is your appetite during the first half-hour after having woken in the mornings?

Very poor ☐ 1
Fairly poor ☐ 2
Fairly good ☐ 3
Very good ☐ 4

7. During the first half-hour after having woken in the morning, how tired do you feel?

Very tired ☐ 1
Fairly tired ☐ 2
Fairly refreshed ☐ 3
Very refreshed ☐ 4

8. When you have no commitments the next day, at what time do you go to bed compared to your usual bedtime?

Seldom or never later ☐ 4
Less than one hour later ☐ 3
1-2 hours later ☐ 2
More than two hours later ☐ 1

9. You have decided to engage in some physical exercise. A friend suggests that you do this one hour twice a week and the best time for him is between 7:00-8:00 a.m. Bearing in mind nothing else but your own "feeling best" rhythm, how do you think you would perform?

Would be on good form ☐ 4
Would be on reasonable form ☐ 3
Would find it difficult ☐ 2
Would find it very difficult ☐ 1

10. At what time in the evening do you feel tired and as a result in need of sleep?

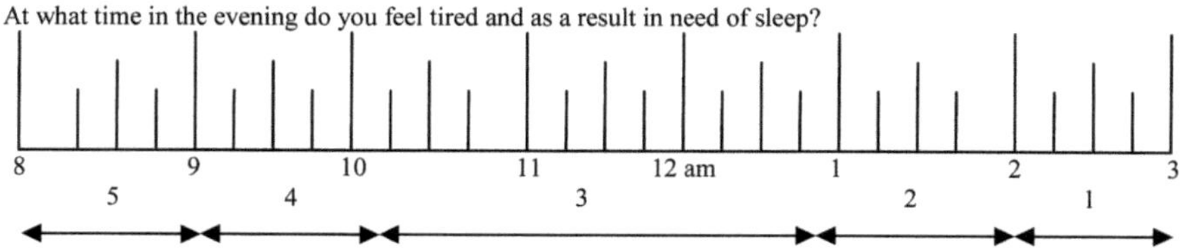

11. You wish to be at your peak performance for a test which you know is going to be mentally exhausting and lasting for two hours. You are entirely free to plan your day and considering only your own "feeling best" rhythm which ONE of the four testing times would you choose?

8:00-10:00 a.m. ☐ 6
11:00 a.m.-1:00 p.m. ☐ 4
3:00-5:00 p.m. ☐ 2
7:00-9:00 p.m. ☐ 0

12. If you went to bed at 11 p.m. at what level of tiredness would you be?

Not at all tired ☐ 0
A little tired ☐ 2
Fairly tired ☐ 3
Very tired ☐ 5

13. For some reason you have gone to bed several hours later than usual, but there is no need to get up at any particular time the next morning. Which ONE of the following events are you most likely to experience?

Will wake up at usual time and will NOT fall asleep ☐ 4
Will wake up at usual time and will doze thereafter ☐ 3
Will wake up at usual time but will fall asleep again ☐ 2
Will NOT wake up until later than usual ☐ 1

14. One night you have to remain awake between 4-6 a.m. in order to carry out a night watch. You have no commitments the next day. Which ONE of the following alternatives will suit you best?

Would NOT go to bed until watch was over ☐ 1
Would take a nap before and sleep after ☐ 2
Would take a good sleep before and nap after ☐ 3
Would take ALL sleep before watch ☐ 4

15. You have to do two hours of hard physical work. You are entirely free to plan your day and considering only your own "feeling best" rhythm which ONE of the following times would you choose?

8:00-10:00 a.m. ☐ 4
11:00 a.m.-1:00 p.m. ☐ 3
3:00-5:00 p.m. ☐ 2
7:00-9:00 p.m. ☐ 1

16. You have decide to engage in hard physical exercise. A friend suggests that you do this for one hour twice a week and the best time for him is between 10-11 p.m. Bearing in mind nothing else but your own "feeling best" rhythm how well do you think you would perform?

Would be on good form ☐ 1
Would be on reasonable form ☐ 2
Would find it difficult ☐ 3
Would find if very difficult ☐ 4

17. Suppose that you can choose your own work hours. Assume that you worked a FIVE hour day (including breaks) and that your job was interesting and paid by results. Which FIVE CONSECUTIVE HOURS would you select?

12 1 2 3 4 5 6 7 8 9 10 11 12 1 2 3 4 5 6 7 8 9 10 11 12
Midnight Noon Midnight
1 5 4 3 2 1

18. At what time of the day do you think that you reach your "feeling best" peak?

12 1 2 3 4 5 6 7 8 9 10 11 12 1 2 3 4 5 6 7 8 9 10 11 12
Midnight Noon Midnight
1 5 4 3 2 1

19. One hears about "morning" and "evening" types of people. Which ONE of these types do you consider yourself to be?

Definitely a "morning" type ☐ 6
Rather more a "morning" than an evening type ☐ 4
Rather more an "evening" than a "morning" type ☐ 2
Definitely an "evening" type ☐ 0

References

1. Horne, J. A., & Östberg, O. (1976). A self-assessment questionnaire to determine morningness-eveningness in human circadian rhythms. *International Journal of Chronobiology, 4*, 97–110.
2. Smith, C. S., Reilly, C., & Midkiff, K. (1989). Evaluation of three circadian rhythm questionnaires with suggestions for an improved measure of morningness. *Journal of Applied Psychology, 74*(5), 728–738.
3. Neubauer, A. C. (1992). Psychometric comparison of two circadian rhythm questionnaires and their relationship with personality. *Personality and Individual Differences, 13*(2), 125–131.

Representative Studies Using Scale

Ayalon, L., Borodkin, K., Dishon, L., Kanety, H., & Dagan, Y. (2007). Circadian rhythm sleep disorders following mild traumatic brain injury. *Neurology, 68*(14), 1136–1140.

Rybak, Y. E., McNeely, H. E., Mackenzie, B. E., Jain, U. R., & Levitan, R. D. (2006). An open trial of light therapy in adult attention-deficit/hyperactivity disorder. *Journal of Clinical Psychiatry, 67*(10), 1527–1535.

Motivation and Energy Inventory (MEI)

55

Purpose The MEI is a 27-item scale created to assess fatigue and lassitude. The scale was initially developed for the purpose of evaluating interventions to improve motivation and energy in patients with depression, though with further evaluation, its clinical applications could be extended to other patient groups [1]. The MEI assesses three factors: mental or cognitive energy, social motivation, and physical energy.

Population for Testing The scale was initially validated in a population of patients experiencing a major depressive episode. Participant ages ranged from 18 to 76 years.

Administration The scale is a self-report, paper-and-pencil measure requiring between 5 and 10 min for completion.

Reliability and Validity Researchers Fehnal and colleagues [1] have evaluated the scale's psychometric properties and demonstrated an internal consistency ranging from .75 to .89. Scores on the MEI were moderately correlated with results obtained on the HAM-D (Chap. 42), a scale to evaluate symptoms of depression, and each of the three subscales was found to be sensitive to changes in depressive symptoms resulting from treatment with antidepressants.

Obtaining a Copy A copy of the scale can be found in the original article published by developers [1].

Direct correspondence to:
S.E. Fehnel
Email: sfehnel@rti.org

Scoring Respondents use scales ranging from 0 (indicating that the behavior is never present) to 5 or 6 (a behavior or feeling that is present very frequently or all of the time). Items 3–11, 13–15, 17, and 18 are reverse-scored in order to ensure that higher scores indicate greater levels of motivation and energy. To find total scores for the three subscales, sum the items that belong to each.

A. Shahid et al. (eds.), *STOP, THAT and One Hundred Other Sleep Scales*,
DOI 10.1007/978-1-4419-9893-4_55, © Springer Science+Business Media, LLC 2012

The Motivation and Energy Inventory (MEI)
For each question below, please check one box to indicate the way you have been feeling during the past 4 weeks. When answering, please try to consider every day of the week (including weekends), as well as every setting that applies to you such as work, home, school, etc.

1. During the past 4 weeks, how often did you feel enthusiastic when you began your day?

□	□	□	□	□	□
Never	Less than one day a week	1 or 2 days a week	3 or 4 days a week	5 or 6 days a week	Every day or nearly every day

2. During the past 4 weeks, how often did you feel satisfied with what you accomplished during the day?

□	□	□	□	□	□
Never	Less than one day a week	1 or 2 days a week	3 or 4 days a week	5 or 6 days a week	Every day or nearly every day

3. During the past 4 weeks, how often did you have trouble getting out of bed in the morning because you didn't want to face the day?

□	□	□	□	□	□
Never	Less than one day a week	1 or 2 days a week	3 or 4 days a week	5 or 6 days a week	Every day or nearly every day

4. During the past 4 weeks, how often did you run out of energy before the end of the day?

□	□	□	□	□	□
Never	Less than one day a week	1 or 2 days a week	3 or 4 days a week	5 or 6 days a week	Every day or nearly every day

5. During the past 4 weeks, how often did you have trouble finishing things you started because you lost interest in them?

□	□	□	□	□	□	□
0	1	2	3	4	5	6
Never			About half of the time			All of the time

6. During the past 4 weeks, how often did you feel overwhelmed even by small tasks?

□	□	□	□	□	□	□
0	1	2	3	4	5	6
Never			About half of the time			All of the time

7. During the past 4 weeks, how often did you procrastinate or put things off until another day?

□	□	□	□	□	□	□
0	1	2	3	4	5	6
Never			About half of the time			All of the time

8. During the past 4 weeks, how often did you have trouble remembering information (such as people's names, where you put things, or what you needed from the grocery store)?

□	□	□	□	□	□	□
0	1	2	3	4	5	6
Never			About half of the time			All of the time

9. During the past 4 weeks, how often did you have problems concentrating?

□	□	□	□	□	□	□
0	1	2	3	4	5	6
Never			About half of the time			All of the time

10. During the past 4 weeks, how often did you have trouble making minor decisions?

□	□	□	□	□	□	□
0	1	2	3	4	5	6
Never			About half of the time			All of the time

11. During the past 4 weeks, how often did you avoid social conversations with others?

□	□	□	□	□	□	□
0	1	2	3	4	5	6
Never			About half of the time			All of the time

12. During the past 4 weeks, how often did you take advantage of opportunities to get to know other people better?

□	□	□	□	□	□	□
0	1	2	3	4	5	6
Never			About half of the time			All of the time

13. During the past 4 weeks, how much of the time did you prefer to be alone?

□	□	□	□	□	□	□
0	1	2	3	4	5	6
Never			About half of the time			All of the time

14. During the past 4 weeks, how much of the time did you have trouble focusing your attention on your work or other activities?

□	□	□	□	□	□	□
0	1	2	3	4	5	6
Never			About half of the time			All of the time

15. During the past 4 weeks, how much of the time did you have trouble keeping things organized?

□	□	□	□	□	□	□
0	1	2	3	4	5	6
Never			About half of the time			All of the time

16. During the past 4 weeks, how much of the time were you able to keep up with chores around the house such as laundry, cleaning, and doing the dishes?

□	□	□	□	□	□	□
0	1	2	3	4	5	6
Never			About half of the time			All of the time

17. During the past 4 weeks, how much of the time did you feel physically tired during the day?

□	□	□	□	□	□	□
0	1	2	3	4	5	6
Never			About half of the time			All of the time

18. During the past 4 weeks, how much of the time did you feel exhausted?

□	□	□	□	□	□	□
0	1	2	3	4	5	6
Never			About half of the time			All of the time

19. During the past 4 weeks, how much of the time did you feel energetic?

□	□	□	□	□	□	□
0	1	2	3	4	5	6
Never			About half of the time			All of the time

20. During the past 4 weeks, how much of the time did you feel motivated?

□	□	□	□	□	□	□
0	1	2	3	4	5	6
Never			About half of the time			All of the time

21. During the past 4 weeks, how often did you call, e-mail, or write letters to friends or family members?

□	□	□	□	□	□
Never	Less than once a week	1 or 2 times a week	3 or 4 times a week	5 or 6 times a week	At least 7 times a week

22. During the past 4 weeks, how often did you get together with friends or family members who don't live with you?

□	□	□	□	□	□
Never	Less than once a week	1 or 2 times a week	3 or 4 times a week	5 or 6 times a week	At least 7 times a week

23. During the past 4 weeks, how often did you engage in recreational activities or hobbies?

□	□	□	□	□	□
Never	Less than once a week	1 or 2 times a week	3 or 4 times a week	5 or 6 times a week	At least 7 times a week

24. During the past 4 weeks, how often did you exercise (for example by walking, swimming, or practicing yoga)?

□	□	□	□	□	□
Never	Less than once a week	1 or 2 times a week	3 or 4 times a week	5 or 6 times a week	At least 7 times a week

25. During the past 4 weeks, to what extent were you interested in sexual activity?

□	□	□	□	□
Not at all interested	A little interested	Somewhat interested	Quite interested	Extremely interested

26. During the past 4 weeks, to what extent were you interested in taking on additional tasks or projects?

□	□	□	□	□
Not at all interested	A little interested	Somewhat interested	Quite interested	Extremely interested

27. During the past 4 weeks, to what extent were you interested in learning or trying new things?

□	□	□	□	□
Not at all interested	A little interested	Somewhat interested	Quite interested	Extremely interested

29. During the past 4 weeks, to what extent were you interested in talking with others?

□	□	□	□	□
Not at all interested	A little interested	Somewhat interested	Quite interested	Extremely interested

30. During the past 4 weeks, to what extent were you interested in social activities like visiting friends, going out to dinner, or parties?

□	□	□	□	□
Not at all interested	A little interested	Somewhat interested	Quite interested	Extremely interested

Reference

1. Fehnel, S. E., Bann, C. M., Hogue, S. L., Kwong, W. J., Mahajan, S. S. (2004). The development and psychometric evaluation of the motivation and energy inventory. Qual Life Res. *13*, 1321–1336.

Representative Studies Using Scale

Gross, P. K., Nourse, R., Wasser, T. E., & Bukenya, D. (2007). Safety and efficacy of buproprion extended release in treating a community sample of Hispanic and African American adults with major depressive disorder: an open-label study. *Journal of Clinical Psychiatry, 9*(2), 108–112.

Multidimensional Dream Inventory (MDI)

56

Purpose The 12-item scale was designed to assess individual differences in four separate domains of dream experience: vividness, usefulness, recall, and importance (the degree to which dreams feel personally relevant). Developers intended the scale to function as a tool for "studying the consequences and correlates of dreams" [1] – a measure providing insight into the nature and function of personal differences in dreaming.

Population for Testing The scale has been validated with individuals aged 17–50 years.

Administration A short, self-report, paper-and-pencil measure, the MDI requires less than 5 min for administration.

Reliability and Validity Developers Kallmeyer and Chang [1] have analyzed the scale's psychometric properties and have found an internal consistency ranging from .64 to .73. They also demonstrated that the scale's four factors – labeled importance, vividness, usefulness, and recall – account for 66.7% of the variance.

Obtaining a Copy An example of the scale can be found in the original article published by developers [1].

Direct correspondence to:
Edward C. Chang
Department of Psychology,
Northern Kentucky University
Highland Heights, KY 41099, USA

Scoring Using a 5-point, Likert-type scale, respondents indicate the degree to which they agree with a variety of statements about dreaming. The scale ranges from 1, meaning "strongly disagree," to 5, "strongly agree." Higher scores denote a greater endorsement of each of the scale's four factors, indicating a higher degree of importance, vividness, usefulness, and recall ascribed by the respondent to his or her dreams.

A. Shahid et al. (eds.), *STOP, THAT and One Hundred Other Sleep Scales*,
DOI 10.1007/978-1-4419-9893-4_56, © Springer Science+Business Media, LLC 2012

Multidimensional Dream Inventory

1 = Strongly Agree
5 = Strongly Disagree

1	I think dreams can have personal meaning	1	2	3	4	5
2	My dreams have colours	1	2	3	4	5
3	I believe that dreams can predict the future	1	2	3	4	5
4	I remember my dreams in the morning at least once a week	1	2	3	4	5
5	I feel that every dream has a specific meaning	1	2	3	4	5
6	My dreams have sound	1	2	3	4	5
7	I have dreams that help me deal with problems in waking life	1	2	3	4	5
8.	I often remember my dreams when I wake up	1	2	3	4	5
9.	I believe that dreams reveal something about the dreamer's personality	1	2	3	4	5
10.	I often feel emotions when I dream	1	2	3	4	5
11.	If I had a dream that "gave me advice," I would follow that advice	1	2	3	4	5
12.	I remember my dreams when I wake up, but I often forget them quickly	1	2	3	4	5

Reference

1. Kallmeyer, R. J., & Chang, E. C. (1997). The multidimensional dream inventory: preliminary evidence for validity and reliability. *Perceptual and Motor Skills, 85*, 803–808.

Representative Studies Using Scale

None.

57 Multidimensional Fatigue Inventory (MFI)

Purpose The MFI is a 20-item scale designed to evaluate five dimensions of fatigue: general fatigue, physical fatigue, reduced motivation, reduced activity, and mental fatigue. By limiting the length of the questionnaire, developers hoped to accommodate those individuals who might find larger measures especially tiring while still obtaining enough detailed information to examine multiple facets of fatigue.

Population for Testing The scale has been validated in a variety of participant populations, including cancer patients (mean age of 61 years), army recruits (mean age of 21 years), psychology students (mean age of 24 years), and individuals participating in a study of chronic fatigue syndrome (mean age of 39 years).

Administration The MFI is a self-report, pencil-and-paper measure requiring between 5 and 10 min for completion.

Reliability and Validity In an initial psychometric evaluation [1], developers reported an internal consistency ranging from .53 to .93. The scale was also found to be sensitive to differences between the participant groups.

Obtaining a Copy An example of the questionnaire format is included in the original article published by developers [1].

For a complete copy, direct correspondence to:
E.M.A. Smets
Academic Medical Centre,
University of Amsterdam
Department of Medical Psychology
Amsterdam, the Netherlands

Scoring Respondents use a scale ranging from 1 to 7 to indicate how aptly certain statements regarding fatigue represent their experiences. Several positively phrased items are reverse-scored. Higher total scores correspond with more acute levels of fatigue.

A. Shahid et al. (eds.), *STOP, THAT and One Hundred Other Sleep Scales*,
DOI 10.1007/978-1-4419-9893-4_57, © Springer Science+Business Media, LLC 2012

amc

MFI® MULTIDIMENSIONAL FATIGUE INVENTORY

Instructions:

By means of the following statements we would like to get an idea of how you have been feeling **lately**. There is, for example, the statement:

"I FEEL RELAXED"

If you think that this is **entirely true**, that indeed you have been feeling relaxed lately, please, place an **X** in the extreme left box; like this:

yes, that is true ☒1 ☐2 ☐3 ☐4 ☐5 **no, that is not true**

The more you **disagree** with the statement, the more you can place an **X** in the direction of "no, that is not true". Please do not miss out a statement and place only one **X** in a box for each statement.

1	I feel fit.	**yes, that is true**	☐1	☐2	☐3	☐4	☐5	**no, that is not true**
2	Physically, I feel only able to do a little.	**yes, that is true**	☐1	☐2	☐3	☐4	☐5	**no, that is not true**
3	I feel very active.	**yes, that is true**	☐1	☐2	☐3	☐4	☐5	**no, that is not true**
4	I feel like doing all sorts of nice things.	**yes, that is true**	☐1	☐2	☐3	☐4	☐5	**no, that is not true**
5	I feel tired.	**yes, that is true**	☐1	☐2	☐3	☐4	☐5	**no, that is not true**
6	I think I do a lot in a day.	**yes, that is true**	☐1	☐2	☐3	☐4	☐5	**no, that is not true**
7	When I am doing something, I can keep my thoughts on it.	**yes, that is true**	☐1	☐2	☐3	☐4	☐5	**no, that is not true**
8	Physically I can take on a lot.	**yes, that is true**	☐1	☐2	☐3	☐4	☐5	**no, that is not true**
9	I dread having to do things.	**yes, that is true**	☐1	☐2	☐3	☐4	☐5	**no, that is not true**
10	I think I do very little in a day.	**yes, that is true**	☐1	☐2	☐3	☐4	☐5	**no, that is not true**
11	I can concentrate well.	**yes, that is true**	☐1	☐2	☐3	☐4	☐5	**no, that is not true**
12	I am rested.	**yes, that is true**	☐1	☐2	☐3	☐4	☐5	**no, that is not true**
13	It takes a lot of effort to concentrate on things.	**yes, that is true**	☐1	☐2	☐3	☐4	☐5	**no, that is not true**
14	Physically I feel I am in a bad condition.	**yes, that is true**	☐1	☐2	☐3	☐4	☐5	**no, that is not true**
15	I have a lot of plans.	**yes, that is true**	☐1	☐2	☐3	☐4	☐5	**no, that is not true**
16	I tire easily.	**yes, that is true**	☐1	☐2	☐3	☐4	☐5	**no, that is not true**
17	I get little done.	**yes, that is true**	☐1	☐2	☐3	☐4	☐5	**no, that is not true**
18	I don't feel like doing anything.	**yes, that is true**	☐1	☐2	☐3	☐4	☐5	**no, that is not true**
19	My thoughts easily wander.	**yes, that is true**	☐1	☐2	☐3	☐4	☐5	**no, that is not true**
20	Physically I feel I am in an excellent condition.	**yes, that is true**	☐1	☐2	☐3	☐4	☐5	**no, that is not true**

Thank you very much for your cooperation

Printed with Permission from the authors Smets et al.[1].

Reference

1. Smets, E. M. A., Garssen, B., Bonke, B., & De Haes, J. C. J. M. (1995). The multidimensional fatigue inventory (MFI) psychometric qualities of an instrument to assess fatigue. *Journal of Psychosomatic Research, 39*(5), 315–325.

Representative Studies Using Scale

Lou, J. S., Kearns, G., Oken, B., Sexton, G., & Nutt, J. (2001). Exacerbated physical fatigue and mental fatigue in Parkinson's disease. *Movement Disorders, 16*(2), 190–196.

Rupp, I., Boshuizen, H. C., Jacobi, C. E., Dinant, H. J., van den Bos, G. A. M. (2004). Impact of fatigue on health-related quality of life in rheumatoid arthritis. *Arthritis & Rheumatism, 51*(4), 578–585.

58 Munich Chronotype Questionnaire (MCTQ)

Purpose The instrument was developed in order to assess individuals' chronotypes – diurnal preferences that manifest in personal sleep-wake rhythms. Consisting of 19 questions, the scale examines wake and sleep schedules (on both work and free days), energy levels throughout the day, sleep latency and inertia, and exposure to daylight. Individuals are also asked to subjectively rate themselves as one of seven possible chronotypes ranging from extreme early (preferring to rise much earlier than others) to extreme late. This information is combined to determine the time of day at which the respondent is likely to feel most alert, placing them objectively in a chronotype category. Though potentially a valuable tool for clinical purposes, the instrument has primarily been used in research to investigate how chronotype relates to age, sex, and external environment (e.g., exposure to daylight, community).

Population for Testing The scale has been validated in adults of college age and older.

Administration Requiring between 5 and 10 min for completion, developers have created a Web site where individuals can take the self-report questionnaire and have their results sent to them by email. A second version of the questionnaire designed specifically for shift workers is also available.

Reliability and Validity Zavada and colleagues [1] conducted a large-scale study in which they compared the Horne-Ostberg Morningness-Eveningness Questionnaire (MEQ; (Chap. 54) to the MCTQ. They found that MEQ scores correlated highly with the midpoint of sleep on free days reported on the MCTQ ($r = .70$), and that a respondent's sleep schedule on free days is a good predictor of that individual's chronotype.

Obtaining a Copy The questionnaire is available online at: http://chrono.biol.rug.nl/mctq-en.html

Direct correspondence to:
Dr. M.C.M. Gordijn
P.O. Box 14, 9750 AA
Haren, the Netherlands.
Email: tvrbiol@rug.nl

Scoring The scale is scored electronically by the Web site at which it is available. Total scores can range from 16 to 86, with the lowest values representing extreme-late chronotypes. However, personal scores are not available through the questionnaire's Web site, which has been constructed for the sole purpose of the authors' research. Rather, individuals completing questionnaires at the site receive an email providing statistical comparisons of themselves to others in their subjective chronotype. Thus, the Web site itself is of limited clinical or diagnostic utility and arrangements must be made with developers in order to make further use of the instrument.

A. Shahid et al. (eds.), *STOP, THAT and One Hundred Other Sleep Scales*,
DOI 10.1007/978-1-4419-9893-4_58, © Springer Science+Business Media, LLC 2012

Munich ChronoType Questionnaire (MCTQ)

Please enter your age, gender, etc. This information is important for our evaluations

Age:_____ female male Height:_____ Weight:_____

On work days…

I have to get up at… _____o'clock
I need… _____min to wake up
I regularly wake up… before the alarm with the alarm

From… _____o'clock I am fully awake
At around… _____o'clock, I have an energy dip
On nights before workdays, I go to bed at _____o'clock…
…and it then takes me… _____min to fall asleep
If I get the chance, I like to take a siesta/nap…
Correct I then sleep for…_____min
Not correct I would feel terrible afterwards

On free days (please only judge normal free days, i.e., without parties etc)…

My dream would be to sleep until… _____o'clock
I normally wake up at… _____o'clock
If I wake up at around the normal (workday) alarm time, I try to get back to sleep…
Correct Not correct

If I get back to sleep, I sleep for another… _____min
I need… _____min to wake up
From… _____o'clock I am fully awake
At around… _____o'clock, I have an energy dip
On nights before free days, I go to bed at _____o'clock…
…and it then takes me… _____min to fall asleep
If I get the chance, I like to take a siesta/nap…
Correct I then sleep for…_____min
Not correct I would feel terrible afterwards

Once I am in bed, I would like to read for… _____min…
…but I generally fall asleep after no more than… _____min

I prefer to sleep in a completely dark room Correct Not Correct
I wake up more easily when morning light shines into my room Correct Not Correct
How long per day do you spend on average outside (really outside) exposed to daylight?
On work days:_____hrs. _____min On free days: _____hrs _____min

Self Assessment
After you have answered the preceding questions, you should have a feeling to which chronotype (time-of-day-type) you belong to. If, for example, you like (and manage) to sleep quite a bit longer on free days than on workdays, or if you cannot get out of bed on Monday mornings, even without a Sunday-night-party, then you are more a late go to bed early type. If, however, you regularly wake up and feel perky once you jump out of bed. and if you would rather than to an evening concert then you are an early type. In the following questions, you should categorise yourself and your family members.

Please tick only one possibility!

Description of categories:

extreme	early type = 0
Moderate	early type = 1
Slight	early type = 2
	Normal type = 3
Slight	late type = 4
Moderate	late type = 5
Extreme	late type = 6

I am…	0	1	2	3	4	5	6
As a child, I was…	0	1	2	3	4	5	6
As a teenager, I was…	0	1	2	3	4	5	6

In case you are older than 65: in the middle of my life, I was…

0 1 2 3 4 5 6

My parents are/were...

Mother...	0	1	2	3	4	5	6
Father...	0	1	2	3	4	5	6

My siblings are/were ...(please underline **Brother** or **Sister**)

Brother/Sister	0	1	2	3	4	5	6
Brother/Sister	0	1	2	3	4	5	6
Brother/Sister	0	1	2	3	4	5	6
Brother/Sister	0	1	2	3	4	5	6
Brother/Sister	0	1	2	3	4	5	6
Brother/Sister	0	1	2	3	4	5	6
Brother/Sister	0	1	2	3	4	5	6

My partner (girl/boy friend, spouse, significant other) is/was...

	0	1	2	3	4	5	6

References

1. Zavada, A., Gordijn, M. C., Beersma, D. G., Daan, S., & Roenneberg, T. (2005). Comparison of the Munich Chronotype Questionnaire with the Horne-Ostberg's Morningness-Eveningness Score. *Chronobiology International, 22*(2), 267–278.
2. Roenneberg, T, Wirz-Justice, A., Merrow, M. Life between clocks: daily temporal patterns of human chronotypes. J Biol Rhythms 2003;18(1):80–90.

Representative Studies Using Scale

Kantermann, T., Juda, M., Merrow, M., & Roenneberg, T. (2007). The human circadian clock's seasonal adjustment is disrupted by daylight saving time. *Current Biology, 17*(22), 1996–2000.

59 Normative Beliefs About Aggression Scale

Purpose This 20-item, Likert-type questionnaire was developed to study attitudes toward aggression in children and young adults. The first section of the scale presents short scenarios in which one child behaves in a verbally or physically aggressive manner toward a second child. The respondent is asked to rate the acceptability of several different aggressive responses on the part of the second child. In the second section, individuals indicate how acceptable they find generally aggressive behaviors (e.g., insulting or pushing others). As sleep disturbances in children often occur in tandem with behavioral issues like aggression [1], such an instrument possesses considerable clinical and research utility in the sleep medicine field.

Population for Testing The scale has been validated with a population ranging from 6 to 30 years of age.

Administration Respondents give self-report answers to questions posed by an interviewer. The testing process requires 5–10 min.

Reliability and Validity Developers have found an internal consistency ranging from .65 to .85 [2].

Obtaining a Copy Use of the scale requires the permission of its developers.

Direct correspondence to:
L.R. Huesmann
Research Center for Group Dynamics
P.O. Box 1248, 426 Thompson Street
Ann Arbor, Michigan 48106–1248, USA
Email: huesmann@umich.edu

Scoring For each question, respondents use a scale ranging from 1 ("perfectly OK") to 4 ("really wrong") to indicate the acceptability of certain aggressive behaviors. For several items, the wording has been changed from positive to negative, and scoring is reversed (4 is "perfectly OK," while 1 is "really wrong"). This encourages respondents to attend to each question carefully, and prevents them from answering with a set response. Scores are tallied and an average score is found for the scale as a whole, giving a General Approval of Aggression score. Additionally, scores are given on several different subscales by calculating the average of just the items included in that category. Subscales include Approval of Retaliation (Strong and Weak) and Approval of Retaliation (Against Males/Against Females).

References

1. Blunden, S., Lushington, K., & Kennedy, D. (2001). Cognitive and behavioural performance in children with sleep-related obstructive breathing disorders. *Sleep Medicine Reviews, 5*(6), 447–461.
2. Huesmann, L. R., Guerra, N. G., Miller, L., & Zelli, A. (1992). The role of social norms in the development of aggression. In H. Zumkley & A. Fraczek (Eds.), *Socialization and aggression* (139–151). New York: Springer.

A. Shahid et al. (eds.), *STOP, THAT and One Hundred Other Sleep Scales*,
DOI 10.1007/978-1-4419-9893-4_59, © Springer Science+Business Media, LLC 2012

Representative Studies Using Scale

Henry, D., Guerra, N., Huesmann, R., Tolan, P., VanAcker, R., & Eron, L. (2000). Normative influences on aggression in urban elementary school classrooms. *American Journal of Community Psychology, 28*(1), 59–81.

Souweidane, V., & Huesmann, L. R. (1999). The influence of American urban culture on the development of normative beliefs about aggression in Middle-Eastern immigrants. *American Journal of Community Psychology, 27*(2), 239–254.

Parkinson's Disease Sleep Scale (PDSS)

60

Purpose As sleep disturbances affect the majority of individuals with Parkinson's disease, Chaudhuri and colleagues created an instrument to evaluate sleep quality in this patient population. The 15-item scale assesses sleep onset and maintenance, restlessness, nightmares and hallucinations, nocturia, motor symptoms, refreshment, and daytime sleepiness.

Population for Testing The scale has been validated with Parkinson's patients aged 38–89 years.

Administration Requires approximately 5 min for completion. The instrument is a self-report, pencil-and-paper measure, though caregivers may also respond as proxies.

Reliability and Validity The developers [1] completed a psychometric evaluation of the instrument and found a test-retest reliability of .94. Additionally, patients diagnosed with more advanced stages of the disease receive significantly lower scores on the scale than those in early stages (indicating more acute sleep disturbances).

Obtaining a Copy A copy can be found in the original article published by developers [1].

Direct correspondence to:
K. R. Chaudhuri
Department of Neurology, King's College Hospital
Denmark Hill, London SE5 9RS

Scoring The instrument uses a visual analogue scale – a 100-mm line extending between two extremes on which respondents place marks meant to represent their experiences with sleep. Scores are found by measuring the distance, to the closest 0.1 cm, between the start of the line and the respondent's mark. Lower scores indicate that sleep issues are "always" present and that sleep quality is "awful," while higher scores mean that sleep difficulties are "never" present. As results are converted to centimeters, total scores can range from 0 to 150. However, individuals responding to visual analogue scales are often reluctant to make use of the highest and lowest extremes. Developers suggest that items 1, 3, 14, and 15 may be particularly important for identifying individuals who require further screening.

A. Shahid et al. (eds.), *STOP, THAT and One Hundred Other Sleep Scales*,
DOI 10.1007/978-1-4419-9893-4_60, © Springer Science+Business Media, LLC 2012

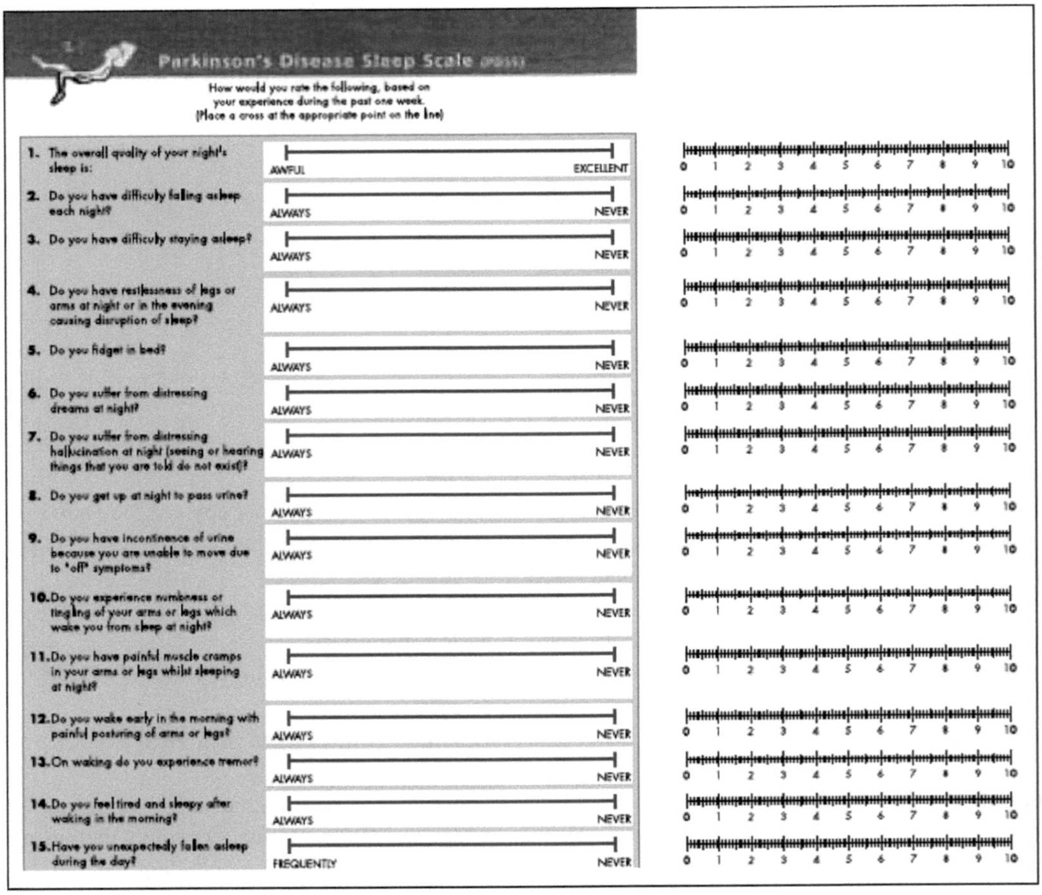

Parkinson's Disease Sleep Scale (PDSS)

How would you rate the following, based on your experience during the past one week.
(Place a cross at the appropriate point on the line)

Item	Anchor (0)	Anchor (10)	Scale
1. The overall quality of your night's sleep is:	AWFUL	EXCELLENT	0 1 2 3 4 5 6 7 8 9 10
2. Do you have difficulty falling asleep each night?	ALWAYS	NEVER	0 1 2 3 4 5 6 7 8 9 10
3. Do you have difficulty staying asleep?	ALWAYS	NEVER	0 1 2 3 4 5 6 7 8 9 10
4. Do you have restlessness of legs or arms at night or in the evening causing disruption of sleep?	ALWAYS	NEVER	0 1 2 3 4 5 6 7 8 9 10
5. Do you fidget in bed?	ALWAYS	NEVER	0 1 2 3 4 5 6 7 8 9 10
6. Do you suffer from distressing dreams at night?	ALWAYS	NEVER	0 1 2 3 4 5 6 7 8 9 10
7. Do you suffer from distressing hallucination at night (seeing or hearing things that you are told do not exist)?	ALWAYS	NEVER	0 1 2 3 4 5 6 7 8 9 10
8. Do you get up at night to pass urine?	ALWAYS	NEVER	0 1 2 3 4 5 6 7 8 9 10
9. Do you have incontinence of urine because you are unable to move due to "off" symptoms?	ALWAYS	NEVER	0 1 2 3 4 5 6 7 8 9 10
10. Do you experience numbness or tingling of your arms or legs which wake you from sleep at night?	ALWAYS	NEVER	0 1 2 3 4 5 6 7 8 9 10
11. Do you have painful muscle cramps in your arms or legs whilst sleeping at night?	ALWAYS	NEVER	0 1 2 3 4 5 6 7 8 9 10
12. Do you wake early in the morning with painful posturing of arms or legs?	ALWAYS	NEVER	0 1 2 3 4 5 6 7 8 9 10
13. On waking do you experience tremor?	ALWAYS	NEVER	0 1 2 3 4 5 6 7 8 9 10
14. Do you feel tired and sleepy after waking in the morning?	ALWAYS	NEVER	0 1 2 3 4 5 6 7 8 9 10
15. Have you unexpectedly fallen asleep during the day?	FREQUENTLY	NEVER	0 1 2 3 4 5 6 7 8 9 10

Reproduced from Chaudhuri et al [1] with permission from BMJ Publishing Group Ltd.

Reference

1. Chaudhuri, K. R., Pal, S., DiMarco, A., Whately-Smith, S., Bridgman, K., Mathew, R. Pezzela, F. R., Forbes, A., Högl, B., & Trenkwalder, C. (2002). The Parkinson's disease sleep scale: a new instrument for assessing sleep and nocturnal disability in Parkinson's disease. *Journal of Neurology, Neurosurgery, & Psychiatry, 73*(6), 629–635.

Representative Studies Using Scale

Dhawan, V., Dhoat, S., Williams, A., DiMarco, A., Pal, S., Forbes, A., Tobias, A., Martinez-Martin, P., & Ray, C. K. (2006). The range and nature of sleep dysfunction in untreated Parkinson's disease (PD). A comparative controlled clinical study using the Parkinson's disease sleep scale and selective polysomnography. *Journal of Neurological Sciences, 248*(1–2), 158–162.

Hjort, N., Ostergaard, K., & Dupont, E. (2004). Improvement of sleep quality in patients with advanced Parkinson's disease treated with deep brain stimulation of the subthalamic nucleus. *Movement Disorders, 19*(2), 196–199.

61 Pediatric Daytime Sleepiness Scale (PDSS)

Purpose Consisting of 8 questions, the scale is designed as a brief measure for evaluating subjective experiences of daytime sleepiness in young students. While no time reference is specifically identified by the questionnaire, items query feelings of drowsiness in a variety of settings over the course of the day. The measure was initially designed to be used in research, but may also possess clinical and screening utility.

Population for Testing The scale was designed for middle-school students aged 11–15 years.

Administration A self-report measure completed with paper and pencil, the scale requires approximately 5 min for completion.

Reliability and Validity A validation study conducted by developers Drake and colleagues [1] demonstrated an internal consistency of .80.

Obtaining a Copy A copy of the scale can be found in the original article published by developers [1].

Direct correspondence to:
Christopher L. Drake, Senior Bioscientific Staff
Sleep Disorders and Research Center, Henry Ford Hospital
2799 West Grand Blvd.
Detroit, MI 48202, USA
Telephone: 313-916-4455
Email: cdrake1@hfhs.org

Scoring Using a Likert-type scale, respondents indicate how frequently they experience drowsiness or alertness in certain situations. Responses are coded on a scale from 0 ("seldom") to 4 ("always"), except for item 3 for which the scale is reversed. Higher scores on the scale are indicative of more acute daytime sleepiness.

A. Shahid et al. (eds.), *STOP, THAT and One Hundred Other Sleep Scales*,
DOI 10.1007/978-1-4419-9893-4_61, © Springer Science+Business Media, LLC 2012

Pediatric Daytime Sleepiness Scale (PDSS)

Pediatric Daytime Sleepiness Scale (PDSS)
Please answer the following questions as honestly as you can by circling one answer only:

1. How often do you fall asleep or get drowsy during class periods?
Always Frequently Sometimes Seldom Never

2. How often do you get sleepy or drowsy while doing your homework?
Always Frequently Sometimes Seldom Never

*3. Are you usually alert most of the day?
Always Frequently Sometimes Seldom Never

4. How often are you ever tired and grumpy during the day?
Always Frequently Sometimes Seldom Never

5. How often do you have trouble getting out of bed in the morning?
Always Frequently Sometimes Seldom Never

6. How often do you fall back to sleep after being awakened in the morning?
Very often Often Sometimes Seldom Never

7. How often do you need someone to awaken you in the morning?
Always Frequently Sometimes Seldom Never

8. How often do you think that you need more sleep?
Very often Often Sometimes Seldom Never

Scoring
4 3 2 1 0
*Reverse score this item

Reference

1. Drake, C., Nickel, C., Burduvali, E., Roth, T., Jefferson, C., & Badia, P. (2003). The pediatric daytime sleepiness scale (PDSS): sleep habits and school outcomes in middle-school children. *Sleep, 26* (4), 455–458.

Representative Studies Using Scale

Beebe, D. W., Lewin, D., Zeller, M., McCabe, M., MacLeod, K., Daniels, S. R., & Amin, R. (2007). Sleep in overweight adolescents: shorter sleep, poorer sleep quality, sleepiness, and sleep-disordered breathing. *Journal of Pediatric Psychiatry, 32*(1), 69–79.

Perez-Chada, D., Perez-Lloret, S., Videla, A. J., Cardinali, D., Bergna, M. A., Fernández-Acquier, M., Larrateguy, L., Zabert, G. E., & Drake, C. (2007). Sleep disordered breathing and daytime sleepiness are associated with poor academic performance in teenagers. A study using the pediatric daytime sleepiness scale (PDSS). *Sleep, 30*(12), 1698–1703.

62 Pediatric Quality of Life Inventory (PedsQL) Multidimensional Fatigue Scale

Purpose Though numerous versions of the PedsQL have been developed as measures of health-related quality of life in pediatric patient populations, the PedsQL Multidimensional Fatigue Scale is the first of these scales to deal specifically with subjective experiences of fatigue. Composed of 18 items, the instrument possesses three subscales: general fatigue, sleep and rest fatigue, and cognitive fatigue. Both self-report and parental-report versions have been created to address issues of cross-informant discrepancies.

Population for Testing A parental version can be completed for children aged 2 through 18, while the child self-report version has been validated with youth aged 5–18 years.

Administration Both the self-report and caregiver report forms are pencil-and-paper measures requiring between 10 and 15 min for completion. The scale should be read aloud to children 7 and younger and to those too fatigued or ill to complete the instrument themselves. As symptoms and experiences of fatigue may vary widely within such a large age range, slightly different versions exist for children 2–4, 5–7, 8–12, and 13–18 in order to ensure age-appropriateness.

Reliability and Validity In a psychometric evaluation conducted by Varni and colleagues [1], researchers demonstrated an internal consistency ranging from 77 to 93, and found that scores on the fatigue scale significantly differentiated between patient samples and healthy controls.

Obtaining a Copy The instrument is under copyright and can be obtained from publishers MAPI Research Trust at their Web site: http://www.mapi-trust.org/

Direct correspondence to:
James W. Varni
Center for Child Health Outcomes, Children's Hospital and Health Center
3020 Children's Way, San Diego
CA 92123, USA
Email: jvarni@chsd.org

Scoring Respondents use a Likert-type scale to indicate how frequently certain fatigue-related symptoms and complaints trouble them. The scale ranges from "never" (which receives a score of 100) and "almost always" (which receives 0). Higher scores indicate a better health-related quality of life and less acute fatigue. Total and subscale scores are obtained by averaging scores on each relevant item.

A. Shahid et al. (eds.), *STOP, THAT and One Hundred Other Sleep Scales*,
DOI 10.1007/978-1-4419-9893-4_62, © Springer Science+Business Media, LLC 2012

ID#____________________

Date:____________________

PedsQL™

Multidimensional Fatigue Scale

Standard Version

PARENT REPORT for **CHILDREN** (ages **8-12**)

DIRECTIONS

On the following page is a list of things that might be a problem for **your child**. Please tell us **how much of a problem** each one has been for **your child** during the **past ONE month** by circling:

0 if it is **never** a problem
1 if it is **almost never** a problem
2 if it is **sometimes** a problem
3 if it is **often** a problem
4 if it is **almost always** a problem

There are no right or wrong answers.
If you do not understand a question, please ask for help.

PedsQL 2

*In the past **ONE month,** how much of a **problem** has this been for your child …*

GENERAL FATIGUE *(problems with…)*	Never	Almost Never	Some-times	Often	Almost Always
1. Feeling tired	0	1	2	3	4
2. Feeling physically weak (not strong)	0	1	2	3	4
3. Feeling too tired to do things that he/she likes to do	0	1	2	3	4
4. Feeling too tired to spend time with his/her friends	0	1	2	3	4
5. Trouble finishing things	0	1	2	3	4
6. Trouble starting things	0	1	2	3	4

SLEEP/REST FATIGUE *(problems with…)*	Never	Almost Never	Some-times	Often	Almost Always
1. Sleeping a lot	0	1	2	3	4
2. Difficulty sleeping through the night	0	1	2	3	4
3. Feeling tired when he/she wakes up in the morning	0	1	2	3	4
4. Resting a lot	0	1	2	3	4
5. Taking a lot of naps	0	1	2	3	4
6. Spending a lot of time in bed	0	1	2	3	4

COGNITIVE FATIGUE *(problems with…)*	Never	Almost Never	Some-times	Often	Almost Always
1. Difficulty keeping his/her attention on things	0	1	2	3	4
2. Difficulty remembering what people tell him/her	0	1	2	3	4
3. Difficulty remembering what he/she just heard	0	1	2	3	4
4. Difficulty thinking quickly	0	1	2	3	4
5. Trouble remembering what he/she was just thinking	0	1	2	3	4
6. Trouble remembering more than one thing at a time	0	1	2	3	4

PedsQL Parent (8-12) Fatigue
05/01
PedsQL#-Fatigue-PC-usaor

Reference

1. Varni, J. W., Burwinkle, T. M., Katz, E. R., Meeske, K., & Dickinson, P. (2002). The PedsQL in pediatric cancer: reliability and validity of the pediatric quality of life inventory generic core scales, multidimensional fatigue scale, and cancer module. *Cancer, 94*, 2090–2106.

Representative Studies Using Scale

Crabtree, V. M., Varni, J. W., & Gozal, D. (2004). Health-related quality of life and depressive symptoms in children with suspected sleep-disordered breathing. *Sleep, 27*(6), 1131–1138.

Hiscock, J., Canterford, L., Ukoumunne, O. C., & Wake, M. (2007). Adverse associations of sleep problems in Australian preschoolers: national population study. *Pediatrics, 119*(1), 86–93.

Pediatric Sleep Questionnaire (PSQ) 63

Purpose Designed to screen for sleep problems in children. A shorter version is shown (following) which specifically relates to sleep-disordered breathing (SDB) in children. The scale consists of 22 parent-reported items examining snoring and breathing problems, daytime sleepiness, inattention, hyperactivity, and other signs and symptoms of apnea including obesity and nocturnal enuresis.

Population for Testing The scale has been validated with patients aged 2–18 years.

Administration Requiring between 5 and 10 min for completion, the instrument is a self-report measure that solicits responses from parents or caregivers.

Reliability and Validity Developers Chervin and colleagues [1] evaluated the scale against the results of polysomnography and found a sensitivity ranging from .81 to .85, a specificity of .87, an internal consistency of .66 to .89, and a test–retest reliability of .66 to .92.

Obtaining a Copy Questionnaire examples can be found in developers' original published article [1].

Direct correspondence to:
R.D. Chervin
Sleep Disorders Center, University Hospital
8D8702
P.O. Box 0117, 1500 E. Medical Center
Dr Ann Arbor, MI 48109-0117, USA
Email: chervin@umich.edu

Scoring The majority of items are responded to with simple "yes" or "no" answers, and receive scores of 1 or 0 respectively. However, questions concerning inattention and hyperactivity are completed using a Likert-type scale which is later made binary – "does not apply" and "applies just a little" are scored as 0 and "applies quite a bit" and "definitely applies most of the time" receive a score of 1. While this "yes/no" system of scoring ensures that respondents who shy away from the most extreme values of the scale are still counted within applicable categories, it also prevents the instrument from distinguishing between different degrees of disorder severity.

A. Shahid et al. (eds.), *STOP, THAT and One Hundred Other Sleep Scales*,
DOI 10.1007/978-1-4419-9893-4_63, © Springer Science+Business Media, LLC 2012

PEDIATRIC SLEEP QUESTIONNAIRE

Version 070424

Child's Name: ______________________, ______________________ ______.
(Last) (First) (M.I.)

Name of Person Answering Questions: ______________________.

Relation to Child: ______________________.

Your phone number, days: ______________, **and evenings:** ______________.
Area Code Number Area Code Number

Relative's name and number in case we cannot reach you: ______________________.

______________________.
Area Code Number

Instructions:

Please answer the questions on the following pages regarding the behavior of your child during sleep and wakefulness. The questions apply to how your child acts in general, not necessarily during the past few days since these may not have been typical if your child has not been well. If you are not sure how to answer any question, please feel free to ask your husband or wife, child, or physician for help. You should circle the correct response or print your answers neatly in the space provided. A "Y" means "yes," "N" means "no," and "DK" means "don't know." When you see the word "usually" it means "more than half the time" or "on more than half the nights."

GENERAL INFORMATION ABOUT YOUR CHILD:

	Office use only
	GI1
Today's Date: ______________________. (Month Day Year)	GI2
Where are you completing this questionnaire? ______________.	GI3
Date of Child's Birth: ____________________. (Month Day Year)	GI4
Sex: Male or Female? ______________.	GI5
Current Height (feet/inches) : ____________.	GI6
Current Weight (pounds) : __________.	GI7
Grade in school (if applicable): __________.	GI8
Racial/Ethnic Background of your Child (please circle):	GI9
1.) American Indian **2.) Asian-American**	
3.) African-American **4.) Hispanic**	
5.) White/not Hispanic **6.) Other or unknown**	

(continued)

Page 3

A. Nighttime and sleep behavior: WHILE SLEEPING, DOES YOUR CHILD …		Office use only
… ever snore?	Y N DK	A1
… snore more than half the time?	Y N DK	A2
… always snore?	Y N DK	A3
… snore loudly?	Y N DK	A4
… have "heavy" or loud breathing?	Y N DK	A5
… have trouble breathing, or struggle to breathe? HAVE YOU EVER …	Y N DK	A6
… seen your child stop breathing during the night? If so, please describe what has happened:	Y N DK	A7
… been concerned about your child's breathing during sleep?	Y N DK	A8
… had to shake your sleeping child to get him or her to breathe, or wake up and breathe?	Y N DK	A9
… seen your child wake up with a snorting sound? DOES YOUR CHILD …	Y N DK	A11
… have restless sleep?	Y N DK	A12
… describe restlessness of the legs when in bed? … have "growing pains" (unexplained leg pains)? … have "growing pains" that are worst in bed? WHILE YOUR CHILD SLEEPS, HAVE YOU SEEN …	Y N DK Y N DK Y N DK	A13 A13a A13b
… brief kicks of one leg or both legs? … repeated kicks or jerks of the legs at regular intervals (i.e., about every 20 to 40 seconds)? AT NIGHT, DOES YOUR CHILD USUALLY …	Y N DK Y N DK	A14 A14a
… become sweaty, or do the pajamas usually become wet with perspiration?	Y N DK	A15
… get out of bed (for any reason)?	Y N DK	A16

... get out of bed to urinate? If so, how many times each night, on average?	Y N DK ______ times	A17 A17a
Does your child usually sleep with the mouth open?	Y N DK	A21
Is your child's nose usually congested or "stuffed" at night?	Y N DK	A22
Do any allergies affect your child's ability to breathe through the nose? DOES YOUR CHILD ...	Y N DK	A23
... tend to breathe through the mouth during the day?	Y N DK	A24
... have a dry mouth on waking up in the morning?	Y N DK	A25
... complain of an upset stomach at night?	Y N DK	A27
... get a burning feeling in the throat at night?	Y N DK	A29
... grind his or her teeth at night?	Y N DK	A30
... occasionally wet the bed?	Y N DK	A32
Has your child ever walked during sleep ("sleep walking")?	Y N DK	A33
Have you ever heard your child talk during sleep ("sleep talking")?	Y N DK	A34
Does your child have nightmares once a week or more on average?	Y N DK	A35
Has your child ever woken up screaming during the night?	Y N DK	A36
Has your child ever been moving or behaving, at night, in a way that made you think your child was neither completely awake nor asleep? If so, please describe what has happened:	Y N DK	A37
Does your child have difficulty falling asleep at night?	Y N DK	A40
How long does it take your child to fall asleep at night? (a guess is O.K.)	______ minutes	A41
At bedtime does your child usually have difficult "routines" or "rituals," argue a lot, or otherwise behave badly?	Y N DK	A42
DOES YOUR CHILD ... ... bang his or her head or rock his or her body when going to sleep?	Y N DK	A43
... wake up more than twice a night on average?	Y N DK	A44
... have trouble falling back asleep if he or she wakes up at night?	Y N DK	A45

(continued)

… wake up early in the morning and have difficulty going back to sleep?	Y N DK	A46
Does the time at which your child <u>goes to bed</u> change a lot from day to day?	Y N DK	A47
Does the time at which your child <u>gets up from bed</u> change a lot from day to day? WHAT TIME DOES YOUR CHILD USUALLY …	Y N DK	A48
… go to bed during the week?		A49
… go to bed on the weekend or vacation?		A50
… get out of bed on weekday mornings?		A51
… get out of bed on weekend or vacation mornings?		A52

B. Daytime behavior and other possible problems: DOES YOUR CHILD …		Office Use Only
… wake up feeling <u>un</u>refreshed in the morning?	Y N DK	B1
… have a problem with sleepiness during the day?	Y N DK	B2
… complain that he or she feels sleepy during the day?	Y N DK	B3
Has a teacher or other supervisor commented that your child appears sleepy during the day?	Y N DK	B4
Does your child usually take a nap during the day?	Y N DK	B5
Is it hard to wake your child up in the morning?	Y N DK	B6
Does your child wake up with headaches in the morning?	Y N DK	B7
Does your child get a headache at least once a month, on average?	Y N DK	B8
Did your child stop growing at a normal rate at any time since birth? If so, please describe what happened:	Y N DK	B9
Does your child still have tonsils? If not, when and why were they removed?: HAS YOUR CHILD EVER …	Y N DK	B10
… had a condition causing difficulty with breathing?	Y N DK	B11

Page 6

If so, please describe:		
… had surgery? If so, did any difficulties with breathing occur before, during, or after surgery?	Y N DK Y N DK	B12 B12a
… become suddenly weak in the legs, or anywhere else, after laughing or being surprised by something?	Y N DK	B13
… felt unable to move for a short period, in bed, though awake and able to look around?	Y N DK	B15
Has your child felt an irresistible urge to take a nap at times, forcing him or her to stop what he or she is doing in order to sleep?	Y N DK	B16
Has your child ever sensed that he or she was dreaming (seeing images or hearing sounds) while still awake?	Y N DK	B17
Does your child drink caffeinated beverages on a typical day (cola, tea, coffee)? If so, how many cups or cans per day?	Y N DK ______ cups	B18 B18a
Does your child use any recreational drugs? If so, which ones and how often?:	Y N DK	B19
Does your child use cigarettes, smokeless tobacco, snuff, or other tobacco products? If so, which ones and how often?:	Y N DK	B20
Is your child overweight? If so, at what age did this first develop?	Y N DK ______ years	B22 B22a
Has a doctor ever told you that your child has a high-arched palate (roof of the mouth)?	Y N DK	B23
Has your child ever taken Ritalin (methylphenidate) for behavioral problems?	Y N DK	B24
Has a health professional ever said that your child has attention-deficit disorder (ADD) or attention-deficit/hyperactivity disorder (ADHD)?	Y N DK	B25

(continued)

Page 7

C. Other Information

1. If you are currently at a clinic with your child to see a physician, what is the problem that brought you?

2. If your child has long-term medical problems, please list the three you think are most significant.

____.

____.

____.

3. Please list any medications your child currently takes:

Medicine	**Size (mg) or amount per dose**	**Taken when?**
________	________________	________
Effect:	____________________________.	
________	________________	________
Effect:	____________________________.	
________	________________	________
Effect:	____________________________.	
________	________________	________
Effect:	____________________________.	

4. Please list any medication your child has taken in the past if the purpose of the medication was to improve his or her behavior, attention, or sleep:

Medicine	**Size (mg) or amount per dose**	**Taken how often?**	**Dates Taken**
________	____________________	____________	________
Effect:	____.		
________	____________________	____________	________
Effect:	____.		
________	____________________	____________	________
Effect:	____.		
________	____________________	____________	________
Effect:	____.		

5. Please list any sleep disorders diagnosed or suspected by a physician in your child. For each problem, please list the date it started and whether or not it is still present.

6. Please list any psychological, psychiatric, emotional, or behavioral problems diagnosed or suspected by a physician in your child. For each problem, please list the date it started and whether or not it is still present.

(continued)

7. **Please list any sleep or behavior disorders diagnosed or suspected in *your child's* brothers, sisters, or parents:**

<u>**Relative**</u>	<u>**Condition**</u>
____________________	________________________
____________________	________________________
____________________	________________________

D. Additional Comments:

Please use the space below to print any additional comments you feel are important. Please also use this space to describe details regarding any of the above questions.

Instructions:

Please indicate, by checking the appropriate box, how much each statement* applies to this child:

This child often...	Does not apply 0	Applies just a little 1	Applies quite a bit 2	Definitely applies most of the time 3
... does not seem to listen when spoken to directly.				
... has difficulty organizing tasks and activities.				
... is easily distracted by extraneous stimuli.				
... fidgets with hands or feet or squirms in seat.				
... is "on the go" or often acts as if "driven by a motor".				
... interrupts or intrudes on others (e.g., butts into conversations or games.				

* Derived from DSM-IV.

THANK YOU

Reference

1. Chervin, R. D., Hedger, K., Dillon, J. E., & Pituch, K. J. (2000). Pediatric sleep questionnaire (PSQ): validity and reliability of scales for sleep-disordered breathing, snoring, sleepiness, and behavioral problems. *Sleep Medicine, 1*, 21–32.

Representative Studies Using Scale

Archbold, K. H., Pituch, K. J., Panahi, P., & Chervin, R. D. (2002). Symptoms of sleep disturbances among children at two general pediatric clinics. *The Journal of Pediatrics, 140*(1), 97–102.

Chervin, R. D., Archbold, K. H., Dillon, J. E., Pituch, K. J., Panahi, P., Dahl, R. E., & Guilleinault, C. (2002). Associations between symptoms of inattention, hyperactivity, restless legs, and periodic leg movements. *Sleep, 25*(2), 213–218.

63.1 Instructions for Scoring the Pediatric Sleep Questionnaire: Sleep-Related Breathing Disorders (SRBD) Scale

The 22 items of the SRBD Scale are each answered yes = 1, no = 0, or don't know = missing. The number of symptom-items endorsed positively ("yes") is divided by the number of items answered positively or negatively; the denominator therefore excludes items with missing responses and items answered as don't know. The result is a number, a proportion that ranges from 0.0 to 1.0. Scores >0.33 are considered positive and suggestive of high risk for a pediatric sleep-related breathing disorder. This threshold is based on a validity study that suggested optimal sensitivity and specificity at the 0.33 cut-off [1], but this number could be lowered in practice if increased sensitivity is a priority, or raised if increased specificity is a priority. Additional references that support the validity of the SRBD Scale, or employ it in research, are listed below [2–7].

Pediatric Sleep Questionnaire: Sleep-Disordered Breathing Subscale

070129

Child's Name: ______________________ **Study ID #:** __________
Person completing form: ____________________ **Date:** ____/____/____

Please answer these questions regarding the behavior of your child during sleep and wakefulness. The questions apply to how your child acts in general during the past month, not necessarily during the past few days since these may not have been typical if your child has not been well. You should circle the correct response or *print* your answers neatly in the space provided. A "Y" means "yes," "N" means "no," and "DK" means "don't know."

1. WHILE SLEEPING, DOES YOUR CHILD:				
Snore more than half the time?	Y	N	DK	A2
Always snore?	Y	N	DK	A3
Snore loudly?	Y	N	DK	A4
Have "heavy" or loud breathing?	Y	N	DK	A5
Have trouble breathing, or struggle to breathe?	Y	N	DK	A6
2. HAVE YOU EVER SEEN YOUR CHILD STOP BREATHING DURING THE NIGHT?	Y	N	DK	A7
3. DOES YOUR CHILD:				
Tend to breathe through the mouth during the day?	Y	N	DK	A24
Have a dry mouth on waking up in the morning?	Y	N	DK	A25
Occasionally wet the bed?	Y	N	DK	A32
4. DOES YOUR CHILD:				
Wake up feeling unrefreshed in the morning?	Y	N	DK	B1
Have a problem with sleepiness during the day?	Y	N	DK	B2
5. HAS A TEACHER OR OTHER SUPERVISOR COMMENTED THAT YOUR CHILD APPEARS SLEEPY DURING THE DAY?	Y	N	DK	B4
6. IS IT HARD TO WAKE YOUR CHILD UP IN THE MORNING?	Y	N	DK	B6
7. DOES YOUR CHILD WAKE UP WITH HEADACHES IN THE MORNING?	Y	N	DK	B7
8. DID YOUR CHILD STOP GROWING AT A NORMAL RATE AT ANY TIME SINCE BIRTH?	Y	N	DK	B9
9. IS YOUR CHILD OVERWEIGHT?	Y	N	DK	B22
10. THIS CHILD **OFTEN**:				
Does not seem to listen when spoken to directly.	Y	N	DK	C3
Has difficulty organizing tasks and activities.	Y	N	DK	C5
Is easily distracted by extraneous stimuli.	Y	N	DK	C8
Fidgets with hands or feet or squirms in seat.	Y	N	DK	C10
Is "on the go" or often acts as if "driven by a motor".	Y	N	DK	C14
Interrupts or intrudes on others (eg., butts into conversations or games).	Y	N	DK	C18

Thank you!

Reference List

1. Chervin RD, Hedger KM, Dillon JE, Pituch KJ. Pediatric Sleep Questionnaire (PSQ): validity and reliability of scales for sleep-disordered breathing, snoring, sleepiness, and behavioral problems. Sleep Med 2000;1:21–32.
2. Chervin RD, Weatherly RA, Garetz SL et al. Pediatric sleep questionnaire: Prediction of sleep apnea and outcomes. Archives of Otolaryngology-Head & Neck Surgery 2007;133(3):216–222.
3. Chervin RD, Archbold KH, Dillon JE et al. Inattention, hyperactivity, and symptoms of sleep-disordered breathing. Pediatrics 2002;109:449–456.
4. Archbold KH, Pituch KJ, Panahi P, Chervin RD. Symptoms of sleep disturbances among children at two general pediatric clinics. J Pediatr 2002;140:97–102.
5. Chervin RD, Dillon JE, Archbold KH, Ruzicka DL. Conduct problems and symptoms of sleep disorders in children. Journal of the American Academy of Child & Adolescent Psychiatry 2003;42:201–208.
6. Chervin RD, Clarke DF, Huffman JL et al. School performance, race, and other correlates of sleep-disordered breathing in children. Sleep Med 2003; 4:21–27.
7. Chervin RD, Ruzicka DL, Archbold KH, Dillon JE. Snoring predicts hyperactivity four years later. Sleep 2005;28:885–890.

Perceived Stress Questionnaire (PSQ) 64

Purpose Consisting of 30 items, the PSQ was developed as an instrument for assessing the stressful life events and circumstances that tend to trigger or exacerbate disease symptoms. With stress bearing significantly on the quality and consistency of the sleep cycle [1], the PSQ is a potentially valuable tool for evaluating the underlying causes of sleep disturbances. The scale is specifically recommended for clinical settings, though it has been employed in research studies as well.

Population for Testing The PSQ has been validated with a population of in-patients, outpatients, students, and health care workers with a mean age of 31.8 ± 13.9.

Administration The scale is a self-report, pencil-and-paper measure requiring between 10 and 15 min for completion.

Reliability and Validity Developers Levenstein and colleagues [2] conducted a psychometric evaluation of the scale and found an internal consistency ranging from 90 to .92 and a test–retest reliability of .82. Results of the PSQ correlated highly with trait anxiety and with scores on Cohen's Perceived Stress Scale.

Obtaining a Copy A copy can be found in the original article published by developers [2].

Direct correspondence to:
Cesare Balbo 43
00184 Rome, Italy

Scoring In order to complete the PSQ, respondents receive one of two sets of scoring instructions: the general questionnaire queries stressful feelings and experiences over the course of the previous year or two, while the recent questionnaire concerns stress during the last month. Respondents indicate on a scale from 1 ("almost never") to 4 ("usually") how frequently they experience certain stress-related feelings. Higher scores indicate greater levels of stress. A total score is found by tallying each item (questions 1, 7, 10, 13, 17, 21, 25, and 29 are positive and are scored according to the directions accompanying the scale). A PSQ index can be found by subtracting 30 from the raw score and dividing the result by 90, yielding a score between 0 and 1.

A. Shahid et al. (eds.), *STOP, THAT and One Hundred Other Sleep Scales*,
DOI 10.1007/978-1-4419-9893-4_64, © Springer Science+Business Media, LLC 2012

The Perceived Stress Questionnaire

Instructions for the General questionnaire

For each sentence, circle the number that describes how often it applies to you in general, *during the last year or two*. Work quickly, without bothering to check your answers, and be careful to describe your life *in the long run*.

	Almost	Sometimes	Often	Usually
1. You feel rested	1	2	3	4
2. You feel that too many demands are being made on you	1	2	3	4
3. You are irritable or grouchy	1	2	3	4
4. You have too many things to do	1	2	3	4
5. You feel lonely or isolated	1	2	3	4
6. You find yourself in situations of conflict	1	2	3	4
7. You feel you're doing things you really like	1	2	3	4
8. You feel tired	1	2	3	4
9. You fear you may not manage to attain your goals	1	2	3	4
10. You feel calm	1	2	3	4
11. You have too many decisions to make	1	2	3	4
12. You feel frustrated	1	2	3	4
13. You are full of energy	1	2	3	4
14. You feel tense	1	2	3	4
15. Your problems seem to be piling up	1	2	3	4
16. You feel you're in a hurry	1	2	3	4
17. You feel safe and protected	1	2	3	4
18. You have many worries	1	2	3	4
19. You are under pressure from other people	1	2	3	4
20. You feel discouraged	1	2	3	4
21. You enjoy yourself	1	2	3	4
22. You are afraid for the future	1	2	3	4
23. You feel you're doing things because you have to not because you want to	1	2	3	4
24. You feel criticized or judged	1	2	3	4
25. You are lighthearted	1	2	3	4
26. You feel mentally exhausted	1	2	3	4
27. You have trouble relaxing	1	2	3	4
28. You feel loaded down with responsibility	1	2	3	4
29. You have enough time for yourself	1	2	3	4
30. You feel under pressure from deadlines	1	2	3	4

Instructions for the Recent questionnaire

For each sentence, circle the number that describes how often it applied to you *during the last month*.
Work quickly, without bothering to check your answers, and be careful to consider only *the last month*.
Score 5-circled number for items 1, 7, 10, 13, 17, 21, 25, 29
Score circled number for all other items
PSQ Index = (raw score-30)/90.

Note: The 8 items listed above are inverted, i.e., 4=1, 3=2, 2=3, and 1=4.

References

1. Van Reeth, O., Weibel, L., Spiegel, K., Leproult, R., Dugovic, C., & Maccari, S. (2000). Interactions between stress and sleep: from basic research to clinical situations. *Sleep Medicine Reviews, 4*(2), 201–219.
2. Levenstein, S., Prantera, C., Varvo, V., Scribano, M. L., Berto, E., Luzi, C., & Andreoli, A. (1993). Development of the perceived stress questionnaire: a new tool for psychosomatic research. *Journal of Psychosomatic Research, 37*(1), 19–32.

Representative Studies Using Scale

Levenstein, S., Prantera, C., Varvo, V., Scribano, M. L., Andreoli, A., Luzi, C., Arcà, M., Berto, E., Milite, G., & Marcheggiano, A. (2000). Stress and exacerbation in ulcerative colitis: a prospective study of patients enrolled in remission. *American Journal of Gastroenterology, 95*, 1213–1220.

Öhman, L., Bergdahl, J., Nyberg, L., & Nilsson, L. G. (2007). Longitudinal analysis of the relation between moderate long-term stress and health. *Stress and Health, 23*(2), 131–138.

65 Personal Health Questionnaire (PHQ)

Purpose The PHQ is a 10-item scale intended to evaluate symptoms of depression as defined by the International Classification of Diseases-10. The questionnaire is a simple and inexpensive screening tool for clinical depression, designed to improve rates of diagnosis among primary care physicians. With its proven psychometric properties, it is also suitable for use in research.

Population for Testing The scale has been validated with a population of primary care patients between the ages of 18 and 65 years.

Administration The PHQ is a self-report, paper-and-pencil measure requiring no more than 5 min for completion.

Reliability and Validity The scale's psychometric properties have been analyzed by Rizzo and colleagues [1]. Their research indicates an internal consistency of .79 and a test–retest reliability ranging from 38 to 62. Additionally, they found that a cutoff score of 9 yields a sensitivity of .78 and a specificity of .83. Approximately one-third of those individuals scoring above 9 were considered false positives. Researchers were also hoping the measure could be used to screen for individuals who might benefit from treatment with antidepressants: in this regard, a cutoff score of 10 provided good sensitivity (.84) and specificity (.78).

Obtaining a Copy A copy of the scale can be found in an article published by Rizzo and colleagues [1].

Scoring Respondents rate the frequency with which they have experienced each depressive symptom over the previous two weeks: scales range from 0 ("never") to 2 ("most days"). Total scores fall between 0 and 20, with higher scores indicating more acute depressive symptoms. A cutoff score of 9 is recommended for identifying individuals at high risk of experiencing clinical depression.

A. Shahid et al. (eds.), *STOP, THAT and One Hundred Other Sleep Scales*,
DOI 10.1007/978-1-4419-9893-4_65, © Springer Science+Business Media, LLC 2012

PERSONAL HEALTH QUESTIONNAIRE

This questionnaire asks you how you have been feeling in the past 2 weeks. Check the reply that most nearly applies to you in the following questions.

	Not at all	Occasionally	Most days in past 2 weeks
1. Have you been feeling sad or depressed most of the day?	☐	☐	☐
2. Have you lost interest in things you generally enjoy?	☐	☐	☐
3. Do you get tired easily, or lack energy?	☐	☐	☐
4. Loss of condence or self-esteem ?	☐	☐	☐
5. Had difficulty concentrating?	☐	☐	☐
6. Had sleep disturbance of any kind?	☐	☐	☐
7. Had decreased appetite with weight loss? **or** Noticed increased appetite with weight gain?	☐	☐	☐
8. Noticed that you are slowed up? **or** Inability to keep still?	☐	☐	☐
9. Unreasonable feelings of self-reproach or guilt?	☐	☐	☐
10. Thoughts of death, or thoughts of taking your own life?	☐	☐	☐

If you have reported at least 4 of these symptoms, how long have you had such symptoms?
☐ Less than 1 month, ☐ 1 month to 1 year, ☐ More than 1 year, ☐ More than one year but getting worse recently.

Rizzo et al. [1].

Reference

1. Rizzo, R., Piccinelli, N., Mazzi, M. A., Bellantuono, C., & Tansella, M. (2000). The personal health questionnaire: a new screening instrument for detection of ICD-10 depressive disorders in primary care. *Psychological Medicine, 30*, 831–840.

Representative Studies Using Scale

Bellantuono, C., Mazzi, M. A., Tansella, M., Rizzo, R., & Goldberg, D. (2002). The identification of depression and the coverage of antidepressant drug prescriptions in Italian general practice. *Journal of Affective Disorders, 72*(1), 53–59.

Husain, N., Creed, F., & Tomenson, B. (2000). Depression and social stress in Pakistan. *Psychological Medicine, 30*, 395–402.

66 Pictorial Sleepiness Scale Based on Cartoon Faces

Purpose The scale was developed as an alternative to traditional subjective measures of sleepiness. Where most self-report questionnaires require at least minimal literacy skills, the pictorial faces scale is accessible to a much wider population. Children, individuals new to the English language, and adults not proficient in reading are all capable of completing the scale.

Population for Testing The scale has been validated with individuals aged 4–73.

Administration Requiring approximately 3 min for administration, the scale is a self-report, paper-and-pencil measure.

Reliability and Validity In an initial validation study [1], developers found that results on the pictorial faces scale correlated highly with median scores obtained on the Karolinska Sleepiness Scale (Chap. 47) and the Stanford Sleepiness Scale (Chap. 91). In terms of the suitability of the cartoon faces used on the scale, 99% of participants were able to rank each face in the correct order of sleepiness.

Obtaining a Copy An example of the faces used can be found in the original article published by developers [1].

Direct correspondence to:
C.C. Maldonado
School of Physiology, University of Witwatersrand
Private Bag 3, Wits 2050, South Africa
Email: sleep@physiology.wits.ac.za

Scoring Respondents are presented with five faces indicating varying degrees of sleepiness, and are asked to select the face most representative of their current state. Likert-type values can be assigned to each face, allowing researchers to draw comparisons between and within subjects.

A. Shahid et al. (eds.), *STOP, THAT and One Hundred Other Sleep Scales*,
DOI 10.1007/978-1-4419-9893-4_66, © Springer Science+Business Media, LLC 2012

Pictorial Sleepiness Scale Based on Cartoon Faces

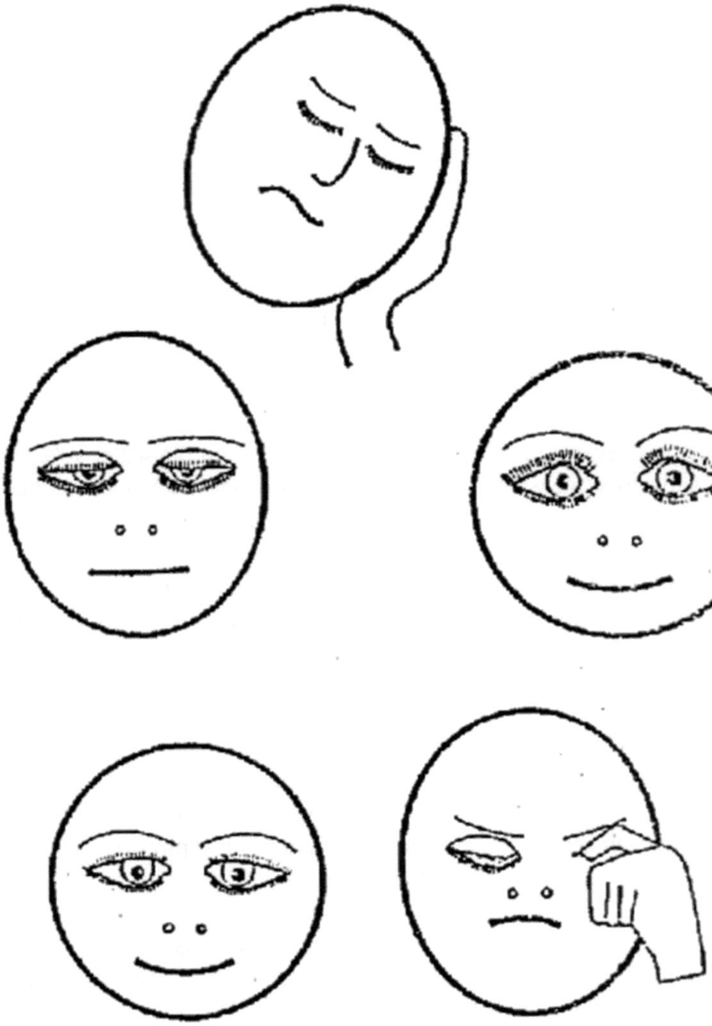

Reference

1. Maldonado, C. C., Bentley, A. J., & Mitchell, D. (2004). A pictorial sleepiness scale based on cartoon faces. *Sleep, 27*(3), 541–548.

Representative Studies Using Scale

None.

Pittsburgh Sleep Quality Index (PSQI)

67

Purpose As psychiatric disorders are often associated with sleep disturbances, the PSQI was designed to evaluate overall sleep quality in these clinical populations. Each of the questionnaire's 19 self-reported items belongs to one of seven subcategories: subjective sleep quality, sleep latency, sleep duration, habitual sleep efficiency, sleep disturbances, use of sleeping medication, and daytime dysfunction. Five additional questions rated by the respondent's roommate or bed partner are included for clinical purposes and are not scored.

Population for Testing The developers' initial psychometric analysis of the instrument was conducted with individuals aged 24–83 years [1]. The questionnaire has been validated with a variety of clinical populations, including: patients with major depressive disorder, disorders of initiating and maintaining sleep, disorders of excessive somnolence, cancer [2], and fibromyalgia [3].

Administration A self-report, pencil-and-paper measure, the instrument should require between 5 and 10 min for completion.

Reliability and Validity Though there have been a variety of studies assessing the psychometric properties of the scale, the developers' initial evaluation [1] found an internal reliability of $\alpha = .83$, a test–retest reliability of .85 for the global scale, a sensitivity of 89.6%, and a specificity of 86.5%.

Obtaining a Copy A copy can be found in the original article published by developers [1].

Direct correspondence to:
Dr. C.F. Reynolds
Western Psychiatric Institute and Clinic, University of Pittsburgh
3811 O'Hara St.
Pittsburgh, PA 15213, USA

Scoring A detailed guide to scoring is included in the original published article [1]. The questionnaire consists of a combination of Likert-type and open-ended questions (later converted to scaled scores using provided guidelines). Respondents are asked to indicate how frequently they have experienced certain sleep difficulties over the past month and to rate their overall sleep quality. Scores for each question range from 0 to 3, with higher scores indicating more acute sleep disturbances. Developers have suggested a cut-off score of 5 for the global scale as it correctly identified 88.5% of the patient group in their validation study.

A. Shahid et al. (eds.), *STOP, THAT and One Hundred Other Sleep Scales*,
DOI 10.1007/978-1-4419-9893-4_67, © Springer Science+Business Media, LLC 2012

Subject's Initials________________ID#____________________________Date__________________Time______AM PM

PITTSBURGH SLEEP QUALITY INDEX

INSTRUCTIONS:
The following questions relate to your usual sleep habits during the past month only. Your answers should indicate the most accurate reply for the majority of days and nights in the past month. Please answer all questions.

1. During the past month, what time have you usually gone to bed at night?

   BED TIME ___________

2. During the past month, how long (in minutes) has it usually taken you to fall asleep each night?

   NUMBER OF MINUTES ___________

3. During the past month, what time have you usually gotten up in the morning?

   GETTING UP TIME ___________

4. During the past month, how many hours of actual sleep did you get at night? (This may be different than the number of hours you spent in bed.)

   HOURS OF SLEEP PER NIGHT ___________

For each of the remaining questions, check the one best response. Please answer all questions.

5. During the past month, how often have you had trouble sleeping because you . . .

a) Cannot get to sleep within 30 minutes

Not during the past month_____	Less than once a week_____	Once or twice a week_____	Three or more times a week_____

b) Wake up in the middle of the night or early morning

Not during the past month_____	Less than once a week_____	Once or twice a week_____	Three or more times a week_____

c) Have to get up to use the bathroom

Not during the past month_____	Less than once a week_____	Once or twice a week_____	Three or more times a week_____

d) Cannot breathe comfortably

Not during the past month_____	Less than once a week_____	Once or twice a week_____	Three or more times a week_____

e) Cough or snore loudly

Not during the past month_____	Less than once a week_____	Once or twice a week_____	Three or more times a week_____

f) Feel too cold

Not during the past month_____	Less than once a week_____	Once or twice a week_____	Three or more times a week_____

g) Feel too hot

Not during the past month_____	Less than once a week_____	Once or twice a week_____	Three or more times a week_____

h) Had bad dreams

Not during the past month_____	Less than once a week_____	Once or twice a week_____	Three or more times a week_____

i) Have pain

Not during the past month_____	Less than once a week_____	Once or twice a week_____	Three or more times a week_____

j) Other reason(s), please describe____

____

How often during the past month have you had trouble sleeping because of this?

Not during the past month_____	Less than once a week_____	Once or twice a week_____	Three or more times a week_____

6. During the past month, how would you rate your sleep quality overall?

Very good ___________

Fairly good ___________

Fairly bad ___________

Very bad ___________

7. During the past month, how often have you taken medicine to help you sleep (prescribed or "over the counter")?

Not during the past month_____ Less than once a week_____ Once or twice a week_____ Three or more times a week_____

8. During the past month, how often have you had trouble staying awake while driving, eating meals, or engaging in social activity?

Not during the past month_____ Less than once a week_____ Once or twice a week_____ Three or more times a week_____

9. During the past month, how much of a problem has it been for you to keep up enough enthusiasm to get things done?

No problem at all __________

Only a very slight problem __________

Somewhat of a problem __________

A very big problem __________

10. Do you have a bed partner or room mate?

No bed partner or room mate __________

Partner/room mate in other room __________

Partner in same room, but not same bed __________

Partner in same bed __________

If you have a room mate or bed partner, ask him/her how often in the past month you have had . . .

a) Loud snoring

Not during the past month_____ Less than once a week_____ Once or twice a week_____ Three or more times a week_____

b) Long pauses between breaths while asleep

Not during the past month_____ Less than once a week_____ Once or twice a week_____ Three or more times a week_____

c) Legs twitching or jerking while you sleep

Not during the past month_____ Less than once a week_____ Once or twice a week_____ Three or more times a week_____

d) Episodes of disorientation or confusion during sleep

Not during the past month_____	Less than once a week_____	Once or twice a week_____	Three or more times a week_____

e) Other restlessness while you sleep; please describe________________________________

____

Not during the past month_____	Less than once a week_____	Once or twice a week_____	Three or more times a week_____

Buysse et al. [1].

References

1. Buysse, D. J., Reynolds, C. F., Charles, F., Monk, T. H., Berman, S. R., & Kupfer, D. J. (1989). The Pittsburgh sleep quality index: a new instrument for psychiatric practice and research. *Psychiatry Research, 28*(2), 193–213.
2. Dudley, W. N. (2004). Psychometric evaluation of the Pittsburgh sleep quality index in cancer patients. *Journal of Pain and Symptom Management, 27*(2), 140–148.
3. Osorio, C. D., Gallinaro, A. L., Lorenzi-Filho, G., & Lage, L. G. (2006). Sleep quality in patients with fibromyalgia using the Pittsburgh sleep quality index. *Journal of Rheumatology, 33*(9), 1863–1865.

Representative Studies Using Scale

Dolberg, O. T., Hirschmann, S., & Grunhaus, L. (1998). Melatonin for the treatment of sleep disturbances in major depressive disorder. *American Journal of Psychiatry, 155*, 1119–1121.

Jennings, J. R., Muldoon, M. F., Hall, M. Buysse, D. J., & Manuck, S. B. (2007). Self-reported sleep quality is associated with the metabolic structure. *Sleep, 30*(2), 219–223.

68 Profile of Mood States (POMS)

Purpose Consisting of 65 items, the POMS was designed to evaluate individuals within seven different mood domains: fatigue-inertia, anger-hostility, vigor-activity, confusion-bewilderment, depression-dejection, tension-anxiety, and friendliness. The scale has been recommended for evaluating affective changes over the course of brief treatment or assessment period. Sleep specialists are likely to find the fatigue-inertia scale particularly relevant.

Population for Testing Developers recommend the scale for individuals ages 18 and older.

Administration The self-report, pencil-and-paper measure requires between 5 and 10 min for completion. In order to purchase the scale, users must have completed graduate-level courses in psychometric measurement, or must be able to prove they possess equivalent levels of training or experience. A wide range of modified and alternative versions have been created, including an adolescent form [1] and a brief form that consists of only 30 items [2].

Reliability and Validity Numerous studies examining the scale's validity have been conducted in a variety of patient populations. Research examining the factor structure of the scale demonstrated considerable support for most of the POMS' seven factors – the fatigue-inertia subscale was found to have particular integrity [3]. Additionally, McNair and colleagues [2] reported an internal consistency ranging from .84 to .95.

Obtaining a Copy The questionnaire is under copyright and can be ordered online or by telephone from Multi-Health Systems Inc.
Telephone: 1 800 268-6011

Scoring The POMS-F requires respondents to indicate how well each item describes their mood over the past week using a five-point scale ranging from "not at all" to "extremely." The instrument is available in a quick-scoring format, where respondent's answers automatically transfer through onto the scoring template. Normative data and T-score conversions are available for each subscale in an accompanying manual.

Note: Many experts feel this scale has been superceded by subsequent scales.

References

1. Terry, P. C., Lane, A. M., Lane, H. J., & Keohane, L. (1999). Development and validation of a mood measure for adolescents. *Journal of Sports Sciences, 17*(11), 861–872.
2. McNair, D., Lorr, M., & Droppleman, L. (1971). *Manual for the Profile of Mood States*. San Diego: Educational and Industrial Testing Service.
3. Norcross, J. C., Guadagnoli, E., & Prochaska, J. O. (1984). Factor structure of the profile of mood states (POMS): two partial replications. *Journal of Clinical Psychology, 40*(5), 1270–1277.

A. Shahid et al. (eds.), *STOP, THAT and One Hundred Other Sleep Scales*,
DOI 10.1007/978-1-4419-9893-4_68,

Representative Studies Using Scale

Blesch, K. S., Paice, J. A., Wickham, R., Harte, N., Schnoor, D. K., Purl, S., Rehwalt, M, Kopp, P. L, Manson, S., & Coveny, S. B. (1991). Correlates of fatigue in people with breast or lung cancer. *Oncology Nursing Forum, 18*, 81–87.

Schwartz, A. L., Nail, L. M., Chen, S., Meek, P., Barsevick, A. M., King, M. E., & Jones, L. S. (2000). Fatigue patterns observed in patients receiving chemotherapy and radiotherapy. *Cancer Investigation, 18*, 11–19.

Dinges, D. F., Pack, F., Williams, K., Gillen, K. A., Powell, J. W., Ott, G. E., Aptowicz, C., & Pack, A. I. (1997). Cumulative sleepiness, mood disturbance, and psychomotor vigilance performance decrements during a week of sleep restricted to 4–5 hours per night. *Sleep, 20*, 267–277.

Psychosocial Adjustment to Illness Scale (PAIS)

69

Purpose Designed to assess the social and psychological factors associated with living with an illness, the 46-item PAIS is a semi-structured interview meant to evaluate seven domains of functioning related to adjustment to illness: health care orientation (attitudes, perceptions, and expectations regarding one's health care), vocational environment, domestic environment, sexual relationships, extended family relationships, social environment, and psychological distress.

Population for Testing The PAIS has been validated with a variety of patient populations with mean ages ranging from 39.6 ± 12.1 years to 59.8 ± 8.4 years. Normative data are available for a variety of patient groups including patients with lung cancer, those undergoing renal dialysis, and burn patients [1].

Administration The scale, requiring between 20 and 30 min for completion, is administered in the form of a semi-structured interview by a trained clinician or interviewer. A self-report, pencil-and-paper version is also available for large-scale research purposes.

Reliability and Validity In a review summarizing the scale's psychometric properties, scale developer Derogatis [2] reports an internal consistency ranging from .12 (for a domain that was later rewritten) to .93 and an interrater reliability of .33 to .86. Additionally, high correlations were observed between the Global Adjustment to Illness Scale and total adjustment scores on the PAIS.

Obtaining a Copy Sample items are included in the original article published by developers [2].

For a complete version, contact:
Clinical Psychometric Research, 1228
Wine Spring Lane, Towson, MD 21204, USA
Telephone: 1-800-245-0277

Scoring Each of the instrument's 46 items is scored on a scale from 0 to 3, where 0 indicates the greatest adjustment to an illness and 3 denotes the most dysfunctional. The interview format offers suggested questions in order to elicit the responses required for each item, though some interviews may deviate from this structure slightly. Responses for the interview format are rated by a professional clinician or trained interviewer, and a total score is calculated and can then be compared to available normative data.

References

1. Derogatis, L. R. & Derogatis, M. A. (1990). *PAIS & PAIS-SR: Administration, scoring & procedures manual-II* (2nd ed.). Baltimore: Clinical Psychometric Research.
2. Derogatis, L. R. (1986). The psychosocial adjustment to illness scale (PAIS). *Journal of Psychosomatic Research, 30*(1), 77–91.

A. Shahid et al. (eds.), *STOP, THAT and One Hundred Other Sleep Scales*,
DOI 10.1007/978-1-4419-9893-4_69, © Springer Science+Business Media, LLC 2012

Representative Studies Using Scale

Moser, D. K., & Dracup, K. (2004). Role of spousal anxiety and depression in patients' psychosocial recovery after a cardiac event. *Psychosomatic Medicine, 66*, 527–532.

Goodwin, P. J., Ennis, M., Bordeleau, L. J., Pritchard, K. I., Trudeau, M. E., Koo, J., & Hood, N. (2004). Health-related quality of life and psychosocial status in breast cancer prognosis: analysis of multiple variables. *Journal of Clinical Oncology, 22*(20), 4184–4192.

70 Quebec Sleep Questionnaire (QSQ)

Purpose The QSQ is a 32-item scale designed to assess health-related quality of life in patients with Obstructive Sleep Apnea (OSA). The instrument evaluates the impact of apnea in five different domains: hypersomnolence, daytime symptoms, nighttime symptoms, emotions, and social interactions. Developers Lacasse and colleagues [1] created the questionnaire for use in clinical trials as a method for evaluating treatment-induced changes. It was originally developed and validated in French (French-Canadian). This English version was provided by the authors, which they obtained from a translation/back-translation process.

Population for Testing The scale has been validated for obstructive sleep apnea patients with a mean age of 55 ± 10.

Administration Requiring between 10 and 15 min for completion, the questionnaire is a self-report, paper-and-pencil measure.

Reliability and Validity Developers Lacasse and colleagues [1] performed an initial psychometric evaluation of the scale and found a test–retest reliability ranging from .82 to .91 and an internal consistency of .68 to .94. The tool was also sensitive to changes in health-related quality of life induced by treatment with CPAP. In order to allow other researchers to properly interpret changes seen over the course of treatment, developers also calculated minimal clinically important differences for each domain: 1.8 for hypersomnolence, 2.0 for daytime symptoms, 1.5 for nocturnal symptoms, 1.1 for emotions, and 2.5 for social interactions.

Obtaining a Copy The scale is not provided in the original article.

Direct correspondence to:
Y. Lacasse
Centre de Pneumologie, Hopital Laval
2725 Chemin Ste-Foy
Ste-Foy, Quebec, Canada
G1V 4G5
Email: yves.lacasse@med.ulaval.ca

Scoring Respondents use a seven-point Likert-type scale to answer a variety of questions regarding their experiences with OSA. Scores range from 1 to 7, with higher scores indicating better quality of life. Mean scores can be calculated for each domain, while a total score can also be obtained by averaging scores achieved on all 32 items.

A. Shahid et al. (eds.), *STOP, THAT and One Hundred Other Sleep Scales*,
DOI 10.1007/978-1-4419-9893-4_70, © Springer Science+Business Media, LLC 2012

QUEBEC SLEEP QUESTIONNAIRE

This questionnaire has been designed to find out how you have been doing and feeling over the last 4 weeks. You will be questioned about the impact that sleep apnea may have had on your daily activities, your emotional functioning, and your social interactions, and about any symptoms it might have caused.

During the last 4 weeks :	All the time	A large amount of the time	A moderate to large amount of the time	A moderate amount of the time	A small to moderate amount of the time	A small amount of the time	Not at all
1. Have you had to force yourself to do your activities?	1	2	3	4	5	6	7
2. Have you disturbed everyone at night while staying with friends?	1	2	3	4	5	6	7
3. Have you felt like not wanting to do things together with your partner, children or friends?	1	2	3	4	5	6	7
4. Have you woken up more than once per night to urinate?	1	2	3	4	5	6	7
5. Have you been feeling depressed?	1	2	3	4	5	6	7
6. Have you been feeling anxious or fearful about what was wrong?	1	2	3	4	5	6	7
7. Have you needed to nap during the day?	1	2	3	4	5	6	7

During the last 4 weeks :	All the time	A large amount of the time	A moderate to large amount of the time	A moderate amount of the time	A small to moderate amount of the time	A small amount of the time	Not at all
8. Have you been feeling impatient?	1	2	3	4	5	6	7
9. Have you woken up often (more than twice) during the night?	1	2	3	4	5	6	7

During the last 4 weeks :	A very large amount	A large amount	A moderate to large amount	A moderate amount	A small to moderate amount	A small amount	None
10. Have you had difficulty with trying to remember things?	1	2	3	4	5	6	7
11. Have you had difficulty with trying to concentrate?	1	2	3	4	5	6	7
12. Have you been upset about being told that your snoring was bothersome or irritating?	1	2	3	4	5	6	7
13. Have you felt guilty about your relationship with family members or close personal friends?	1	2	3	4	5	6	7
14. Have you noticed a decrease in your performance at work?	1	2	3	4	5	6	7
15. Have you been concerned about heart problems or premature death?	1	2	3	4	5	6	7

During the last 4 weeks, how much of a problem have you had with :	A very large problem	A large problem	A moderate to large problem	A moderate problem	A small to moderate problem	A small problem	No problem
16. Having to fight to stay awake during the day?	1	2	3	4	5	6	7
17. Feeling decreased energy?	1	2	3	4	5	6	7
18. Feeling excessive fatigue?	1	2	3	4	5	6	7
19. Feeling that ordinary activities require an extra effort to perform or complete?	1	2	3	4	5	6	7
20. Falling asleep if not stimulated or active?	1	2	3	4	5	6	7
21. Difficulty with a dry or sore mouth/throat upon awakening?	1	2	3	4	5	6	7
22. Difficulty returning to sleep if you wake up in the night?	1	2	3	4	5	6	7
23. Feeling that you lack energy?	1	2	3	4	5	6	7

During the last 4 weeks, how much of a problem have you had with :	A very large problem	A large problem	A moderate to large problem	A moderate problem	A small to moderate problem	A small problem	No problem
24. Concern about the times you stop breathing at night?	1	2	3	4	5	6	7
25. Loud snoring?	1	2	3	4	5	6	7
26. Difficulties with attention?	1	2	3	4	5	6	7
27. Falling asleep suddenly?	1	2	3	4	5	6	7
28. Waking up at night feeling like you were choking?	1	2	3	4	5	6	7
29. Waking up in the morning feeling unrefreshed and/or tired?	1	2	3	4	5	6	7
30. A feeling that your sleep is restless?	1	2	3	4	5	6	7
31. Difficulty staying awake while reading?	1	2	3	4	5	6	7
32. Fighting the urge to fall asleep while driving?	1	2	3	4	5	6	7

Reference

1. Lacasse, Y., Bureau, M-P, Sériès, F. (2004). A new standardised and self-administered quality of life questionnaire specific to obstructive sleep apnoea. *Thorax, 59*, 494–499.

Representative Studies Using Scale

None.

71 Resistance to Sleepiness Scale (RSS)

Purpose Quite similar to the Epworth Sleepiness Scale (ESS; Chap. 29), the RSS is a 12-item scale created to assess daytime sleepiness by asking individuals to rate their likelihood of falling asleep in a variety of situations. However, the RSS is different in that it explicitly queries involuntary experiences of somnolence, while the ESS does not specify such situations. Items are divided into two categories: those situations in which falling asleep is considered appropriate and those in which it is not.

Population for Testing The scale has been validated with patients experiencing disordered sleep aged 18–71 years.

Administration A self-report, paper-and-pencil measure, the RSS requires approximately 5 min for completion.

Reliability and Validity A preliminary psychometric evaluation [1] found an internal consistency of .94 – quite a bit higher than the consistency found for the ESS in the same study (α=.86).

Obtaining a Copy An example of the scale's items can be found in an article published by Violani and colleagues [1].

Direct correspondence to:
C. Violani
Telephone: +39-06-49917646
Email: cristiano.violani@uniroma1.it

Scoring Respondents use a Likert-type scale ranging from 0 ("would never doze") to 3 ("high chance of dozing") to rate their likelihood of sleeping in situations that range from working at a desk to lying down while reading. Higher scores indicate a greater degree of daytime sleepiness.

A. Shahid et al. (eds.), *STOP, THAT and One Hundred Other Sleep Scales*,
DOI 10.1007/978-1-4419-9893-4_71, © Springer Science+Business Media, LLC 2012

RESISTANCE TO SLEEPINESS SCALE

(Rome Sleepiness Scale, Violani et al., 1997)

Name and Surname.. Gender...........Age...............
Occupation... Date and time |_|_|_|_|_|_|_|h.|_|_|:|_|_|

Please assess the likelihood of falling asleep or dozing involuntarily in the situations described below. When responding, imagine that you do not want to fall sleep in these situations and that you are not especially tired. Refer to your present circumstances rather than the past. In case you have not recently experienced one of the situations described below, imagine yourself in the situation, and respond accordingly.

For each situation, choose the appropriate score from the following scale:

ASSESSMENT SCALE. In the situation considered...

0 = I would never fall asleep unless I wanted to
1 = I might fall asleep involuntarily, but it would happen only rarely
2 = I would probably fall asleep involuntarily, rather often
3 = I would fall asleep unwillingly, very often

SITUATION	**Rating Score**
1) Lying down, reading a book or a magazine........................	|_|
2) Sitting in the stalls, at a theatre or cinema........................	|_|
3) Sitting to watch TV........................	|_|
4) At home, after dinner, during a meeting with friends........................	|_|
5) As a passenger in a car, after travelling for over 1 hour........................	|_|
6) Driving at night, on a motorway........................	|_|
7) In the afternoon, in an armchair........................	|_|
8) Sitting in a waiting-room........................	|_|
9) Sitting, after a lunch, without having had any alcohol........................	|_|
10) Sitting, listening to someone........................	|_|
11) Sitting in a train, bus or plane for more than 1 hour........................	|_|
12) In the afternoon, studying or working, sitting at a writing-desk........................	|_|

Reference

1. Violani, C., Lucidi, F., Robusto, E., Devoto, E., Zucconi, M., & Strambi, L. F. (2003). The assessment of daytime sleep propensity: a comparison between the Epworth Sleepiness Scale and a newly developed Resistance to Sleepiness Scale. *Clinical Neurophysiology, 114*, 1027–1033.

Representative Studies Using Scale

None

72 Restless Legs Syndrome Quality of Life Questionnaire (RLSQoL)

Purpose The RLSQoL is an 18-item scale initially designed to assess quality of life in patients with restless legs syndrome [1]. It has since been employed as an outcome measure in a variety of studies evaluating interventions to improve symptoms of restless legs syndrome. The scale queries the impact of restless legs syndrome on daily activity, morning and evening activity, concentration, sexual activity, and work.

Population for Testing The scale has been validated in a population of restless legs syndrome patients aged 26–87 years.

Administration The RLSQoL is a self-report, paper-and-pencil measure requiring between 5 and 10 min for completion.

Reliability and Validity According to a psychometric evaluation study conducted by developers [1], the RLSQoL possesses an internal consistency of .92 and a test–retest reliability ranging from .79 to .84. The scale was found to be responsive to changes in symptoms and it has been shown to distinguish between individuals with mild, moderate, and severe conditions.

Obtaining a Copy A copy of the scale can be found in the original article published by developers [1].

Direct correspondence to:
Linda Abetz
Email: linda.abetz@adelphi.co.uk

Scoring The scoring process for the RLSQoL is relatively complicated for a scale of its kind. Items 1–5, 7–10, and 13 use scales ranging from 1 to 5, with lower scores indicating a greater frequency and interference of restless legs syndrome. The total score for these items is converted to a value between 0 and 100 using an algorithm provided along with the scale. Items 6 and 16–18 require respondents to indicate how many days in the previous month or hours in the previous day they have been able to complete certain activities or have had their daily functioning interfered with. These items are scored as continuous variables (for example, ranging from 0 to 28 days for questions regarding number of days per month). Items 11, 12, 14, and 15 are categorical variables, where a response of "yes" receives (a 1), a response of "no" receives (a 2), and a response of "no because of other reasons" receives (a 3). Additional information regarding scoring procedures and mean scores can be found in the original article published by developers.

A. Shahid et al. (eds.), *STOP, THAT and One Hundred Other Sleep Scales*,
DOI 10.1007/978-1-4419-9893-4_72, © Springer Science+Business Media, LLC 2012

RLS Quality of Life Questionnaire

The following are some questions on how your Restless Legs Syndrome might affect your quality of life. Answer each of the items below in relation to your life experience in the past 4 weeks. Please mark only one answer for each question.

In the past four weeks:

1. How distressing to you were your restless legs?
☐ Not at all ☐A little ☐Some ☐Quite a bit ☐A lot
2. How often in the past 4 weeks did your restless legs disrupt your routine evening activities?
☐ Never ☐A few times ☐Sometimes ☐Most of the time ☐ All the time
3. How often in the past 4 weeks did restless legs keep you from attending your evening social activities?
☐ Never ☐ A few times ☐ Sometimes ☐ Most of the time ☐ All the time
4. In the past 4 weeks how much trouble did you have getting up in the morning due to restless legs?
☐ None ☐ A little ☐ Some ☐Quite a bit ☐ A lot
5. In the past 4 weeks how often were you late for work or your first appointments of the day due to restless legs?
☐ Never ☐ A few times ☐ Sometimes ☐ Most of the time ☐ All the time
6. How many days in the past 4 weeks were you late for work or your first appointments of the day due to restless legs?
Write in number of days: ___
7. How often in the past 4 weeks did you have trouble concentrating in the afternoon?
☐ Never ☐ A few times ☐ Sometimes ☐ Most of the time ☐ All the time
8. How often in the past 4 weeks did you have trouble concentrating in the evening?
☐ Never ☐ A few times ☐ Sometimes ☐ Most of the time ☐ All the time
9. In the past 4 weeks how much was your ability to make good decisions affected by sleep problems?
☐ None ☐ A little ☐ Some ☐ Quite a bit ☐ A lot
10. How often in the past 4 weeks would you have avoided traveling when the trip would have lasted more than two hours?
☐ Never ☐ A few times ☐ Sometimes ☐ Most of the time ☐ All the time
11. In the past 4 weeks how much interest did you have in sexual activity?
☐ None ☐ A little ☐ Some ☐ Quite a bit ☐ A lot
☐ Prefer not to answer
12. How much did restless legs disturb or reduce your sexual activities?
☐ None ☐ A little ☐ Some ☐ Quite a bit ☐ A lot
☐ Prefer not to answer
13. In the past 4 weeks how much did your restless legs disturb your ability to carry out your daily activities, for example carrying out a satisfactory family, home, social, school or work life?
☐ Not at all ☐ A little ☐ Some ☐ Quite a bit ☐ A lot
14. Do you currently work full or part time (paid work, unpaid or volunteer)?
(mark one box)
☐ YES If Yes please answer questions #15 through #18
☐ NO, because of my RLS – Please go to the next page
☐ NO, due to other reasons – Please go to the next page
15. How often did restless legs make it difficult for you to work a full day in the past 4 weeks?
☐ Never ☐ A few times ☐ Sometimes ☐ Most of the time ☐ All the time
16. How many days in the past 4 weeks did you work less than you would like due to restless legs?
Write in number of days: ___
17. On the average, how many hours did you work in the past 4 weeks?
Write in number of hours per day: ___
18. On days you worked less than you would like, on average about how many hours less did you work due to your restless legs.
Write in number of hours per day: ___

Reference

1. Abetz, L., Vallow, S. M., Kirsch, J., Allen, R. P., Washburn, T., & Earley, C. J. (2005). Validation of the restless legs syndrome quality of life questionnaire. *Value in Health, 8*(2), 157–167.

Representative Studies Using Scale

Morgan, J. C., & Sethi, K. D. (2007). Efficacy and safety of pramipexole in restless legs syndrome. *Current Neurology and Neuroscience Reports, 7*(4), 273–277.

Richards–Campbell Sleep Questionnaire (RCSQ)

73

Purpose This five-item, visual analogue scale was designed as an outcome measure for assessing the perception of sleep in critically ill patients [1]. The scale evaluates perceptions of depth of sleep, sleep onset latency, number of awakenings, time spent awake, and overall sleep quality.

Population for Testing The scale has been validated in a population of critical care patients between the ages of 55 and 79 years.

Administration The scale is a self-report, paper-and-pencil measure requiring approximately 2 min for completion. Developers chose a visual analogue format to minimize the physical exertion and manual dexterity required to complete the scale [1]. Richards and colleagues also recommend that the directions and scale items should be read aloud to respondents as initial testing suggested that patients tended to experience some difficulties when no assistance was given.

Reliability and Validity In a psychometric evaluation of the RCSQ [1], researchers found an internal consistency of .90 and demonstrated that scores on the scale have a correlation of .58 with the same sleep variables as measured by PSG.

Obtaining a Copy A copy of the scale's items can be found in the original article published by developers [1].

Scoring For each item, respondents are given a visual analogue scale and are asked to place a mark on the line indicating where their own experiences fit between two extremes (for example, the degree to which they received a "good night's sleep" or "a bad night's sleep"). Scale lines extend from 0 to 100 mm, and scores are calculated by measuring where responses fall on each line. A total score is obtained by summing each score out of 100 and dividing the total by five. Lower scores indicate a poorer quality of sleep.

A. Shahid et al. (eds.), *STOP, THAT and One Hundred Other Sleep Scales*,
DOI 10.1007/978-1-4419-9893-4_73, © Springer Science+Business Media, LLC 2012

Richards Campbell Sleep Questionnaire

Code Number ____________	Date ____________

Each of these questions is answered by placing an "X" on the answer line. Place your "X" **anywhere** on the line that you feel **best** describes your sleep last night. The following are examples of the type of questions you are to answer.

EXAMPLE A

Right now I feel:

Very Sleepy X____ Not sleepy at all

If you were very sleepy, you would place an "X" as is shown at the beginning of the line next to the words "**Very Sleepy**

EXAMPLE B

Right now I feel:

Very Sleepy ____ Not sleepy at all

If you were somewhat sleepy, you would place an "X" near the center of the line. Mark the answer line near the center to indicate the answer "**Somewhat Sleepy**."

EXAMPLE C

Right now I feel:

Very Sleepy ____ Not sleepy at all

If you were not sleepy at all, you would place an "X" at the end of the line next to the words "**Not Sleepy At All**."

Please turn to the next page

You are now ready to begin to answer the questions. Place your "X" **anywhere** on the answer line that you feel **best** describes your sleep last night.

1. My sleep last night was:

Deep Sleep	________________	Light Sleep

2. Last night, the first time I got to sleep, I:

Fell Asleep Almost Immediately	________________	Just Never Could Fall Asleep

3. Last night I was:

Awake Very Little	________________	Awake All Night Long

4. Last night, when I woke up or was awakened, I:

Got Back To Sleep Immediately	________________	Couldn't Get Back To Sleep

5. I would describe my sleep last night as:

A Good Night's Sleep	________________	A Bad Night's Sleep

Richards Campbell Sleep Questionnaire

Scoring Directions

1. Scores may range from 0 (indicating the worst possible sleep) to 100 (indicating the best sleep).

   100 ________________ 0

2. A score for each question is given based on the length of the line in millimeters from the 0 point to the cross of the patient's "X".
3. The Total Sleep Score is derived by adding the individual scores for each question and dividing by five.

Reference

1. Richards, K. C., O'Sullivan, P. S., & Phillips, R. L. (2000). Measurement of sleep in critically ill patients. *Journal of Nursing Measurements, 8*(2), 131–144.

Representative Studies Using Scale

Nicholás, A., Aizpitarte, E., Irruarizaga, A., Vázquez, M., Margall, A., & Asiain, C. (2008). Perception of night-time sleep by surgical patients in an intensive care unit. *Nursing in Critical Care, 13*(1), 25–33.

Bourne, R. S., Mills, G. H., & Minelli, C. (2008) Melatonin therapy to improve nocturnal sleep in critically ill patients: encouraging results from a small randomised controlled trial. *Critical Care, 12*(2), R52.

Note: It should be noted that a once off use of a visual analogue scale is highly suspect. When used on a reported basis for a single subject it can be very informative.

School Sleep Habits Survey

74

Purpose The School Sleep Habits Survey is an eight-page, 63-item questionnaire designed to assess the sleep/wake habits and typical daytime functioning of high school students. As a thorough method for data collection, the survey allows researchers and clinicians alike to gather valuable demographic and behavioral information, including: sleep schedule regularity, school performance, daytime sleepiness, behavior problems, depressive mood, and bed times, rise times, and total sleep times for both weeknights and weekends [1].

Population for Testing The survey was originally administered to 3,000 high school students, grades 9–12.

Administration Requiring approximately 20 min for completion, the scale is a self-report, paper-and-pencil measure.

Reliability and Validity As a general survey designed for data collection and not diagnostic or evaluative purposes, the scale's psychometric properties have been analyzed only minimally. In a study by Carskadon and colleagues [2], researchers evaluated three of the survey's subscales. The sleepiness scale was found to have an internal consistency of .70, the sleep/wake problem behaviors scale had an internal consistency of .75, and the depressive mood scale had an internal consistency of .79 – a finding in line with the results of a previous study conducted by the subscale's original developers [3].

Obtaining a Copy The scale is available online from the Sleep for Science Sleep Research Lab: http://www.sleepforscience.org/contentmgr/showdetails.php/id/93.

Direct correspondence to:
Amy R. Wolfson
College of the Holy Cross, Department of Psychology
Worcester, MA 01610, USA
Email: awolfson@holycross.edu

Scoring In addition to collecting demographic information, the survey queries respondents about their sleeping and waking behaviors over the course of the previous 2 weeks. Each section of the survey employs a different response method. The section relating to sleepiness asks respondents to indicate whether or not they had struggled to remain awake in 10 different situations on a scale ranging from 1 ("no") to 4 ("both struggled to stay awake and fallen asleep"). Total scores on this scale can range from 10 to 40, with higher scores indicating greater sleepiness. The sleep/wake problem behaviors scale queries the frequency of 10 different behaviors using a scale that ranges from 5 ("everyday") to 1 ("never"), with possible total scores ranging from 10 to 50. Finally, the depressive mood scale consists of six items, with a response scale ranging from 1 ("not at all") to 3 ("somewhat too much"). Higher scores on this scale indicate more acute depressive symptoms. These subscales may be used separately to aid in diagnosis or they can be considered in relation to other survey information collected.

A. Shahid et al. (eds.), *STOP, THAT and One Hundred Other Sleep Scales*,
DOI 10.1007/978-1-4419-9893-4_74, © Springer Science+Business Media, LLC 2012

Bradley Hospital

School Sleep Habits Survey

INSTRUCTIONS

Please answer the questions on the following pages as accurately and honestly as you can. There are no right or wrong answers.

- **When you mark a response, please be sure to mark it neatly.**
- **Darken the bubbles as completely as possible using a pencil.**
- **Avoid stray marks and treat forms gently.**
- **Do not spend too much time on any one answer. Your first impression is usually best.**
- **Answer each question in the order that it appears. Do not go back and check your answers.**
- **Place an X beside any item that YOU DO NOT UNDERSTAND or that DOES NOT APPLY TO YOU or for which you CANNOT GIVE A TRUTHFUL ANSWER.**
- **Be sure to complete BOTH SIDES of every page.**

1. Today's Date:

Month	Day		Year	
○ Jan				
○ Feb				
○ Mar	⓪	⓪	⓪	⓪
○ April	①	①	①	①
○ May	②	②	②	②
○ June	③	③	③	③
○ July		④	④	④
○ Aug		⑤	⑤	⑤
○ Sept		⑥	⑥	⑥
○ Oct		⑦	⑦	⑦
○ Nov		⑧	⑧	⑧
○ Dec		⑨	⑨	⑨

2. Birth Date:

Month	Day		Year	
○ Jan				
○ Feb				
○ Mar	⓪	⓪	⓪	⓪
○ April	①	①	①	①
○ May	②	②	②	②
○ June	③	③	③	③
○ July		④	④	④
○ Aug		⑤	⑤	⑤
○ Sept		⑥	⑥	⑥
○ Oct		⑦	⑦	⑦
○ Nov		⑧	⑧	⑧
○ Dec		⑨	⑨	⑨

3. What time is it now? __________ ○ A.M. ○ P.M.

4. What is your sex?
○ Male
○ Female

5. What is your height?______ **feet** ______ **inches**

6. What is your weight?______ **pounds**

7. What is your age in years?
○ 9 ○ 10 ○ 11 ○ 12 ○ 13 ○ 14 ○ 15 ○ 16 ○ 17 ○ 18 ○ 19

8. What grade are you in?
○ 4 ○ 5 ○ 6 ○ 7 ○ 8 ○ 9 ○ 10 ○ 11 ○ 12

FOR OFFICE USE ONLY

3				5			6		
⓪	⓪	⓪	⓪	⓪	⓪	⓪	⓪	⓪	⓪
①	①	①	①	①	①	①	①	①	①
②	②	②	②	②	②	②	②	②	②
③	③	③	③	③	③	③	③	③	③
④	④	④	④	④	④	④	④	④	④
⑤	⑤	⑤	⑤	⑤	⑤	⑤	⑤	⑤	⑤
⑥	⑥	⑥	⑥	⑥	⑥	⑥	⑥	⑥	⑥
⑦	⑦	⑦	⑦	⑦	⑦	⑦	⑦	⑦	⑦
⑧	⑧	⑧	⑧	⑧	⑧	⑧	⑧	⑧	⑧
⑨	⑨	⑨	⑨	⑨	⑨	⑨	⑨	⑨	⑨

00381
DO NOT WRITE IN THIS AREA

9. What best describes your racial/ethnic background?
- ◯ White/Caucasian
- ◯ Black/African American
- ◯ Hispanic/Latino
- ◯ Asian/Asian American
- ◯ Native American/Amerindian
- ◯ Multiracial (please specify) ____________
- ◯ Other (please specify) ____________

10. In the last two weeks, have you slept in the same bed?
- ◯ Every night
- ◯ Almost every night
- ◯ A few nights
- ◯ Not at all

11. Who lives in your home other than you? Please indicate yes or no for every category below:

	Yes	No
Mother/step-mother	◯	◯
Father/step-father	◯	◯
Older brother(s)/sister(s)	◯	◯
Younger brother(s)/sister(s)	◯	◯
Other family member(s)	◯	◯

12. Does your mother work outside of the home?
- ◯ Yes
- ◯ No

If yes, mark each label that best describes her work:

◯ Day shift	◯ Full time
◯ Evening shift	◯ Part time
◯ Night shift (graveyard)	◯ One job
◯ Changing shifts	◯ More than one job

13. Does your father work outside of the home?
- ◯ Yes
- ◯ No

If yes, mark each label that best describes his work:

◯ Day shift	◯ Full time
◯ Evening shift	◯ Part time
◯ Night shift (graveyard)	◯ One job
◯ Changing shifts	◯ More than one job

14. Are your grades in school mostly?:

◯ A's	◯ C's
◯ A's and B's	◯ C's and D's
◯ B's	◯ D's
◯ B's and C's	◯ D's and F's

15. What is the highest grade in school you expect to complete? (mark one)
- ◯ May not finish high school
- ◯ Will finish high school
- ◯ Will get a college degree
- ◯ Will get a degree beyond college

16. Do you have any disabilities or chronic illnesses (for example, asthma, diabetes, deafness, loss of the use of a limb, etc.)?
- ◯ Yes
- ◯ No

If yes, please specify: ____________

17. Compared to other people your age, would you say that your health is:
- ◯ Poor
- ◯ Fair
- ◯ Good
- ◯ Excellent

18. Do you have attention deficit hyperactivity disorder (ADHD) or a learning disability?
- ◯ Yes
- ◯ No

19. Do you take Ritalin or some other medication to help with concentration or a learning problem?
- ◯ Yes
- ◯ No

20. Do you have an individualized education program or receive special help for difficulties with school work?
- ◯ Yes
- ◯ No

21. During the last two weeks, how many days did you stay home from school because you were:

a. sick?	⓪ ① ② ③ ④ ⑤ ⑥ ⑦ ⑧ ⑨ ⑩
b. other?	⓪ ① ② ③ ④ ⑤ ⑥ ⑦ ⑧ ⑨ ⑩

Why did you stay home from school?

____

FOR OFFICE USE ONLY	21	
	⓪	⓪
	①	①
	②	②
	③	③
	④	④
	⑤	⑤
	⑥	⑥
	⑦	⑦
	⑧	⑧
	⑨	⑨

ID NUMBER			
⓪	⓪	⓪	⓪
①	①	①	①
②	②	②	②
③	③	③	③
④	④	④	④
⑤	⑤	⑤	⑤
⑥	⑥	⑥	⑥
⑦	⑦	⑦	⑦
⑧	⑧	⑧	⑧
⑨	⑨	⑨	⑨

There are no right or wrong answers. Be careful to choose the **one** answer that **best** describes the way your sleep has been in the last two school weeks (unless otherwise instructed).

The next set of questions has to do with your usual schedule on days when you have school.

22. What time do you usually go to bed on school days?

List ONE time, not a range.

______________ ○ A.M. ○ P.M.

23. There are many reasons for doing things at one time or another. What is the main reason you usually go to bed at this time on school days? (mark one)

- ○ My parents have set my bedtime
- ○ I feel sleepy
- ○ I finish my homework
- ○ My TV shows are over
- ○ My brother(s) or sister(s) go to bed
- ○ I finish socializing
- ○ I get home from my job
- ○ Other: ______________

24. What time do you usually wake up on school days?

______________ ○ A.M. ○ P.M.

25. What is the main reason you usually wake up at this time on school days? (choose one)

- ○ Noises or my pet wakes me up
- ○ My alarm clock wakes me up
- ○ My parents or other family members wake me up
- ○ I need to go to the bathroom
- ○ I don't know, I just wake up
- ○ Other: ______________

26. What time do you usually leave home on school days?

______________ ○ A.M. ○ P.M.

27. How do you usually get to school?

- ○ Walk
- ○ Take the bus
- ○ Get a ride with parent
- ○ Get a ride with friend(s)
- ○ Drive my car

28. Figure out how long you usually sleep on a normal school night and fill it in here. [Do not include time you spend awake in bed. Remember to mark hours and minutes, even if minutes are zero.]

________ hours ________ minutes

29. On school days, after you go to bed at night, about how long does it usually take you to fall asleep?

________ minutes

The next set of questions has to do with your usual schedule on days when you do not have school, such as on the weekend.

30. What time do you usually go to bed on weekends?

______________ ○ A.M. ○ P.M.

31. There are many reasons for doing things at one time or another. What is the main reason you usually go to bed at this time on weekends? (choose one)

- ○ My parents have set my bedtime
- ○ I feel sleepy
- ○ I finish my homework
- ○ My TV shows are over
- ○ My brother(s) or sister(s) go to bed then
- ○ I finish socializing
- ○ I get home from my job
- ○ Other: ______________

FOR OFFICE USE ONLY

22 Hour Min. **24 Hour Min.** **26 Hour Min.**

28 Hour Min. **29 Minutes** **30 Hour Min.**

00381

DO NOT WRITE IN THIS AREA

32. What time do you usually wake up on weekends?

________________ ◯ A.M. ◯ P.M.

33. What is the main reason you usually wake up at this time on weekends? (choose one)
- ◯ Noises or my pet wakes me up
- ◯ My alarm clock wakes me up
- ◯ My parents wake me up
- ◯ I need to go to the bathroom
- ◯ I don't know, I just wake up
- ◯ Other: ________________

34. Figure out how long you usually sleep on a night when you do not have school the next day (such as a weekend night) and fill it in here. [Do not include time you spend awake in bed. Remember to mark hours and minutes, even if minutes are zero.]

________ hours ________ minutes

35. On weekends, after you go to bed at night, about how long does it usually take you to fall asleep?

________ minutes

36. Some people wake up during the night. Others never do. How many times do you usually wake up at night?
- ◯ Never
- ◯ Once
- ◯ 2 or 3 times
- ◯ More than 3 times
- ◯ I have no idea

37. People sometimes feel sleepy during the daytime. During your daytime activities, how much of a problem do you have with sleepiness (feeling sleepy, struggling to stay awake)?
- ◯ No problem at all
- ◯ A little problem
- ◯ More than a little problem
- ◯ A big problem
- ◯ A very big problem

38. Some people take naps in the daytime every day, others never do. When do you nap? (mark all that apply.)
- ◯ I never nap.
- ◯ I sometimes nap on school days.
- ◯ I sometimes nap on weekends.
- ◯ I never nap unless I am sick.

39. Can you figure out how much sleep you need? Fill out below how much sleep you think you would need each night to feel your best every day. [Remember to mark hours and minutes, even if minutes are zero.]

________ hours ________ minutes

40. In general, do you feel you usually get . . .
- ◯ too much sleep?
- ◯ enough sleep?
- ◯ too little sleep?

41. Do you consider yourself to be . . .
- ◯ a good sleeper?
- ◯ a poor sleeper?

42. How often do you think that you get enough sleep?
- ◯ Always
- ◯ Usually
- ◯ Sometimes
- ◯ Rarely
- ◯ Never

FOR OFFICE USE ONLY

32 Hour Min.

0	0	0	0
1	1	1	1
	2	2	2
	3	3	3
	4	4	4
	5	5	5
	6		6
	7		7
	8		8
	9		9

34 Hour Min.

0	0	0	0
1	1	1	1
	2	2	2
	3	3	3
	4	4	4
	5	5	5
	6		6
	7		7
	8		8
	9		9

35 Minutes

0	0	0
1	1	1
2	2	2
3	3	3
4	4	4
5	5	5
6	6	6
7	7	7
8	8	8
9	9	9

39 Hour Min.

0	0	0	0
1	1	1	1
	2	2	2
	3	3	3
	4	4	4
	5	5	5
	6		6
	7		7
	8		8
	9		9

ID Number

0	0	0	0
1	1	1	1
2	2	2	2
3	3	3	3
4	4	4	4
5	5	5	5
6	6	6	6
7	7	7	7
8	8	8	8
9	9	9	9

Questions 43 to 46 are about things that have happened in the last two weeks.

43. During the last two weeks, have you struggled to stay awake (fought sleep) or fallen asleep in the following situations? (Mark <u>one</u> answer for <u>every</u> item.)

Both struggled to stay awake and fallen asleep
Fallen asleep
Struggled to stay awake
No

- in a face-to-face conversation with another person? ○○○○
- traveling in a bus, train, plane or car? ○○○○
- attending a performance (movie, concert, play)? ○○○○
- watching television or listening to the radio or stereo? ○○○○
- reading, studying or doing homework? ○○○○
- during a test? ○○○○
- in a class at school? ○○○○
- while doing work on a computer or typewriter? ○○○○
- playing video games? ○○○○
- driving a car? ○○○○

Do you drive? ○ Yes
○ No

44. During the last two weeks, how often did you . . . (<u>Mark one answer for every item</u>.)

Every day
Several times every day
Once or twice a day
Never

a. drink soda with caffeine [like Coke, Pepsi; <u>not</u> like root beer, orange soda or Sprite]? ○○○○
b. drink coffee or tea with caffeine? ○○○○
c. use tobacco? [cigarettes, cigar, chewing tobacco, etc.]? ○○○○
d. drink alcohol [beer, wine, liquor]? ○○○○
e. use drugs [like marijuana, cocaine]? ○○○○
please specify type:

____

45. In the last two weeks, how often have you . . . (<u>Mark one answer for every item</u>.)

Never
Once
Twice
Several times
Everyday/night

a. felt satisfied with your sleep? ○○○○○
b. arrived late to class because you overslept? ○○○○○
c. fallen asleep in a morning class? ○○○○○
d. fallen asleep in an afternoon class? ○○○○○
e. awakened too early in the morning and couldn't get back to sleep? ○○○○○
f. stayed up until at least 3 a.m.? ○○○○○
g. stayed up all night? ○○○○○
h. slept in past noon? ○○○○○
i. felt tired, dragged out, or sleepy during the day? ○○○○○
j. needed more than one reminder to get up in the morning? ○○○○○
k. had an extremely hard time falling asleep? ○○○○○
l. had nightmares or bad dreams during the night? ○○○○○
m. gone to bed because you just could not stay awake any longer? ○○○○○
n. done dangerous things without thinking? ○○○○○
o. had a good night's sleep? ○○○○○

46. During the last two weeks, how often were you bothered or trouble by the following?

Much
Somewhat
Not at all

a. Feeling too tired to do things ○○○
b. Having trouble going to sleep or staying asleep ○○○
c. Feeling unhappy, sad, or depressed ○○○
d. Feeling hopeless about the future ○○○
e. Feeling nervous or tense ○○○
f. Worrying too much about things ○○○

ID Number

0	0	0	0
1	1	1	1
2	2	2	2
3	3	3	3
4	4	4	4
5	5	5	5
6	6	6	6
7	7	7	7
8	8	8	8
9	9	9	9

Questions 47 - 56 have to do with how you might organize the timing of various activities if you were free to plan your day according to when you feel your best. Please answer the questions based on your body's "feeling best" times.

47. Imagine: School is cancelled! You can get up whenever you want to. When would you get out of bed? Between:
- ◯ 5:00 and 6:30 a.m.
- ◯ 6:30 and 7:45 a.m.
- ◯ 7:45 and 9:45 a.m.
- ◯ 9:45 and 11:00 a.m.
- ◯ 11:00 a.m. and noon

48. Is it easy for you to get up in the morning?
- ◯ No way!
- ◯ Sort of.
- ◯ Pretty easy.
- ◯ It's a cinch!

49. Gym class is set for 7:00 in the morning. How do you think you'll do?
- ◯ My best!
- ◯ Okay.
- ◯ Worse than usual.
- ◯ Awful!

50. The bad news: You have to take a two-hour test. The good news: You can take it when you think you'll do your best. What time is that?
- ◯ 8:00 to 10:00 a.m.
- ◯ 11:00 a.m. to 1:00 p.m.
- ◯ 3:00 p.m. to 5:00 pm.
- ◯ 7:00 p.m. to 9:00 p.m.

51. When do you have the most energy to do your favorite things?
- ◯ Morning! I am tired in the evening.
- ◯ Morning more than evening.
- ◯ Evening more than morning.
- ◯ Evening! I am tired in the morning.

52. Your parents have decided to let you set your own bed time. What time would you pick? Between:
- ◯ 8:00 and 9:00 p.m.
- ◯ 9:00 and 10:15 p.m.
- ◯ 10:15 p.m. and 12:30 a.m.
- ◯ 12:30 and 1:45 a.m.
- ◯ 1:45 and 3:00 a.m.

53. How alert are you in the first half hour you're up?
- ◯ Out of it.
- ◯ A little dazed.
- ◯ Okay.
- ◯ Ready to take on the world.

54. When does your body start to tell you it's time for bed (even if you ignore it)? Between:
- ◯ 8:00 and 9:00 p.m.
- ◯ 9:00 and 10:15 p.m.
- ◯ 10:15 p.m. and 12:30 a.m.
- ◯ 12:30 and 1:45 a.m.
- ◯ 1:45 and 3:00 a.m.

55. Say you had to get up at 6:00 a.m. every morning: What would it be like?
- ◯ Awful!
- ◯ Not so great.
- ◯ Okay (if I have to).
- ◯ Fine, no problem!

56. When you wake up in the morning how long does it take for you to be totally "with it"?
- ◯ 0 to 10 minutes
- ◯ 11 to 20 minutes
- ◯ 21 to 40 minutes
- ◯ More than 40 minutes

57. Would you say that your growth in height:
- ◯ Has not begun to spurt ("spurt" means faster growth than usual)
- ◯ Has barely started
- ◯ Is definitely underway
- ◯ Seems complete
- ◯ I don't know

58. Would you say that your other signs of physical maturation:
- ◯ Have not yet started to show
- ◯ Have barely started to show
- ◯ Are definitely underway
- ◯ Seem complete
- ◯ I don't know

0 0	0 0	0 0	0 0	0 0	0 0	0 0	0 0
1 1	1 1	1 1	1 1	1 1	1 1	1 1	1 1
2 2	2 2	2 2	2 2	2 2	2 2	2 2	2 2
3 3	3 3	3 3	3 3	3 3	3 3	3 3	3 3
4 4	4 4	4 4	4 4	4 4	4 4	4 4	4 4
5 5	5 5	5 5	5 5	5 5	5 5	5 5	5 5
6 6	6 6	6 6	6 6	6 6	6 6	6 6	6 6
7 7	7 7	7 7	7 7	7 7	7 7	7 7	7 7
8 8	8 8	8 8	8 8	8 8	8 8	8 8	8 8
9 9	9 9	9 9	9 9	9 9	9 9	9 9	9 9

00381

DO NOT WRITE IN THIS AREA

59. During the last week, did you work at a job for pay? (If no, skip to number 60.)
◯ Yes ◯ No

What kind of job? ______________________

How many days did you work at the following times?
in the morning before school .... ⓪ ① ② ③ ④ ⑤
in the afternoon after school .... ⓪ ① ② ③ ④ ⑤
in the evening on days that you have school .. ⓪ ① ② ③ ④ ⑤
on the weekend .... ⓪ ① ②

How many hours did you work at your paying job this week?

during the school week: _________ **hours**

during the weekend: _________ **hours**

During the last two weeks, have you struggled to stay awake (fought sleep) or fallen asleep at your job?
◯ no ◯ struggled to stay awake
◯ fallen asleep ◯ both struggled to stay awake and fallen asleep

If you did not have your job, would you go to bed:
◯ earlier than you do. ◯ the same as you do.
◯ later than you do.

If you did not have your job, would you wake up:
◯ earlier than you do. ◯ the same as you do.
◯ later than you do.

60. During the last week, did you engage in organized sports or a regularly scheduled physical activity? (If no, skip to number 61.)
◯ Yes ◯ No

What kind of sport? ______________________

How many days did you practice at the following times?
in the morning before school .... ⓪ ① ② ③ ④ ⑤
in the afternoon after school .... ⓪ ① ② ③ ④ ⑤
in the evening on days that you have school .. ⓪ ① ② ③ ④ ⑤
on the weekend .... ⓪ ① ②

How many hours did you practice this week?

during the school week: _________ **hours**

during the weekend: _________ **hours**

During the last two weeks, have you struggled to stay awake (fought sleep) or fallen asleep during practice?
◯ no ◯ struggled to stay awake
◯ fallen asleep ◯ both struggled to stay awake and fallen asleep

If you did not have your sports activity, would you go to bed:
◯ earlier than you do. ◯ the same as you do.
◯ later than you do.

If you did not have your sports activity, would you wake up:
◯ earlier than you do. ◯ the same as you do.
◯ later than you do.

61. During the last week, did you participate in organized extracurricular activities? (For example, committees, clubs, volunteer work, musical groups, church groups, etc.) (If no, skip to number 62.)
◯ Yes ◯ No

What kind of activity? ______________________

How many days did you participate at the following times?
in the morning before school .... ⓪ ① ② ③ ④ ⑤
in the afternoon after school .... ⓪ ① ② ③ ④ ⑤
in the evening on days that you have school .. ⓪ ① ② ③ ④ ⑤
on the weekend .... ⓪ ① ②

How many hours did you participate this week?

during the school week: _________ **hours**

during the weekend: _________ **hours**

During the last two weeks, have you struggled to stay awake (fought sleep) or fallen asleep during this participation?
◯ no ◯ struggled to stay awake
◯ fallen asleep ◯ both struggled to stay awake and fallen asleep

If you did not have your organized activity, would you go to bed:
◯ earlier than you do. ◯ the same as you do.
◯ later than you do.

If you did not have your organized activity, would you wake up:
◯ earlier than you do. ◯ the same as you do.
◯ later than you do.

62. During the last week, did you study/do homework?
◯ Yes ◯ No (If no, skip to number 63.)

How many days did you study at the following times?
in the morning before school .... ⓪ ① ② ③ ④ ⑤
in the afternoon after school .... ⓪ ① ② ③ ④ ⑤
in the evening on days that you have school .. ⓪ ① ② ③ ④ ⑤
on the weekend .... ⓪ ① ②

How many hours did you study this week?

during the school week: _________ **hours**

during the weekend: _________ **hours**

During the last two weeks, have you struggled to stay awake (fought sleep) or fallen asleep during studying?
◯ no ◯ struggled to stay awake
◯ fallen asleep ◯ both struggled to stay awake and fallen asleep

If you did not have your homework, would you go to bed:
◯ earlier than you do. ◯ the same as you do.
◯ later than you do.

If you did not have your homework, would you wake up:
◯ earlier than you do. ◯ the same as you do.
◯ later than you do.

FOR OFFICE USE ONLY
ID NUMBER

⓪	⓪	⓪	⓪
①	①	①	①
②	②	②	②
③	③	③	③
④	④	④	④
⑤	⑤	⑤	⑤
⑥	⑥	⑥	⑥
⑦	⑦	⑦	⑦
⑧	⑧	⑧	⑧
⑨	⑨	⑨	⑨

63. Below are some ways that people get hurt or injured. If you answer Yes in the first column to any item, please fill in an answer to each of the follow-up questions. IN THE PAST 6 MONTHS:

	Were you injured this way?	IF YES, then: Were you treated by a doctor or nurse for the injury?	Did this injury limit your physical activity?	Had you been drinking alcohol or using drugs at the time of the injury?	Where did the injury occur? H = home W = work S = school O = other
	Yes No	Yes No	Yes No	Yes No	
A. By being in a physical fight with someone?	Ⓨ Ⓝ	If Yes: Ⓨ Ⓝ	Ⓨ Ⓝ	Ⓨ Ⓝ	Ⓗ Ⓦ Ⓢ Ⓞ
B. By getting cut?	Ⓨ Ⓝ	If Yes: Ⓨ Ⓝ	Ⓨ Ⓝ	Ⓨ Ⓝ	Ⓗ Ⓦ Ⓢ Ⓞ
C. By a gun, BB gun, or pellet gun?	Ⓨ Ⓝ	If Yes: Ⓨ Ⓝ	Ⓨ Ⓝ	Ⓨ Ⓝ	Ⓗ Ⓦ Ⓢ Ⓞ
D. By being hit by something, like a rock or glass?	Ⓨ Ⓝ	If Yes: Ⓨ Ⓝ	Ⓨ Ⓝ	Ⓨ Ⓝ	Ⓗ Ⓦ Ⓢ Ⓞ
E. By nearly drowning?	Ⓨ Ⓝ	If Yes: Ⓨ Ⓝ	Ⓨ Ⓝ	Ⓨ Ⓝ	Ⓗ Ⓦ Ⓢ Ⓞ
F. By falling?	Ⓨ Ⓝ	If Yes: Ⓨ Ⓝ	Ⓨ Ⓝ	Ⓨ Ⓝ	Ⓗ Ⓦ Ⓢ Ⓞ
G. By being burned by fire, chemicals, electricity, or hot liquids?	Ⓨ Ⓝ	If Yes: Ⓨ Ⓝ	Ⓨ Ⓝ	Ⓨ Ⓝ	Ⓗ Ⓦ Ⓢ Ⓞ
H. By an animal bite or serious insect bite?	Ⓨ Ⓝ	If Yes: Ⓨ Ⓝ	Ⓨ Ⓝ	Ⓨ Ⓝ	Ⓗ Ⓦ Ⓢ Ⓞ
I. While driving a car, truck, or bus?	Ⓨ Ⓝ	If Yes: Ⓨ Ⓝ	Ⓨ Ⓝ	Ⓨ Ⓝ	Ⓗ Ⓦ Ⓢ Ⓞ
J. While riding in a car, truck, or bus?	Ⓨ Ⓝ	If Yes: Ⓨ Ⓝ	Ⓨ Ⓝ	Ⓨ Ⓝ	Ⓗ Ⓦ Ⓢ Ⓞ
K. While riding a bicycle, skateboard, rollerblades, or rollerskates?	Ⓨ Ⓝ	If Yes: Ⓨ Ⓝ	Ⓨ Ⓝ	Ⓨ Ⓝ	Ⓗ Ⓦ Ⓢ Ⓞ
L. While riding a moped, motorcycle, all-terrain vehicle (ATV), or snowmobile?	Ⓨ Ⓝ	If Yes: Ⓨ Ⓝ	Ⓨ Ⓝ	Ⓨ Ⓝ	Ⓗ Ⓦ Ⓢ Ⓞ
M. During a team sport, athletic activity, or exercise?	Ⓨ Ⓝ	If Yes: Ⓨ Ⓝ	Ⓨ Ⓝ	Ⓨ Ⓝ	Ⓗ Ⓦ Ⓢ Ⓞ
N. By being hit by a moving vehicle while walking?	Ⓨ Ⓝ	If Yes: Ⓨ Ⓝ	Ⓨ Ⓝ	Ⓨ Ⓝ	Ⓗ Ⓦ Ⓢ Ⓞ
O. By drinking or eating a dangerous substance?	Ⓨ Ⓝ	If Yes: Ⓨ Ⓝ	Ⓨ Ⓝ	Ⓨ Ⓝ	Ⓗ Ⓦ Ⓢ Ⓞ
P. By being physically attacked?	Ⓨ Ⓝ	If Yes: Ⓨ Ⓝ	Ⓨ Ⓝ	Ⓨ Ⓝ	Ⓗ Ⓦ Ⓢ Ⓞ
Q. Injured in some other way?	Ⓨ Ⓝ	If Yes: Ⓨ Ⓝ	Ⓨ Ⓝ	Ⓨ Ⓝ	Ⓗ Ⓦ Ⓢ Ⓞ

If yes to Q, please describe how you were injured: ______________________

____

FOR OFFICE USE ONLY
⓪ ① ② ③ ④ ⑤ ⑥ ⑦ ⑧ ⑨
⓪ ① ② ③ ④ ⑤ ⑥ ⑦ ⑧ ⑨

00381

DO NOT WRITE IN THIS AREA

R8492-PFI-54321

References

1. Wolfson, A. R., Carskadon, M. A. (1998). Sleep schedules and daytime functioning in adolescents. *Child Development, 69*(4), 875–887.
2. Carskadon, M. A., Seifer, R., & Acebo, C. (1991). Reliability of six scales in a sleep questionnaire for adolescents. *Sleep Research, 20*, 421.
3. Kandel, D. B., & Davies, M. (1982). Epidemiology of depressive mood in adolescents. *Archives of General Psychiatry, 39*, 1205–1212.

Representative Studies Using Scale

Russo, P. M., Bruni, O., Fabio, L., Ferri, R., & Violani, C. (2007). Sleep habits and circadian preference in Italian children and adolescents. *Journal of Sleep Research, 16*(2), 163–169.

Yang, C. K., Kim, J. K., Patel, S. R., & Lee J. H. (2005). Age-related changes in sleep/wake patterns among Korean teenagers. *Pediatrics, 115*(1), 250–256.

75 Self-Efficacy Measure for Sleep Apnea (SEMSA)

Purpose The SEMSA was developed in response to research indicating that cognitive factors like self-efficacy can significantly predict compliance with continuous positive airway pressure (CPAP), even in the first week of treatment [1]. The scale consists of 26 items and evaluates three cognitive subscales: the perceived risk of obstructive sleep apnea, CPAP outcome expectations, and treatment self-efficacy. By examining these cognitive issues prior to treatment, clinicians can identify those patients with low levels of self-efficacy and initiate educational interventions to improve treatment outcomes.

Population for Testing The scale has been evaluated in a study of participants with a mean age of 47.7 ± 12.3 years.

Administration The SEMSA is a self-administered, paper-and-pencil measure requiring approximately 15 min for completion.

Reliability and Validity In a psychometric evaluation conducted by Weaver and colleagues [2], the scale was found to have an internal consistency of .92 and a test–retest reliability ranging from .68 to .77.

Obtaining a Copy An example of the scale's items can be found in the original article published by developers [2].

Direct correspondence to:
Terri E. Weaver
University of Pennsylvania School of Nursing
420 Guardian Drive
Philadelphia, PA 19104-6096, USA
Email: tew@nursing.upen.edu

Scoring Respondents use a four-point, Likert-type scale ranging from 1 to 4 to indicate their agreement with statements regarding the risks of OSA, their expectations for treatment, and their dedication to CPAP therapy. For each of the instrument's subscales, resulting scores indicate different things. High scores on the perceived risk scale denote greater perceived risks of OSA; high scores on the outcome expectations scale denote more positive beliefs about treatment; high scores on the treatment self-efficacy scale denote a greater willingness to engage in CPAP treatment despite certain obstacles. These three scores can be used to target specific patient cognitions that could potentially hinder treatment outcomes.

A. Shahid et al. (eds.), *STOP, THAT and One Hundred Other Sleep Scales*,
DOI 10.1007/978-1-4419-9893-4_75, © Springer Science+Business Media, LLC 2012

Self-Efficacy Measure for Sleep Apnea (SEMSA)

Here are some sample questions from the scale.

My chances of having high blood pressure compared to people my own age and sex who do not have sleep apnea are:

Very low	Low	High	Very high
❑	❑	❑	❑

My chances of falling asleep while driving compared to people my own age and sex who do not have sleep apnea are:

Very low	Low	High	Very high
❑	❑	❑	❑

If I use CPAP then I will not snore.

Not at all true	Barely true	Somewhat true	Very true
❑	❑	❑	❑

If I do not use CPAP I will be less alert during the day.

Not at all true	Barely true	Somewhat true	Very true
❑	❑	❑	❑

I would use CPAP, even if I have to wear a tight mask on my face at night.

Not at all true	Barely true	Somewhat true	Very true
❑	❑	❑	❑

I would use CPAP, even if it made my nose stuffy.

Not at all true	Barely true	Somewhat true	Very true
❑	❑	❑	❑

References

1. Stepnowky, C. J., Marler, M. R., & Ancoli-Israel, S. (2002). Determinants of nasal CPAP compliance. *Sleep Medicine, 3*(3), 239–247.
2. Weaver, T. E., Maislin, G., Dinges, D. F., Younger, J., Cantor, C., McCloskey, S., & Pack, A. I. (2003). Obstructive sleep apnea risk: instrument development and patient perceptions of obstructive sleep apnea risk, treatment benefit, and volition to use continuous positive airway pressure. *Sleep, 26*(6), 727–732.

Representative Studies Using Scale

Olsen, S., Smith, S., Oei, T., & Douglas, J. (2008). Health belief models predicts adherence to CPAP before experience with CPAP. *European Respiratory Journal, 32*(3), 710–717.

Baron, K. G., Smith, T. W., Czajkowski, L. A., Gunn, H. E., & Joes, H. R. (2009). Relationship quality and CPAP adherence in patients with obstructive sleep apnea. *Behavioral Sleep Medicine, 7*(1), 22–36.

76 SF-36 Health Survey

Purpose Consisting of 36 items, the SF-36 is a brief survey designed to assess functional health and well-being in a variety of age, disease, and control populations [1]. Each question relates to one of eight domains: physical functioning, role-physical, bodily pain, general health perceptions, vitality, social functioning, role-emotional, and mental health. Results from these subscales contribute to scores for overall physical and mental health. As the scale is sensitive to change, its developers recommend it particularly for assessing treatment outcomes. The most recent version, Version 2.0, was designed to improve the wording and layout of the survey and to simplify its use.

Population for Testing The survey is intended for adults 18 and older.

Administration The SF-36 is a self-report measure requiring between 5 and 10 min for completion. QualityMetric, an organization created by the survey's developers, has made the survey available in a variety of formats. It can be administered by interview, online, by fax, and using traditional pencil and paper. In order to use the SF-36, permission must be obtained from QualityMetric. Licenses are granted following the submission and review of a "Survey Information Request Form." A short-form version is also available.

Reliability and Validity Though a number of studies examining the scale's psychometric properties have been conducted, one of the largest involved a sample of more than 3,000 participants [2]. Researchers found an internal consistency ranging from .78 to .93, and demonstrated powerful item-discriminant validity – for 99.5% of all tests, items were highly correlated with the scales to which they belonged. The SF-36's user manual [3] also lists subscale reliability scores as ranging from .68 to .93.

Obtaining a Copy The scale is under copyright and can be purchased through QualityMetric at http://www.qualitymetric.com/.

Scoring Respondents use Likert-type scales to rate the quality of their health and to indicate how it has affected their daily functioning over the course of the past month. The scale uses norm-based scoring where scores of 50 are considered average, with scores of 0 being the lowest and 100 being the highest. Each item is weighted equally, so it is not necessary to standardize them. User's manuals that describe the scoring process in detail can be purchased from QualityMetric, along with scoring software that will perform calculations electronically.

References

1. Ware, J. E. *SF-36® Health Survey Update*. Retrieved June 19, 2009, from http://www.sf-36.org/tools/sf36.shtml.
2. McHorney, C. A., Ware, J. E., Lu, J. F. R., & Sherbourne, C. D. (1994). The MOS 36-Item Short-Form Health Survey (SF-36): III. tests of data quality, scaling assumptions and reliability across diverse patient groups. *Medical Care, 32*(1), 40–66.

A. Shahid et al. (eds.), *STOP, THAT and One Hundred Other Sleep Scales*,
DOI 10.1007/978-1-4419-9893-4_76, © Springer Science+Business Media, LLC 2012

3. Ware, J. E., Kosinski, M., & Keller, S. K. (1994). *SF-36 Physical and Mental Health Summary Scales: A User's Manual.* Boston: The Health Institute.

Representative Studies Using Scale

Baldwin, C. M., Griffith, K. A., Nieto, F. J., O'Connor, G. T., Walsleben, J. A., & Redline, S. (2001). The association of sleep-disordered breathing and sleep symptoms with quality of life in the sleep heart health study. *Sleep, 24*(1), 96–105.

Manocchia, M., Keller, S., & Ware, J. E. (2001). Sleep problems, health-related quality of life, work functioning and health care utilization among the chronically ill. *Quality of Life Research, 10*(4), 331–345.

Ramsawh, H. J., Stein, M. B., Belik, S. L., Jacobi, F., & Sareen, J. (2009). Relationship of anxiety disorders, sleep quality, and functional impairment in a community sample. *Journal of Psychiatric Research, 43*(10), 926–933.

77 Sleep-50 Questionnaire

Purpose The SLEEP-50 consists to 50 items designed to screen for a variety of sleep disorders in the general population. The scale consists of nine subscales, reflecting some of the most common disorders and complaints related to sleep and the factors required for diagnosis with the *DSM-IV*: sleep apnea, insomnia, narcolepsy, restless legs/periodic leg movement disorder, circadian rhythm sleep disorder, sleepwalking, nightmares, factors influencing sleep, and the impact of sleep complaints on daily functioning [1].

Population for Testing The scale has been validated in a population of sleep clinic patients with a mean age of 47.6 ± 12.2 years and in a group of college students with a mean age of 22.3 ± 3.4 years.

Administration The SLEEP-50 is a self-report, paper-and-pencil measure requiring between 5 and 10 min for administration.

Reliability and Validity In an evaluation of the scale's psychometric properties, Spoormaker and colleagues [1] found an internal consistency of .85 and a test–retest reliability of .78. Additionally, ten factors were able to explain 67.5% of the variance and, in terms of predictive validity, individuals found to possess certain sleep disorders scored significantly higher on those subscales of the questionnaire than other participants.

Obtaining a Copy A copy of the scale can be found in the original article published by developers [1].

Direct correspondence to:
Victor I. Spoormaker
Department of Clinical Psychology,
Utrecht University
P. O. Box 80.140
3508 TC Utrecht, The Netherlands
Email: v.i.spoormaker@fss.uu.nl

Scoring For each item, respondents are provided with a scale ranging from 1 ("not at all") to 4 ("very much") and are asked to indicate the extent to which the statement has matched their experience over the previous month. Total scores can be calculated for each subscale. In order to diagnose a sleep disorder using the questionnaire, developers recommend that respondents should meet a cutoff score for that subscale while also endorsing a score of at least 3 or 4 on the relevant impact scale. For their own analyses, Spoormaker and colleagues [1] used cutoff points that optimized the sensitivity and specificity of specific subscales. A list of these points can be found in the original article.

A. Shahid et al. (eds.), *STOP, THAT and One Hundred Other Sleep Scales*,
DOI 10.1007/978-1-4419-9893-4_77,

SLEEP-50

Please read every statement below and indicate to what extent it applied to you during the last four weeks.

	not at all	a little	rather much	very much
1. I am told that I snore	o	o	o	o
2. I sweat during the night	o	o	o	o
3. I am told that I hold my breath when sleeping	o	o	o	o
4. I am told that I wake up gasping for air	o	o	o	o
5. I wake up with a dry mouth	o	o	o	o
6. I wake up during the night while coughing / being short of breath	o	o	o	o
7. I wake up with a sour taste in my mouth	o	o	o	o
8. I wake up with a headache	o	o	o	o
9. I have difficulty in falling asleep	o	o	o	o
10. Thoughts go through my head and keep me awake	o	o	o	o
11. I worry and find it hard to relax	o	o	o	o
12. I wake up during the night	o	o	o	o
13. After waking up during the night, I fall asleep slowly	o	o	o	o
14. I wake up early and cannot get back to sleep	o	o	o	o
15. I sleep lightly	o	o	o	o
16. I sleep too little	o	o	o	o
17. I see dreamlike images when falling asleep or waking up	o	o	o	o
18. I sometimes fall asleep on a social occasion	o	o	o	o
19. I have sleep attacks during the day	o	o	o	o
20. With intense emotions, my muscles sometimes collapse during the day	o	o	o	o
21. I sometimes cannot move when falling asleep or waking up	o	o	o	o
22. I am told that I kick my legs when I sleep	o	o	o	o
23. I have cramp or pain in my legs during the night	o	o	o	o
24. I feel little shocks in my legs during the night	o	o	o	o
25. I cannot keep my legs at rest when falling asleep	o	o	o	o

Continued

	not at all	a little	rather much	very much
26. I would rather go to bed at a different time	o	o	o	o
27. I go to bed at very different times (more than 2 hours difference)	o	o	o	o
28. I do shift work	o	o	o	o
29. I sometimes walk when I am sleeping	o	o	o	o
30. I sometimes wake up in a different place than where I fell asleep	o	o	o	o
31. I sometimes find evidence of having performed an action during the night I do not remember	o	o	o	o
32. I have frightening dreams (if not, go to 37)	o	o	o	o
33. I wake up from these dreams	o	o	o	o
34. I remember the content of these dreams	o	o	o	o
35. I can orientate quickly after these dreams	o	o	o	o
36. I have physical symptoms during or after these dreams (e.g. movements, sweating, heart palpitations, shortness of breath)	o	o	o	o
37. It is too light in my bedroom during the night	o	o	o	o
38. It is too noisy in my bedroom during the night	o	o	o	o
39. I drink alcoholic beverages during the evening	o	o	o	o
40. I smoke during the evening	o	o	o	o
41. I use other substances during the evening (e.g. sleep or other medication)	o	o	o	o
42. I feel sad and depressed	o	o	o	o
43. I have no pleasure or interest in daily occupations	o	o	o	o
44. I feel tired at getting up	o	o	o	o
45. I feel sleepy during the day and struggle to remain alert	o	o	o	o
46. I would like to have more energy during the day	o	o	o	o
47. I am told that I am easily irritated	o	o	o	o
48. I have difficulty in concentrating at work or school	o	o	o	o
49. I worry whether I sleep enough	o	o	o	o
50. Generally, I sleep badly	o	o	o	o

A. I rate my sleep as ____ (1 = very bad, 10 = very good)

B. I sleep ____ hours, mostly from ____ to ____

Reference

1. Spoormaker, V. I., Verbeek, I., van den Bout, J., & Klip, E. C. (2005). Initial validation of the SLEEP-50 questionnaire. *Behavioral Sleep Medicine, 3*(4), 227–246.

Representative Studies Using Scale

None.

78 Sleep Beliefs Scale (SBS)

Purpose The SBS is a revised version of the Sleep Hygiene Awareness and Practice Scale. Possessing a simplified scoring method, the SBS consists of the nine most salient questions from the previous scale, along with 11 relevant additions. The scale requires respondents to indicate how certain behaviors (e.g., drug consumption, daytime and evening activities) can influence the quality and quantity of an individual's sleep. Since the tool assesses the beliefs and attitudes of a respondent, it may be relevant for both clinical and research purposes – as a means for evaluating an educational program, for example, or as an instrument for examining sleep beliefs in treatment and clinical populations.

Population for Testing The scale has been validated with university students aged 18–33 years. However, as sleep habits and behaviors often change dramatically with age, future studies featuring older participant populations may be valuable.

Administration Requiring between 5 and 10 min for completion, the SBS is a simple, self-report measure administered with pencil and paper.

Reliability and Validity Initial psychometric evaluations [1] have demonstrated an internal consistency of .71. The scale's potential uses with older adults still need to be evaluated.

Obtaining a Copy A copy can be found in the original article published by developers [1].

Direct correspondence:
Ana Adan
Department of Psychiatry and Clinical Psychobiology
School of Psychology,
University of Barcelona
Passeig Vall d'Hebrón 171, 08035
Barcelona, Spain

Scoring Each item of the SBS requires respondents to indicate how certain behaviors affect the sleep quality and quantity of most individuals. Respondents choose one of three options: "positive effect," "negative effect," or "neither effect." For most items, the behaviors examined possess a negative effect – questions 5, 9, 15, and 19, however, are positive. Correct responses are tallied and can be compared to the responses of other research populations and participants, or can be used to evaluate a change in beliefs over time.

A. Shahid et al. (eds.), *STOP, THAT and One Hundred Other Sleep Scales*,
DOI 10.1007/978-1-4419-9893-4_78, © Springer Science+Business Media, LLC 2012

APPENDIX 1. THE SLEEP BELIEFS SCALE

This is a survey of the effects of selected behaviours upon sleep. We are interested in knowing your opinion about whether any of these behaviours may influence the quality and/or quantity of sleep. For the following list of behaviours, please indicate whether you believe they produce a "positive" effect, a "negative" effect, or "neither'' effect on sleep (this is the central list below). Please do not make reference to how they influence your sleep in particular, but to the effects you think these behaviours have on people in general. Please answer ALL the statements by checking the appropriate box, even if you are not completely sure of the answer.

	Positive effect	Neither effect	Negative effect
1. Drinking alcohol in the evening	□	□	□
2. Drinking coffee or other substances with caffeine after dinner	□	□	□
3. Doing intense physical exercise before going to bed	□	□	□
4. Taking a long nap during the day	□	□	□
5. Going to bed and waking up always at the same hour	□	□	□
6. Thinking about one's engagements for the next day before falling asleep	□	□	□
7. Using sleep medication regularly	□	□	□
8. Smoking before falling asleep	□	□	□
9. Diverting one's attention and relaxing before bedtime	□	□	□
10. Going to bed 2 h later than the habitual hour	□	□	□
11. Going to bed with an empty stomach	□	□	□
12. Using the bed for eating, calling on the phone, studying and other non-sleeping activities	□	□	□
13. Trying to fall asleep without having a sleep sensation	□	□	□
14. Studying or working intensely until late night	□	□	□
15. Getting up when it is difficult to fall asleep	□	□	□
16. Going to bed 2 h earlier than the habitual hour	□	□	□
17. Going to bed immediately after eating	□	□	□
18. Being worried about the impossibility of getting enough sleep	□	□	□
19. Sleeping in a quiet and dark room	□	□	□
20. Recovering lost sleep by sleeping for a long time	□	□	□

Reference

1. Adan, A., Fabbri, M., Natale, V., & Prat, G. (2006). Sleep beliefs scale (SBS) and circadian typology. *Journal of Sleep Research, 15*(2), 125-132.

Representative Studies Using Scale

None.

79 Sleep Disorders Inventory for Students – Adolescent Form (SDIS-A)

Purpose The SDIS-A is composed of 35 items designed to screen for a variety of sleep disorders in adolescents, including: obstructive sleep apnea, periodic limb movement disorder, delayed sleep phase syndrome, excessive daytime sleepiness, narcolepsy, overall sleep disturbance, bruxism, somnambulism, sleep-talking, night terrors, and nocturnal enuresis. Though not a substitute for clinical diagnosis, the instrument is brief and easy to administer, and it addresses the most common sleep complaints faced by youth populations, making it a potential tool for screening.

Population for Testing The adolescent form is indicated for use with youth ages 11–18 years. A second version designed for children 2–10 is also available (Chap. 80).

Administration The pencil-and-paper measure is completed by a parent or caregiver on behalf of the adolescent in question. It requires between 10 and 15 min for completion.

Reliability and Validity Developer Luginbuehl [1] conducted a psychometric evaluation of the questionnaire and found a predictive validity of 96%, an internal consistency of .92, and a test–retest reliability of .86.

Obtaining a Copy The scale is under copyright and is available from publishers Child Uplift Inc. at their website:
http://www.sleepdisorderhelp.com/index.php

Direct correspondence to:
Child Uplift Inc. P.O. Box 146
Fairview, WY

Scoring The majority of questions ask respondents to rate, on a seven-point, Likert-type scale, how frequently their child exhibits certain sleep behaviors. Additional items related to general childhood health issues are presented in a "yes/no" format. Researchers and clinicians hoping to use the scale are first required to purchase a kit containing a technical manual and a computerized scoring program for the scale. Though the manual describes the process of hand-scoring, electronic scoring is recommended as it creates an interpretive read-out that may be more useful for screening purposes. Read-outs provide T-scores and percentiles for each disorder evaluated. Based on normative data, results for each domain are placed in one of three categories: "normal," "caution," and "high risk."

Reference

1. Luginbuehl, M. (2003). The initial development and validation study of the sleep disorders inventory for students. *Sleep, 26*, A399–A400.

Representative Studies Using Scale

None

A. Shahid et al. (eds.), *STOP, THAT and One Hundred Other Sleep Scales*,
DOI 10.1007/978-1-4419-9893-4_79, © Springer Science+Business Media, LLC 2012

80 Sleep Disorders Inventory for Students – Children's Form (SDIS-C)

Purpose Consisting of 30 items, the SDIS-C was created as a screening tool for sleep disorders in children. The scale analyzes obstructive sleep apnea, periodic limb movement disorder, delayed sleep phase syndrome, excessive daytime sleepiness, overall sleep disturbance, bruxism, somnambulism, sleep-talking, night terrors, and nocturnal enuresis. Though not a substitute for a clinical diagnosis, the instrument is easy to administer and addresses the most common sleep complaints faced by youth populations, making it a valuable tool for screening.

Population for Testing The form is indicated for use with children ages 2–10 years. A second version designed for adolescents 11–18 is also available (Chap. 79).

Administration The pencil-and-paper measure is completed by a parent or caregiver on behalf of the child in question. It requires between 10 and 15 min for completion.

Reliability and Validity Developer Luginbuehl [1] conducted a psychometric evaluation of the questionnaire and found a predictive validity of 86%, an internal consistency of .91, and a test–retest reliability of .97.

Obtaining a Copy The scale is under copyright and is available from publishers Child Uplift Inc. at their website:
http://www.sleepdisorderhelp.com/index.php

Direct correspondence to:
Child Uplift Inc. P.O. Box 146
Fairview, WY

Scoring Using a seven-point, Likert-type scale, parents indicate how frequently their child exhibits certain sleep behaviors. Additional items related to general childhood health issues are presented in a "yes/no" format. Researchers and clinicians hoping to use the scale are first required to purchase a kit containing a technical manual and a computerized scoring program for the scale. Though the manual describes the process of hand-scoring, electronic scoring is recommended as it creates an interpretive read-out that may be more useful for screening purposes. Read-outs provide T-scores and percentiles for each disorder evaluated. Based on normative data, results for each domain are placed in one of three categories: "normal," "caution," and "high risk."

Reference

1. Luginbuehl, M. (2003). The initial development and validation study of the sleep disorders inventory for students. *Sleep, 26*, A399–A400.

Representative Studies Using Scale

None

A. Shahid et al. (eds.), *STOP, THAT and One Hundred Other Sleep Scales*,
DOI 10.1007/978-1-4419-9893-4_80, © Springer Science+Business Media, LLC 2012

81 Sleep Disorders Questionnaire (SDQ)

Purpose The SDQ was designed as a tool for the identification of those at high risk for possessing a sleep disorder. The 175-item scale was created by selecting the best and most salient questions from the Sleep Questionnaire and Assessment of Wakefulness (SQAW), a general measure consisting of more than 800 items [1]. The scale was initially intended for use by general practitioners and other health professionals outside the field of sleep medicine, though the questionnaire may function as a diagnostic aid for sleep specialists as well. Developers have also created a smaller, 45-item version of the scale to assess four common sleep disorders: sleep apnea, narcolepsy, psychiatric sleep disorders, and periodic limb movement disorder.

Population for Testing The scale's items were selected using a group of participants attending a sleep disorder clinic. In later psychometric evaluations, researchers selected participants with mean ages of 24.8 ± 8.3 years [2] and 43.6 ± 12.9 years [3].

Administration The scale is a self-report, paper-and-pencil measure requiring approximately 15 min for completion.

Reliability and Validity Developers Douglass and colleagues [2] conducted a psychometric evaluation of the scale and found an average test-retest reliability of .5. In a subsequent study by Douglass and colleagues [3], scale developers examined only 45 of the instrument's initial 175 items, dividing them through into four different scales representing common sleep disorders: sleep apnea, narcolepsy, psychiatric sleep disorder, and periodic limb movement disorder. For these subscales, researchers found an internal consistency of .85 and a test-retest reliability ranging from .75 to .85.

Obtaining a Copy

Direct correspondence to:
Alan B. Douglass
Royal Ottawa Mental Health Centre
1145 Carling Avenue
Sleep Lab, Room 3124
Ottawa, ON K1Z 7K4
Canada

Scoring Respondents use a scale ranging from 1 to 5 to answer questions regarding the frequency of sleep issues (never to always), the degree to which they agree with certain statements (strongly disagree to strongly agree), and the quantity of things like hours of sleep and caffeinated drinks. Higher scores indicate more severe symptoms. Total scores can be calculated for the entire scale, as well as for relevant subscales.

A. Shahid et al. (eds.), *STOP, THAT and One Hundred Other Sleep Scales*,
DOI 10.1007/978-1-4419-9893-4_81, © Springer Science+Business Media, LLC 2012

References

1. Douglass, A. B., Bornstein, R., Nino-Murcia, G., & Keenan, S. (1986). Creation of the "ASDC sleep disorders questionnaire." *Sleep Research, 15*, 117.
2. Douglass, A. B., Bornstein, R., Nin-Murcia, G., Keenan, S., Laughton, M., Zarcone, V., Guillemault, C., Dement, W. C., & Abelseth, D. (1990). Test-retest reliability of the sleep disorders questionnaire. *Sleep Research, 19*, 215.
3. Douglass, A. B., Bornstein, R., Nino-Murcia, G., Keenan, S., Miles, L., Zarcone, V. P., Guilleminault, C., & Dement, W. C. (1994). The sleep disorders questionnaire I: creation and multivariate structure of SDQ. *Sleep, 17*(2), 160–167.

Representative Studies Using Scale

Valipour, A., Lothaller, H., Rauscher, H., Zwick, H., Burghuber, O. C., & Lavie, P. (2007). Gender-related differences in symptoms of patients with suspected breathing disorders in sleep: a clinical population study using the sleep disorders questionnaire. *Sleep, 30*(3), 312–319.

Léger, D., Annesi-Maesano, I., Carat, F., Rugina, M., Chantal, I., Pribil, C., Hasnaoui, A. E., & Bousquet, J. (2006). Allergic rhinitis and its consequences on quality of sleep. *Archives of Internal Medicine, 166*(16), 1744–1748.

82 Sleep Disturbance Scale for Children (SDSC)

Purpose Consisting of 26 Likert-type items, the SDSC was designed both to evaluate specific sleep disorders in children, and to provide an overall measure of sleep disturbance suitable for use in clinical screening and research. Using factor analysis, developers Bruni and colleagues [1] divided items into six categories representing some of the most common sleep difficulties affecting adolescents and children: disorders of initiating and maintaining sleep, sleep breathing disorders, disorders of arousal/nightmares, sleep-wake transition disorders, disorders of excessive somnolence, and sleep hyperhidrosis (nighttime sweating).

Population for Testing The scale has been validated with youth populations aged 6–15 years.

Administration The questionnaire is completed by a parent or caregiver on behalf of the child using pencil and paper. Administration should require between 10 and 15 min.

Reliability and Validity Bruni and colleagues [1] conducted a psychometric evaluation of the SDSC and found an internal consistency ranging from .71 to .79, a test-retest reliability of .71, a diagnostic accuracy of .91.

Obtaining a Copy A copy can be found in the original article published by developers (1996).

Direct correspondence to:
Dr. Oliviero Bruni
Department of Developmental Neurology and Psychiatry
University of Rome
Via dei Sabelli 108-00185
Rome, Italy

Scoring Parents use a five-point, Likert-type scale to indicate how frequently certain behaviors are exhibited by their children: 1 means "never," while five corresponds with "always (daily)." Respondents also offer estimates of sleep quantity and onset time. Higher scores indicate more acute sleep disturbances. To obtain results, scores are tallied for each of the six sleep-disorder categories, and an overall score is calculated. Bruni and colleagues [1] have suggested a total cutoff score of 39 – in their evaluations of the scale, they found that this score corresponded with the upper quartile of their control group and gave a sensitivity of .89 and a specificity of .74.

A. Shahid et al. (eds.), *STOP, THAT and One Hundred Other Sleep Scales,*
DOI 10.1007/978-1-4419-9893-4_82, © Springer Science+Business Media, LLC 2012

***INSTRUCTIONS:** This questionnaire will allow to your doctor to have a better understanding of the sleep-wake rhythm of your child and of any problems in his/her sleep behaviour. Try to answer every question; in answering, consider each question as pertaining to the **past 6 months** of the child's life. Please answer the questions by circling or striking the number ① to ⑤.* Thank you very much for your help.

Name:________________________ Age:________ Date:________

1. How many hours of sleep does your child get on most nights.	① *9-11 hours*	② *8-9 hours*	③ *7-8 hours*	④ *5-7 hours*	⑤ *less than 5 hours*
2. How long after going to bed does your child usually fall asleep	① *less than 15'*	② *15-30'*	③ *30-45'*	④ *45-60'*	⑤ *more than 60'*

	① Never	② Occasionally (once or twice per month or less)	③ Sometimes (once or twice per week)	④ Often (3 or 5 times per week)	⑤ Always (daily)
3. The child goes to bed reluctantly	①	②	③	④	⑤
4. The child has difficulty getting to sleep at night	①	②	③	④	⑤
5. The child feels anxious or afraid when falling asleep	①	②	③	④	⑤
6. The child startles or jerks parts of the body while falling asleep	①	②	③	④	⑤
7. The child shows repetitive actions such as rocking or head banging while falling asleep	①	②	③	④	⑤
8. The child experiences vivid dream-like scenes while falling asleep	①	②	③	④	⑤
9. The child sweats excessively while falling asleep	①	②	③	④	⑤
10. The child wakes up more than twice per night	①	②	③	④	⑤
11. After waking up in the night, the child has difficulty to fall asleep again	①	②	③	④	⑤
12. The child has frequent twitching or jerking of legs while asleep or often changes position during the night or kicks the covers off the bed.	①	②	③	④	⑤
13. The child has difficulty in breathing during the night	①	②	③	④	⑤
14. The child gasps for breath or is unable to breathe during sleep	①	②	③	④	⑤
15. The child snores	①	②	③	④	⑤
16. The child sweats excessively during the night	①	②	③	④	⑤
17. You have observed the child sleepwalking	①	②	③	④	⑤
18. You have observed the child talking in his/her sleep	①	②	③	④	⑤
19. The child grinds teeth during sleep	①	②	③	④	⑤
20. The child wakes from sleep screaming or confused so that you cannot seem to get through to him/her, but has no memory of these events the next morning	①	②	③	④	⑤
21. The child has nightmares which he/she doesn't remember the next day	①	②	③	④	⑤
22. The child is unusually difficult to wake up in the morning	①	②	③	④	⑤
23. The child awakes in the morning feeling tired	①	②	③	④	⑤
24. The child feels unable to move when waking up in the morning	①	②	③	④	⑤
25. The child experiences daytime somnolence	①	②	③	④	⑤
26. The child falls asleep suddenly in inappropriate situations	①	②	③	④	⑤

Disorders of initiating and maintaining sleep (sum the score of the items 1,2,3,4,5,10,11)	
Sleep Breathing Disorders (sum the score of the items 13,14,15)	
Disorders of arousal (sum the score of the items 17,20,21)	
Sleep-Wake Transition Disorders (sum the score of the items 6,7,8,12,18,19)	
Disorders of excessive somnolence (sum the score of the items 22,23,24,25,26)	
Sleep Hyperhydrosis (sum the score of the items 9,16)	
Total score (sum 6 factors' scores)	

Reference

1. Bruni, O., Ottaviano, S., Guidetti, V., Romoli, M., Innocenzi, M., Cortesi, F., & Giannotti, F. (1996). The sleep disturbance scale for children (SDSC): Construction and validation of an instrument to evaluate sleep disturbances in childhood and adolescence. *Journal of Sleep Research, 5*, 251–261.

Representative Studies Using Scale

Carotenuto, M., Bruni, O., Santoro, N., Del Giudice, E. M., Perrone, L., & Pascotto, A. (2006). Waist circumference predicts the occurrence of sleep-disordered breathing in obese children and adolescents: a questionnaire-based study. *Sleep Medicine, 7*(4), 357–361.

Hartshorne, T. S., Heussler, H. S., Dailor, A. N., Williams, G. L., Papadopoulos, D., & Brandt, K. K. (2009). Sleep disturbances in CHARGE syndrome: types and relationships with behavior and caregiver well-being. *Developmental Medicine & Child Neurology, 51*(2), 143–150.

83 Sleep Locus of Control Scale (SLOC)

Purpose The SLOC is an 8-item questionnaire designed to evaluate a respondent's sleep-related locus of control – the degree to which an individual attributes his or her experiences of sleep to chance or to internal, intentional causes. Researchers posit that a chance locus of control may be associated with experiences of learned helplessness, leading individuals to believe that there is nothing they can do to improve their sleep quality [1]. Conversely, studies have shown that internally oriented beliefs about sleep responsibility may lead to greater anxiety about having sleep problems and may increase sleep-onset delay [2]. Thus, beliefs that fall at either extreme of the locus-of-control spectrum may be harmful to sleep quality. The SLOC allows clinicians to identify disruptive cognitions in their patients, improving the quality of treatment interventions.

Population for Testing Developers validated the scale with two sample populations: an insomnia patient group with a mean age of 50.5 ± 11.8 and an adult control group with a mean age of 43.3 ± 15.0.

Administration Requiring 3–5 min for administration, the scale is a self-report, paper-and-pencil measure.

Reliability and Validity The scale's psychometric properties have been evaluated in a study conducted by Vincent and colleagues [3]. Researchers found an internal consistency ranges from .47 to .73. Additionally, the insomnia patient group endorsed both internal and external loci of control to greater extremes than the control group, suggesting that a balance between the two may be ideal.

Obtaining a Copy An example of the scale's items can be found in an article published by Vincent and colleagues [3].

Direct correspondence to:
Norah Vincent
PZ-251
771 Bannatyne Ave., PsycHealth Centre
Winnipeg, Manitoba, Canada
R3E 3N4
Email: nvincent@exchange.hsc.mb.ca

Scoring Using a Likert-type scale that ranges from 1 to 6, respondents indicate the degree to which they agree with certain statements relating to their control over insomnia. Items 3, 4, and 6 are reverse-scored. Total scores can range from 8 to 48 – higher scores correspond with a greater internal locus of control, while lower scores denote attributions to external forces.

A. Shahid et al. (eds.), *STOP, THAT and One Hundred Other Sleep Scales*,
DOI 10.1007/978-1-4419-9893-4_83, © Springer Science+Business Media, LLC 2012

Sleep Locus of Control Scale

1. If I take care of myself, I can avoid insomnia

1	2	3	4	5	6
Strongly disagree					**Strongly agree**

2. Whether I have insomnia is entirely up to me

1	2	3	4	5	6
Strongly disagree					**Strongly agree**

3. Good sleep is largely a matter of luck

1	2	3	4	5	6
Strongly disagree					**Strongly agree**

4. No matter what I do, if I am going to have a sleepless night, I will

1	2	3	4	5	6
Strongly disagree					**Strongly agree**

5. When I have insomnia, I know it is because of something I have done (e.g., not enough time to relax, worrying about things that I can't control, worrying about not sleeping)

1	2	3	4	5	6
Strongly disagree					**Strongly agree**

6. People who never get insomnia are just plain lucky

1	2	3	4	5	6
Strongly disagree					**Strongly agree**

7. People's insomnia results from their own carelessness

1	2	3	4	5	6
Strongly disagree					**Strongly agree**

8. I am directly responsible for my sleep

1	2	3	4	5	6
Strongly disagree					**Strongly agree**

Scoring for Sleep Locus of Control (SLOC) Scale

Internal Sleep Locus = 1+ 2+ 5+ 7+ 8

Chance Sleep Locus = 3 + 4 + 6

Norms for the SLOC

Samples	SLOC subscale	N	*M*	*SD*
University Alumnae[a]	Internal	423	18.39 (range: 5-30)	4.7
	Chance	421	13.14 (range: 4-18)	3.2
University Students[a]	Internal	228	19.27 (range: 6-30)	4.7
	Chance	230	12.64 (range: 3-18	3.0

Age-Based Norms: University Alumnae[a]

Age Range	SLOC subscale	N	*M*	*SD*
18-29	Internal	94	18.51 (range: 9-27)	4.6
	Chance	94	12.8 (range: 4-18)	3.3
30-39	Internal	68	18.82 (range: 10-29)	4.5
	Chance	67	14.10 (range: 8-18)	2.7
40-49	Internal	89	18.52 (range: 8-30)	4.5
	Chance	89	13.36 (range: 5-18)	3.2
50-59	Internal	112	18.06 (range: 5-29)	4.9
	Chance	111	12.91 (range: 5-19)	3.0
60-69	Internal	49	18.59 (range: 8-27)	4.5
	Chance	49	12.81 (range: 7-18)	3.0
>70	Internal	9	15.77 (range: 6-28)	7.7
	Chance	9	11.88 (range 6-18)	3.8

Norms for Insomnia Types: Primary vs. Comorbid Insomnia

Sample	Administration	Insomnia Type	SLOC subscale	N	M	SD
Adult Outpatients (Clinic Referral and Community-Recruited)	In-Person[a]	Primary Insomnia	Internal	49	14.48 (range: 5-22)	4.0
			Chance	50	8.56 (range: 3-16)	3.3
		Comorbid Insomnia	Internal	47	14.17 (range: 5-25)	4.3
			Chance	47	10.29 (range: 5-17)	3.2
	Online[b]	Primary Insomnia	Internal	68	13.60 (range 5-25)	4.6
			Chance	68	10.31 (range: 5-17)	3.2
		Comorbid Insomnia	Internal	77	14.81 (range 7-29)	4.2
			Chance	77	9.75 (range: 3-18)	3.2

Norms for the SLOC for Adults with Chronic Primary and Comorbid Insomnia: Recruitment Differences

Administration	Recruitment	SLOC subscale	N	M	SD
In-Person[a]	Community Recruited	Internal	39	15.51 (range: 8-25)	4.3
		Chance	39	8.97 (range: 3-15)	2.9
	Clinic Referral	Internal	42	13.54 (range: 5-20)	3.8
		Chance	43	9.39 (range: 3-17)	3.6
Online[b]	Community Recruited	Internal	78	14.06 (range 5-25)	4.3
		Chance	78	9.12 (range: 3-16)	3.1
	Clinic Referral	Internal	68	14.40 (range: 6-29)	4.5
		Chance	68	11.06 (range: 5-18)	2.9

a. Vincent N, Sande G, Read C, Giannuzzi T. Sleep locus of control: report on a new scale. Behav Sleep Med. 2004;2(2):79-93.

b. Vincent N, Lewycky S. Logging on for better sleep: a randomized controlled trial of the effectiveness of online treatment for insomnia. Forthcoming 2009.

References

1. Morin, C. M. (1993). *Insomnia: psychological assessment and management.* New York: Guilford Press.
2. Van Egeren, L., Haynes, S.N., Franzen, M., & Hamilton, J. (1983). Presleep cognitions and attributions in sleep-onset insomnia. *Journal of Behavioral Medicine, 6*, 217–232.
3. Vincent, N., Sande, G., Read, C., & Giannuzzi, T. (2004). Sleep locus of control: report on a new scale. *Behavioral Sleep Medicine, 2*(2), 79–93.

Representative Studies Using Scale

None.

84 Sleep Preoccupation Scale (SPS)

Purpose A 22-item, self-report scale, the SPS was designed to assess daytime cognitions in patients with insomnia. Though researchers have frequently focused on nighttime thoughts and preoccupations when attempting to treat disordered sleep, a growing body of research suggests that daytime beliefs about sleep may be just as significant in the experience of insomnia [1]. SPS items evaluate two distinct domains: the cognitive and behavioral consequences of poor sleep (e.g., negative thoughts and perceptions), and the affective consequences (e.g., worry and distress). The tool may be particularly useful for clinicians attempting to identify and treat the origins of sleep issues in their patients.

Population for Testing The scale has been validated with patient and control samples with a mean age of 43 ± 23.

Administration A self-report, paper-and-pencil measure, the scale requires between 10 and 15 min for completion.

Reliability and Validity Developers Ellis and colleagues (2007) conducted a study analyzing the psychometric properties of the scale and found a reliability of .91. Additionally, analysis of variance demonstrated significant differences between the three different samples of sleepers (poor, average, and good).

Obtaining a Copy An example of questionnaire items can be found in the original article published by developers [2].

Direct correspondence to:
J. Ellis
Department of Psychological Medicine, Division of Community Based Science
Gartnaval Royal Hospital
1055 Great Western Road, G12 0XH
Glasgow, United Kingdom
Email: j.ellis@clinmed.gla.ac.uk

Scoring Using a six-point, Likert-type scale, respondents indicate how frequently they experience certain thoughts and behave in specific ways on a typical day – 0 means "never," while 6 denotes "all the time." Higher total scores are indicative of more negative daytime cognitions and feelings about sleep, and are a sign that treatment programs targeting these thought processes may be valuable.

A. Shahid et al. (eds.), *STOP, THAT and One Hundred Other Sleep Scales*,
DOI 10.1007/978-1-4419-9893-4_84, © Springer Science+Business Media, LLC 2012

This questionnaire is designed to find out how often you think about your sleep pattern throughout the day and the kinds of thoughts that you have. Read each statement carefully and circle the answer that best represents how often, **on a typical day** within the last month, you have experienced the thought or feeling, or performed that specific behaviour.

	Never	Hardly At All	Very Infreq-uently	Every Now and Then	Quite Often	Almost All the Time	All the Time
I feel anxious about my sleep pattern	0	1	2	3	4	5	6
I feel anxious about what will happen when I try to sleep tonight	0	1	2	3	4	5	6
I try to get to bed early the next day after a bad night's sleep	0	1	2	3	4	5	6
I find it hard to concentrate during the day after a bad night's sleep	0	1	2	3	4	5	6
My memory appears to be worse after a bad night's sleep	0	1	2	3	4	5	6
I am more sensitive to what other people say after a bad night's sleep	0	1	2	3	4	5	6
I have to make more of an effort with my appearance after a bad night's sleep	0	1	2	3	4	5	6
I am more irritable after a bad night's sleep	0	1	2	3	4	5	6
I become frustrated when I think about my sleep pattern	0	1	2	3	4	5	6
I get upset when others talk about their 'good' sleep patterns	0	1	2	3	4	5	6
I have a lie-in after a bad night's sleep	0	1	2	3	4	5	6
I know that if I have a bad night's sleep, I will also have a bad day	0	1	2	3	4	5	6
I worry about the long-term consequences of poor sleep	0	1	2	3	4	5	6
I cannot perform my daily tasks as well when I have had a bad night's sleep	0	1	2	3	4	5	6
I think of what 'good' sleep would be like	0	1	2	3	4	5	6
I take it easy the next day after a bad night	0	1	2	3	4	5	6

	Never	Hardly At All	Very Infreq-uently	Every Now and Then	Quite Often	Almost All the Time	All the Time
All my problems seem worse after a bad night's sleep	0	1	2	3	4	5	6
I cannot stop dwelling on thoughts of sleep during the day	0	1	2	3	4	5	6
I wonder if my sleep patterns will ever become 'normal'	0	1	2	3	4	5	6
I try to avoid other people when I have had a bad night's sleep	0	1	2	3	4	5	6
I yawn more often after a bad night's sleep	0	1	2	3	4	5	6
My eyes are more sensitive / sore after a bad night's sleep.	0	1	2	3	4	5	6

References

1. Harvey, A. G. (2002). A cognitive model of insomnia. *Behaviour Research and Therapy, 40*, 869–893.
2. Ellis, J., Mitchell, K., & Hogh, H. (2007). Sleep preoccupation in poor sleepers: psychometric properties of the sleep preoccupation scale. *Journal of Psychosomatic Research, 63*(6), 579–585.

Representative Studies Using Scale

Ellis, J., Hampson, S. E., & Cropsley, M. (2007). The role of preoccupation in attributions for poor sleep. *Sleep Medicine, 8*(3), 277–280.

85 Sleep Quality Scale (SQS)

Purpose Consisting of 28 items, the SQS evaluates six domains of sleep quality: daytime symptoms, restoration after sleep, problems initiating and maintaining sleep, difficulty waking, and sleep satisfaction. Developers hoped to create a scale that could be used as an all-inclusive assessment tool – a general, efficient measure suitable for evaluating sleep quality in a variety of patient and research populations.

Population for Testing The scale has been validated in individuals aged 18–59 years.

Administration Requiring between 5 and 10 min for administration, the scale is a simple self-report, pencil-and-paper measure.

Reliability and Validity An initial psychometric evaluation conducted by Yi and colleagues [1] found an internal consistency of .92, a test-retest reliability of .81. The SQS is strongly correlated with results obtained on the Pittsburgh Sleep Quality Index (Chap. 67). Scores achieved by the insomnia sample were significantly higher than those of controls, indicating good construct validity.

Obtaining a Copy A list of the scale's 28 items can be found in the original article published by developers [1].

Direct correspondence to:
Chol Shin
Division of Pulmonary and Critical Care Medicine
Department of Internal Medicine
Korea University Ansan Hospital
516, Gojan 1-dong, Danwon-gu, Ansan-si, Gyeonggi-do 425–707
Republic of Korea
Email: shinchol@pol.net

Scoring Using a four-point, Likert-type scale, respondents indicate how frequently they exhibit certain sleep behaviors (0 = "few," 1 = "sometimes," 2 = "often," and 3 = "almost always"). Scores on items belong to factors 2 and 5 (restoration after sleep and satisfaction with sleep) and are reversed before being tallied. Total scores can range from 0 to 84, with higher scores demoting more acute sleep problems.

A. Shahid et al. (eds.), *STOP, THAT and One Hundred Other Sleep Scales*,
DOI 10.1007/978-1-4419-9893-4_85, © Springer Science+Business Media, LLC 2012

Sleep Quality Scale

The following survey is to know the quality of sleep you had for the last one month. Read the questions and check the closest answer.

Examples

Rarely : None or 1-3 times a month
Sometimes : 1-2 times a week
Often : 3-5 times a week
Almost always : 6-7 times a week

		Rarely	Sometimes	Often	Almost always
1	I have difficulty falling asleep.				
2	I fall into a deep sleep.				
3	I wake up while sleeping.				
4	I have difficulty getting back to sleep once I wake up in middle of the night.				
5	I wake up easily because of noise.				
6	I toss and turn.				
7	I never go back to sleep after awakening during sleep.				
8	I feel refreshed after sleep.				
9	I feel unlikely to sleep after sleep.				
10	Poor sleep gives me headaches.				
11	Poor sleep makes me irritated.				
12	I would like to sleep more after waking up.				
13	My sleep hours are enough.				
14	Poor sleep makes me lose my appetite.				
15	Poor sleep makes hard for me to think.				
16	I feel vigorous after sleep.				
17	Poor sleep makes me lose interest in work or others.				
18	My fatigue is relieved after sleep.				

		Rarely	Sometimes	Often	Almost always
19	Poor sleep causes me to make mistakes at work.				
20	I am satisfied with my sleep.				
21	Poor sleep makes me forget things more easily.				
22	Poor sleep makes it hard to concentrate at work.				
23	Sleepiness interferes with my daily life.				
24	Poor sleep makes me lose desire in all things.				
25	I have difficulty getting out of bed.				
26	Poor sleep makes me easily tired at work.				
27	I have a clear head after sleep.				
28	Poor sleep makes my life painful.				

 Note: This is an English translation from the original Korean scale. A back-translation is in the works.

A number of translated versions such as the two that follow can be found on our website: www.sleepontario.com

♧ 다음은 귀하의 지난 한달 동안의 수면의 질을 알아보기 위한 것입니다. 각 질문과 아래의 보기를 읽고 가장 가깝다고 생각되는 곳에 v표하여 주십시오.

< 보기 >

거의 그렇지 않다 : 한 달 동안 한 번도 없었거나, 월 1 - 3 회

가끔 그렇다 : 일주일에 1 - 2 회

자주 그렇다 : 일주일에 3 - 5 회

거의 항상 그렇다 : 일주일에 6 - 7 회

	지난 한달 동안에	거의 그렇지 않다	가끔 그렇다	자주 그렇다	거의 항상 그렇다
1	잠드는데 어려움이 있다				
2	잠이 깊이 든다				
3	잠을 자다가 깬다				
4	잠을 자다가 깨면 다시 잠드는데 어려움이 있다				
5	소음으로 인해 잠이 쉽게 깬다				
6	잠을 설친다				
7	잠을 자다가 깨면 다시 잠들지 못한다				
8	잠을 자고 일어나면 몸이 개운하다				
9	잠을 자고 일어나도 자고 난 것 같지 않다				
10	잠을 못자기 때문에 머리가 아프다				
11	잠을 못자기 때문에 짜증이 난다				

	지난 한달 동안에	거의 그렇지 않다	가끔 그렇다	자주 그렇다	거의 항상 그렇다
12	잠을 자고 일어날 때 더 자고 싶은 생각이 든다				
13	수면 시간이 충분하다				
14	잠을 못자기 때문에 식욕이 떨어진다				
15	잠을 못자기 때문에 생각하는데 어려움이 있다				
16	잠을 자고 일어나면 활력을 되찾는다				
17	잠을 못자기 때문에 일이나 다른 사람에 대한 관심이 줄어든다				
18	잠을 자고 일어나면 피로가 풀린다				
19	잠은 못자기 때문에 일하는데 실수가 많아진다				
20	전반적으로 수면(잠)에 대해 만족한다				
21	잠을 못자기 때문에 건망증이 심해진다				
22	잠을 못자기 때문에 일에 집중하기가 어렵다				
23	졸음이 일상생활에 지장을 준다				
24	잠을 못자기 때문에 의욕이 떨어진다				
25	잠을 자고 난 후 잠자리에서 일어나기가 어렵다				
26	잠을 못자기 때문에 일할 때 빨리 피로해진다				
27	잠을 자고 일어나면 머리가 맑다				
28	잠을 못자기 때문에 삶이 고통스럽다				

Reference

1. Yi, H., Shin, K., & Shin, C. (2006). Development of the sleep quality scale. *Journal of Sleep Research, 15*(3), 309–316.

Representative Studies Using Scale

Howell, A. J., Digdon, N. L., Buro, K., & Sheptycki, A. R. (2008). Relations among mindfulness, well-being, and sleep. *Personality and Individual Differences, 45*, 773–777.

86 Sleep Timing Questionnaire (STQ)

Purpose The STQ was created in order to obtain an accurate sketch of an individual's typical sleep schedule, allowing sleep technicians to tailor the timing of polysomnographic studies to the patient's specific needs and habits. The questionnaire is meant to function as an alternative to the more time-consuming sleep diary format. Consisting of 18 items, the STQ queries a variety of issues, including preferences for bed and waking times, frequency and length of night awakenings, and stability of sleep schedules.

Population for Testing The scale has been validated with a group of individuals aged 20–82 years.

Administration A self-report, paper-and-pencil measure, the scale requires between 5 and 10 min for completion.

Reliability and Validity In order to ensure that the STQ could produce results similar to those obtained through a more traditional sleep diary, developers Monk and colleagues [1] conducted a psychometric evaluation. Over the course of four studies, developers found a test-retest reliability ranging from .71 to .83, a correlation of .59 to .77 between the STQ and measure of bed timing taken by wrist actigraphy, and a correlation of .84 to .86 between the STQ and a 2-week sleep diary.

Obtaining a Copy A copy of the questionnaire can be found in the original article published by developers [1].

Direct correspondence to:
Timothy Monk
WPIC Room E1123
3811 O'Hara St.
Pittsburgh PA 15213
U.S.A.

Scoring Respondents indicate their earliest and latest typical bed and wake times on both weekends and work nights by filling in blanks. As developers explain, "[t]his part of the questionnaire is less to derive actual data endpoints but more to focus the patient on thinking about their actual bedtimes and waketimes, to avoid them merely responding with a 'boilerplate' response" [1]. Following these responses, participants answer questions regarding their typical bedtimes. Finally, multiple-choice questions ask individuals to estimate, in 15-min increments, how stable their schedules tend to be. These responses combined can then be used to estimate suitable study or research times that will fit the individual's schedule and provide the most accurate results of polysomnography. When an overall score is needed, developers recommend weighting typical weeknight to weekend schedules with a ratio of 5:2, which will provide an average time in bed.

A. Shahid et al. (eds.), *STOP, THAT and One Hundred Other Sleep Scales,*
DOI 10.1007/978-1-4419-9893-4_86,

SLEEP TIMING QUESTIONNAIRE (STQ)

Name____

ID#____

Date____

SLEEP TIMING QUESTIONNAIRE (STQ)

This questionnaire asks about when you normally sleep. We are interested in getting as accurate a picture as we can of the times when you normally go to bed and get up. Please think carefully before giving your answers and be as accurate and as specific as you can be. Please answer in terms of a recent "normal average week," not one in which you traveled, vacationed or had family crises. Thanks.

Please think of GOOD NIGHT TIME as the time at which you are finally in bed and trying to fall asleep.

On the night before a work day or school day,
what is your earliest GOOD NIGHT TIME ?____:____ pm/am

On the night before a work day or school day,
what is your latest GOOD NIGHT TIME ?____:____ pm/am

On the night before a work day or school day,
what is your usual GOOD NIGHT TIME ?____:____ pm/am

How stable (i.e., similar each night) are your GOOD NIGHT TIMES before a work day or school day? (circle one)

0-15 min	16-30 min	31-45 min	46-60 min
61-75 min	76-90 min	91-105 min	106-120 min
2-3 hours	3-4 hours	over 4hours	

On a night before a day off (e.g. a weekend),
what is your earliest GOOD NIGHT TIME ?____:____ pm/am

On a night before a day off (e.g. a weekend),
what is your latest GOOD NIGHT TIME ?____:____ pm/am

On a night before a day off (e.g. a weekend),
what is your usual GOOD NIGHT TIME ?___:____ pm/am

How stable (i.e., similar each night) are your GOOD NIGHT TIMES on a night before a day off (e.g. a weekend)? (circle one)

0-15 mins.	16-30 mins.	31-45 mins.	46-60mins.
61-75 mins.	76-90 mins.	91-105 mins	106-120 mins.
2-3 hours	3-4 hours	over 4 hours	

Please think of GOOD MORNING TIME as the time at which you finally get out of bed and start your day.

Before a work day or school day,
what is your earliest GOOD MORNING TIME ?____:____ am/pm

Before a work day or school day,
what is your latest GOOD MORNING TIME ?____:____ am/pm

Before a work day or school day,
what is your usual GOOD MORNING TIME ?____:____ am/pm

How stable (i.e., similar each night) are your GOOD MORNING TIMES before a work day or school day? (circle one)

0-15 mins.	16-30 mins.	31-45 mins.	46-60 mins.
61-75 mins.	76-90 mins.	91-105 mins	106-120 mins.
2-3 hours	3-4 hours	over 4 hours	

Before a day off (e.g. a weekend),
what is your earliest GOOD MORNING TIME ?____:____ am/pm

Before a day off (e.g. a weekend),
what is your latest GOOD MORNING TIME ?____:____ am/pm

Before a day off (e.g. a weekend),
what is your usual GOOD MORNING TIME ?____:____ am/pm

How stable (i.e., similar each night) are your GOOD MORNING TIMES on a night before a day off (e.g. a weekend)? (circle one)

0-15 mins.	16-30 mins.	31-45 mins.	46-60 mins.
61-75 mins.	76-90 mins.	91-105 mins	106-120 mins.
2-3 hours	3-4 hours	over 4 hours	

These questions are about how much sleep you lose to unwanted wakefulness:

On most nights, how long, on average does it take you to fall asleep after you start trying?
______________minutes

On most nights, how much sleep do you lose, on average, from waking up during the night (e.g. to go to the bathroom)?
______________minutes

Reference

1. Monk, T. H., Buysse, D. J., Kennedy, K. S., Potts, J. M., DeGrazia, J. M., & Miewald, J. M. (2003). Measuring sleep habits without using a diary: the sleep timing questionnaire. *Sleep, 26*(2), 208–212.

Representative Studies Using Scale

Klei, L., Reitz, P., Miller, M., Wood, J., Maendel, S., Gross, D., et al. (2005). Heritability of morningness-eveningness and self-report sleep measures in a family-based sample of 521 Hutterites. *Chronobiology International, 22*(6), 1041–1054.

87 Sleep-Wake Activity Inventory (SWAI)

Purpose Consisting of 59 items, the SWAI was designed to screen for excessive daytime sleepiness in a clinical setting. Specifically, the scale evaluates six domains: excessive daytime sleepiness, distress, social desirability, energy level, ability to relax, and nighttime sleep. In contrast with laboratory measures like the Multiple Sleep Latency Test (MSLT), the SWAI offers a quick, inexpensive method for assessing excessive daytime sleepiness.

Population for Testing The SWAI has been validated with a population of individuals aged 16–81 years.

Administration Requiring between 10 and 15 min for completion, the scale is a self-report, pencil-and-paper measure.

Reliability and Validity Initial psychometric validations conducted by developers [1] have demonstrated an internal consistency ranging from .69 to .89, and have found a significant correlation between the SWAI's excessive daytime sleepiness factor and the results of MSLT.

Obtaining a Copy An example of the scale can be found in the original article published by developers [1].

Direct correspondence to:
Leon Rosenthal
HFH Sleep Disorders Center
2921 West Grand Blvd
Detroit, MI 48202

Scoring The scale examines a respondent's tendency to fall asleep in inappropriate situations. Questions are posed using a Likert-type scale that ranges from 1 (meaning the behavior is always present) to 9 (indicating that it never occurs). Individuals are asked to refer to the previous 7 days when answering. Lower scores are indicative of more acute daytime sleepiness.

A. Shahid et al. (eds.), *STOP, THAT and One Hundred Other Sleep Scales*,
DOI 10.1007/978-1-4419-9893-4_87, © Springer Science+Business Media, LLC 2012

Sleep-Wake Activity Inventory (SWAI)

1. I seem to have very little time for my hobbies.
2. I enjoy my daily activities.
3. I have a lot of control over my schedule.
4. I get drowsy two or more times during the day.
5. I feel resentful when I don't get my way.
6. Even if I am sick, I keep going as usual.
7. I get the blues.
8. My energy level is high.
9. I doze off while watching TV.
10. I hesitate to go out of my way to help someone in trouble.
11. I have difficulty with falling asleep.
12. I am liked by people.
13. I can take a nap anywhere.
14. I feel slowed down.
15. I have been irked when people expressed ideas very different from my own.
16. I seem to have very little control over what happens to me.
17. When I am sleepy, I try to keep it to myself.
18. Even if I take a nap, I sleep well at night.
19. My muscles feel stiff.
20. I have very little control over my work schedule.
21. I have doubts about my ability to succeed in life.
22. I can relax without falling asleep.
23. I feel motivated by my daily activities.
24. I fall asleep during a conversation.
25. I am disliked by people.
26. I insist on having things my own way.
27. I get impatient easily.
28. I have a strong will power.
29. I get drowsy driving a few minutes.
30. My mind seems to be working slower than usual.
31. I resent being asked to return a favor.
32. I feel useless.
33. Even if I'm sleepy, I try to just keep going as usual.
34. I seem to have enough time for my hobbies.
35. It takes me less than 5 minutes to fall asleep.
36. I have felt like rebelling against people in authority even though I knew they were right.
37. I feel uneasy most of the day.
38. I seem to have very little time to relax.
39. I set deadlines or quotas for myself at work or at home.
40. I get drowsy within 10 min when I sit still.
41. My mind seems to be working faster than usual.
42. I would rather sit and daydream than doing anything else.
43. I try to get even, rather than forgive and forget.
44. My life is filled by challenges which need to be met.
45. I fall asleep when visiting with friends.
46. I seem to have a lot of control over what happens to me.
47. I am irritated by people who ask favors of me.
48. When in competition, I try hard to win.
49. My temper is fiery and hard to control.
50. I get sleepy after reading for 15 minutes.
51. I seem to have enough time to relax.
52. If I could get into a movie without paying and be sure I was not seen, I would do it.
53. I doze off when relaxed.
54. I fall asleep when riding as a passenger.
55. My appetite is poor.
56. I like to gossip.
57. I make written lists of what needs to be done.
58. When bored, I tend to drift away.
59. I can feel my heart beating.

Reference

1. Rosenthal, L., Roehrs, T. A., & Roth, T. (1993). The sleep-wake activity inventory: a self-report measure of daytime sleepiness. *Biological Psychiatry, 34*(11), 810–820.

Representative Studies Using Scale

Breslau, N., Roth, T., Rosenthal, L., & Andreski, P. (1997). Daytime sleepiness: an epidemiological study of young adults. *American Journal of Public Health, 87*(10), 1649–1653.

Rosenthal, L., Bishop, C., Guido, P., Syron, M. L., Helmus, T. Rice, F. M., & Roth, T. (1997). The sleep/wake habits of patients diagnosed as having obstructive sleep apnea. *Chest, 111*(6), 1494–1499.

88 Snore Outcomes Survey (SOS)

Purpose Designed to evaluate sleep-related quality of life in patients with sleep-disordered breathing (SDB), the SOS consists of 8 items relating to the intensity, duration, frequency, and impact of SDB symptoms – specifically snoring. An additional, three-item measure called the Spouse/Bed Partner Survey is also included with the scale and can be administered to gain an alternative perspective on snoring habits. The instrument may be useful in both research and clinical settings as a tool for assessing changes in quality of life.

Population for Testing The scale has been validated with SDB patients: Mean age was 46.2 ± 11.6 years.

Administration Respondents use pencil and paper to provide self-report answers. The scale requires approximately 5 min for completion.

Reliability and Validity During scale development, researchers Gliklich and Wang [1] found a test-retest reliability of .86 and an internal consistency of .85. Results on the scale also correlated highly with several previously validated measures: the Epworth Sleepiness Scale, the SF-36, and the Pittsburgh Sleep Quality Index.

Obtaining a Copy An example of the scale's questions can be found in the original article published by developers [1]. All permissions to use this scale must be forwarded to Outcome Sciences, Inc., Cambridge MA.

Direct correspondence to:
Richard E. Gliklich,
Department of Otolaryngology and Clinical Outcomes
Research Unit, Massachusetts Eye and Ear Infirmary
243 Charles St, Boston, MA 02114

Scoring Respondents use several Likert-type scales to answer questions regarding their snoring, with lower scores indicating more acute problems with SDB. Scores are normalized on a scale from 0 to 100.

A. Shahid et al. (eds.), *STOP, THAT and One Hundred Other Sleep Scales*,
DOI 10.1007/978-1-4419-9893-4_88, © Springer Science+Business Media, LLC 2012

Snore Outcomes Survey (SOS)

1. In the past 4 weeks, when you have been asleep, to the best of your knowledge do you snore?
All the time Most of the time Some of the time A little of the time
None of the time Don't know

2. In the past 4 weeks, how would you describe your snoring or how has it been describe to you?
None Mild Moderate Severe Very severe Don't Know

3. My snoring wakes me from sleep and/or makes me tired the next day.
Definitely true Somewhat true Don't Know False Definitely false

4. During the past 4 weeks, how much did your snoring interfere with your normal sleep and your level of energy?
Not at all A little bit Moderately Quite a bit Extremely

5. Does your snoring annoy or bother your spouse/bed partner?
Extremely (sleeps in the other room) Quite a bit Moderately A little bit
Not at all Don't know

6. Compared to one year ago, how would you rate your snoring now?
Much less than a year ago Somewhat less than a year ago
About the same as a year ago Somewhat more than a year ago
Much more than a year ago

7. How would your spouse/bed partner describe your snoring?
Extremely loud Very loud Somewhat loud Soft or quiet
No snoring at all Don't know

8. Please describe when you snore.
I don't snore I snore very rarely I snore only in certain positions
I snore most of the time I snore all of the time

Spouse/Bed Partner Survey (SBPS)

1. How would you describe your spouse/bed partner's snoring?
Extremely loud Very loud Somewhat loud Soft or quiet No snoring at all
Don't know

2. In the past 4 weeks, how would you describe your spouse/bed partner's snoring?
None Mild Moderate Severe Very Severe Don't know

3. In the past 4 weeks, how much has your spouse/bed partner's snoring bothered you?
Extremely (sleeping in the other room) Quite a bit Moderately A little bit
Not at all Don't know

Reference

1. Gliklich, R. E. & Wang, P. C. (2002). Validation of the snore outcomes survey for patients with sleep-disordered breathing. *Archives of Otolaryngology – Head and Neck Surgery, 128*(7), 819–824.

Representative Studies Using Scale

Li, H. Y., Lin, Y., Chen, N. H., Lee, L. A., Fang, T. J., & Wang, P. C. (2008). Improvement in quality of life after nasal surgery alone for patients with obstructive sleep apnea and nasal obstruction. *Archives of Otolaryngology - Head and Neck Surgery, 134*(4), 429–433.

Chuang, L. P., Chen, N. H., Li, H. Y., Lin, S. W., Chou, Y. T., Wang, C. J., Liao, Y. F., & Tsai, Y. H. (2009). Dynamic upper airway changes during sleep in patients with obstructive sleep apnea syndrome. *Acta Oto-Laryngologica*, 1651–2251.

St. Mary's Hospital Sleep Questionnaire

89

Purpose Well-suited for repeated use across the span of a study or treatment period, the scale evaluates the duration and subjective quality of an individual's previous night's sleep. The scale's 14 items query a variety of sleep-related issues, including sleep latency, restlessness, nighttime waking, and morning alertness.

Population for Testing The scale has been validated with patient populations between the ages of 15–80 years.

Administration A self-report, pencil-and-paper measure, the questionnaire requires between 5 and 10 min for completion.

Reliability and Validity In a psychometric evaluation conducted by Ellis and colleagues [1], the scale possessed a test-retest reliability ranging from .70 to .96. Additional research on the part of developers [2] supports the scale as a significant measure of change in sleep.

Obtaining a Copy A copy of the scale can be found in an article published by Ellis and colleagues [1].

Direct correspondence to:
Dr. Priest
Academic Department of Psychiatry
St. Mary's Hospital Medical School
Harrow Road, London W9 3RL, England

Scoring As the scale solicits both Likert-type and fill-in-the-blank responses, the scale's scoring process has not been standardized and will depend on the specific purposes of the research or clinician. Some studies select only one or two of the scale's items to focus on (e.g., sleep latency), while others make use of results obtained on the entire instrument. As a measure designed to detect change, a respondent's results are primarily relevant when viewed in relation to results obtained at different times or by different individuals.

A. Shahid et al. (eds.), *STOP, THAT and One Hundred Other Sleep Scales*,
DOI 10.1007/978-1-4419-9893-4_89,

St. Mary's Hospital Sleep Questionnaire

This questionnaire refers to your sleep over the past 24 hours. Please try and answer every question.

Name:________________________
Today's date: ____/_____/_____
Age:____ Yrs.
Sex: Male/Female (delete whichever inapplicable) (M = 1; F = 2)

At what time did you:

1. Settle down for the night? ____Hrs. ____Mins.
2. Fall asleep last night? ____Hrs. ____Mins.
3. Finally wake this morning? ____Hrs. ____Mins.
4. Get up this morning? ____Hrs. ____Mins.
5. Was your sleep: (tick box)
   1. Very light ☐
   2. Light ☐
   3. Fairly light ☐
   4. Light average ☐
   5. Deep average ☐
   6. Fairly deep ☐
   7. Deep ☐
   8. Very deep ☐

6. How many times did you wake up? (tick box)
   0. Not at all ☐
   1. Once ☐
   2. Twice ☐
   3. Three times ☐
   4. Four times ☐
   5. Five times ☐
   6. Six times ☐
   7. More than six times ☐

How much sleep did you have:

7. Last night? ____Hrs. ____Mins.
8. During the day, yesterday? ____Hrs. ____Mins.
9. How well did you sleep last night? (tick box)
   1. Very badly ☐
   2. Badly ☐
   3. Fairly badly ☐
   4. Fairly well ☐
   5. Well ☐
   6. Very well ☐

If not well, what was the trouble? (e.g., restless, etc.)

1. ________________________________
2. ________________________________
3. ________________________________

10. How clear-headed did you feel after getting up this morning? (tick box)
    1. Still very drowsy indeed ☐
    2. Still moderately drowsy ☐
    3. Still slightly drowsy ☐
    4. Fairly clear-headed ☐
    5. Alert ☐
    6. Very alert ☐
11. How satisfied were you with last night's sleep?
    1. Very unsatisfied ☐
    2. Moderately unsatisfied ☐
    3. Slightly unsatisfied ☐
    4. Fairly satisfied ☐
    5. Completely satisfied ☐
12. Were you troubled by waking early and being unable to get off to sleep again? (tick box)
    1. No ☐
    2. Yes ☐
13. How much difficulty did you have in getting off to sleep last night? (tick box)
    1. None or very little ☐
    2. Some ☐
    3. A lot ☐
    4. Extreme difficulty ☐
14. How long did it take you to fall asleep last night?
    _____Hrs. _____Mins

References

1. Ellis, B. W., Johns, M. W., Lancaster, R., Raptopoulos, P., Angelopoulos, N., & Priest, R. G. (1981). The St. Mary's Hospital sleep questionnaire: a study of reliability. *Sleep, 4*(1), 93–97.
2. Murray, F., Bentley, S., Ellis, B. W., & Dudley, H. (1977). Sleep deprivation in patients undergoing operation: a factor in the stress of surgery. *British Medical Journal, 2*(6101), 1521–1522.

Representative Studies Using Scale

Argyropoulos, S. V., Hicks, J. A., Nash, J. R., Bell, C. J., Rich, A. S., Nutt, D. J., & Wilson, S. J. (2003). Correlation of subjective and objective sleep measurements at different stages of the treatment of depression. *Psychiatry Research, 120*(2), 179–190.

Pien, G. W., Sammel, M. D., Freeman, E. W., Lin, H., & ReBlasis, T. L. (2008). Predictors of sleep quality in women in the postmenopausal transition. *Sleep, 31*(7), 991–999.

90 State-Trait Anxiety Inventory (STAI)

Purpose The STAI is a 40-item questionnaire designed to measure two aspects of anxiety: the temporary and episodic form of anxiety that fluctuates across situations and circumstances, and the stable personality traits that predispose individuals to anxiety in general [1]. Though the scale has been widely used in research, it is also a valuable clinical tool. The STAI's two subscales make it ideal for sleep specialists hoping to identify both current recurring anxiety problems in order to address their influence on sleep quality.

Population for Testing Normative data is available for adults aged 19–69 as well as for high school students [2]. A children's version is also available for ages 6–14 years.

Administration The scale is a self-report, paper-and-pencil measure requiring between 10 and 15 min for completion. Administrators are required to possess at least some university-level training in psychometric testing, or relevant field experience.

Reliability and Validity In 2002, Barnes and colleagues [3] conducted a review study in which they examined all articles published over the previous decade reporting reliability for the STAI. The mean internal consistency was .91 for the state scale and .89 for the trait scale. The mean test-retest reliability for the trait scale was .88. As anticipated, the mean for the state scale was lower (.70), reflecting the transitory nature of the measure. Developers Spielberger and colleagues [4] have also demonstrated good concurrent validity, as scores on the STAI correlate highly with results found on alternative anxiety measures like the Anxiety Scale Questionnaire.

Obtaining a Copy The scale can be purchased from a variety of psychological assessment outlets.

Direct correspondence to the developer:
Charles Spielberger
Email: spielber@cas.usf.edu

Scoring The two subscales of the STAI are completed and scored in much the same way. For the state section, respondents use a four-point, Likert-type scale to indicate how accurately statements regarding tension and anxiety apply to them at that moment. Scales range from 1 ("not at all") to 4 ("very much so"). The trait section offers a similar four-point scale, but instead focuses on how respondents feel in general. The scale for this section ranges from 1("almost never") to 4 ("almost always"). Scores are totaled to provide a global score for each subscale. Normative data, T-scores, and percentiles ranks are available for a variety of age ranges. A scoring key can be purchased alongside testing materials to speed the administration process.

A. Shahid et al. (eds.), *STOP, THAT and One Hundred Other Sleep Scales*,
DOI 10.1007/978-1-4419-9893-4_90, © Springer Science+Business Media, LLC 2012

References

1. Spielberger, C, Gorsuch, R. L., Lushene, R., Vagg, P. R., & Jacobs, G. A. (1983). *Manual for the state-trait anxiety inventory*. Palo Alto: Consulting Psychologists Press.
2. Mindgarden Inc. (2008). *State-trait anxiety inventory for adults*. Retrieved July 11, 2009 from http://www.mindgarden.com/products/staisad.htm.
3. Barnes, L., Harp, D., & Jung, W. S. (2002). Reliability generalization of scores on the Spielberger state-trait anxiety inventory. *Educational and Psychological Measurement, 62*(4), 603–618.
4. Spielberger, C., Sydeman, S., Owen, A., & Marsh, B. (1999). Measuring anxiety and anger with the state-trait anxiety inventory (STAI) and the state-trait anger expression inventory (STAXI). In: Maruish, M. E. (Ed.), *The use of psychological testing for treatment planning and outcomes assessment* (2nd ed.; 993–1021). New Jersey: Lawrence Erlbaum Associates.

Representative Studies Using Scale

Baker, A., Simpson, S., & Dawson, D. (1997). Sleep disruption and mood changes associated with menopause. *Journal of Psychosomatic Research, 43*(4), 359–369.

Schlotz, W., Shulz, P., Hellhammer, J., Stone, A., & Hellhammer, D. (2006). Trait anxiety moderates the impact of performance pressure on salivary cortisol in everyday life. *Psychoneuroendocinology, 31*(4), 459–472.

Spira, A. P., Friedman, L., Aulakh, J. S., Lee, T., Shiekh, J. I., & Yesavage, J. A. (2008). Subclinical anxiety symptoms, sleep, and daytime dysfunction in older adults with primary insomnia. *Journal of Geriatric Psychiatry and Neurology, 21*(2), 149–153.

Stanford Sleepiness Scale (SSS) 91

Purpose The SSS is a subjective measure of sleepiness, frequently used for both research and clinical purposes. Whereas an instrument like the Epworth Sleepiness Scale (Chap. 29) examines general experiences of sleepiness over the course of an entire day, the SSS evaluates sleepiness at specific moments in time. Consisting of only one item, the scale requires respondents to select one of seven statements best representing their level of perceived sleepiness [1]. As a single-item measure, the scale is best suited for repeated use over the course of a research study or treatment intervention.

Population for Testing The scale has no specified population for testing, though its performance has been evaluated exclusively in adults over the age of 18.

Administration The scale is a self-administered, paper-and-pencil measure requiring 1–2 min for completion.

Reliability and Validity In an early examination of the SSS, Hoddes and colleagues [2] found that average scores on the scale were significantly elevated following 24 h of total sleep deprivation. Researchers have found that the scale can be used to predict performance on tasks related to alertness (e.g., reaction time, vigilance tests) following total sleep deprivation; however, the scale is not as sensitive to partial sleep deprivation, which most closely mimics the deficits experienced by those with sleep disorders [3]. Though widely used in research settings, some have taken issue with the scale and its unidimensional quality. In their evaluation of the scale, MacLean and colleagues [4] found that sleepiness as measured by the SSS has at least two dimensions – what they referred to as "activation" and "sleepiness" – and that the descriptors used as each level are often not considered equivalent by respondents.

Obtaining a Copy The scale is freely available online.

Scoring Respondents use a scale from 1 to 7 to indicate their current level of sleepiness. Values are assigned as follows:

1. "Feeling active and vital; alert; wide awake."
2. "Functioning at a high level, but not at peak; able to concentrate."
3. "Relaxed; awake; not at full alertness; responsive."
4. "A little foggy; not at peak; let down."
5. "Fogginess; beginning to lose interest in remaining awake; slowed down."
6. "Sleepiness; prefer to be lying down; fighting sleep; woozy."
7. "Almost in reverie; sleep onset soon; lost struggle to remain awake."

Scores can then be compared longitudinally across different times of day, seasons, and stages of treatment. However, researchers and clinicians

A. Shahid et al. (eds.), *STOP, THAT and One Hundred Other Sleep Scales*,
DOI 10.1007/978-1-4419-9893-4_91, © Springer Science+Business Media, LLC 2012

The Stanford Sleepiness Scale (SSS)

Degree of Sleepiness	Scale Rating
Feeling active, vital, alert, or wide awake	1
Functioning at high levels, but not at peak; able to concentrate	2
Awake, but relaxed; responsive but not fully alert	3
Somewhat foggy, let down	4
Foggy; losing interest in remaining awake; slowed down	5
Sleepy, woozy, fighting sleep; prefer to lie down	6
No longer fighting sleep, sleep onset soon; having dream-like thoughts	7
Asleep	X

should be careful when comparing scores between individuals who may possess different baselines for sleepiness.

References

1. Hoddes, E., Dement, W., & Zarcone, V. (1972). The development and use of the Stanford sleepiness scale (SSS). *Psychophysiology, 9*, 150.
2. Hoddes, E., Zarcone, V., Smythe, H., Phillips, R., & Dement, W.C. (1973). Quantification of sleepiness: a new approach. *Psychophysiology, 10*, 431–436.
3. Broughton, R. (1982). Performance and evoked potential measures of various states of daytime sleepiness. *Sleep, 5*, S135-S146.
4. MacLean, A. W., Fekken, G. C., Saskin, P., & Knowles, J.B. (1992). Psychometric evaluation of the Stanford sleepiness scale. *Journal of Sleep Research, 1*(1), 35–39.

Representative Studies Using Scale

Carskadon, M. A. & Dement, W. C. (2007). Cumulative effects of sleep restriction on daytime sleepiness. *Psychophysiology, 18*(2), 107–113.

Connor, J., Norton, R., Ameratunga, S., Robinson, E., Civil, I., Dunn, R., Bailey, J., & Jackson, R. (2002). Driver sleepiness and risk of serious injury to car occupants: population based case control study. *British Medical Journal, 324*, 1125–1128.

92 STOP-Bang Questionnaire

Purpose Designed to screen for symptoms of obstructive sleep apnea (OSA) in surgical patients in particular and in all individuals in general, the questionnaire consists of four yes/no and four fill-in-the-blank questions primed by the mnemonic "STOP-Bang:" S – "Do you **S**nore loudly (louder than talking or loud enough to be heard through closed doors)?" T – "Do you often feel **T**ired, fatigued, or sleepy during daytime?" O – "Has anyone **O**bserved you stop breathing during your sleep?" P – "Do you have or are you being treated for high blood **P**ressure?" In order to improve the accuracy of the scale B – **BMI**, A – **A**ge, N – **N**eck circumference, and G – **G**ender are recorded. The scale was specifically developed for use in a preoperative setting, where untreated OSA is associated with increased post-operative complications and longer hospital stays [1]. The purpose was also to provide a short, easy to use scale that could be used in the clinical setting.

Population for Testing The scale has been validated with a population of surgical patients with a mean age of 57 ± 16.

Administration The STOP-Bang is a paper-and-pencil measure requiring approximately 1 min for completion.

Reliability and Validity To create the questionnaire, developers Chung and colleagues [1] analyzed a preexisting apnea scale – the Berlin questionnaire – and found that it consisted of four separate factors. Using these factors, the first four yes/no questions of the STOP-Bang were created. Developers also found that the inclusion of factors like **BMI**, **A**ge, **N**eck circumference, and **G**ender greatly increased the sensitivity of the measure and these were then added. The STOP-Bang possesses both sensitivity and specificity greater than 90% in patients with moderate-to-severe OSA.

Obtaining a Copy A copy can be found in the original article published by developers [1].

Direct correspondence to:
Dr. Chung
Room 405, 2 McL, Department of Anesthesia
399 Bathurst Street
Toronto, Ontario, Canada
M5T 2S8

Scoring For the first four yes/no questions, a response of "yes" is given one point. An additional one point is awarded for each of the following conditions: a BMI of more than 35 kg/m^2, an age of 50 years or greater, a neck circumference greater than 40 cm, and a final point for patients who are male. If only the first four items are being scored, a total score of two or more is considered high risk of OSA. When using the complete STOP-Bang, a total score of three or more places the individual at high risk.

A. Shahid et al. (eds.), *STOP, THAT and One Hundred Other Sleep Scales*,
DOI 10.1007/978-1-4419-9893-4_92, © Springer Science+Business Media, LLC 2012

STOP-BANG

STOP

Do you **S**nore?	Yes ❑ No ❑
Do you feel **T**ired, fatigued or sleepy during the day?	Yes ❑ No ❑
Has anyone **O**bserved you stop breathing in your sleep?	Yes ❑ No ❑
Do you have high blood **P**ressure ?	Yes ❑ No ❑

Please count the number of "Yes" responses and put the number in this box ❑

B	A	N	G
BMI	Age	Neck Size	Gender
>35	>50 y	> 40cm > 15.7"	- Male

If height is	ft.in.	4'10"	5'0"	5'2"	5'4"	5'6"	5'8"	5'10"	6'0"	6'2"	6'4"
& weight is >	lbs	167	179	191	204	216	230	250	258	272	287

Then BMI is > 35

姓名 ________ 年齡 ________ 電話 ________ 填表日期 ________

推薦醫生 ________ 推薦醫生電話 ________

STOP BANG 量表

你睡眠時有打鼻鼾嗎? (**S**nore) 是 □ 否□

你白天感覺疲勞或睏倦嗎? (**T**ired) 是 □ 否□

睡眠時有人發現你有呼吸暫停嗎? (**O**bserved stop breathing) 是 □ 否□

你有高血壓嗎? (High blood **P**ressure) 是 □ 否□

請計算以上有多少 “是” 的答案, 並填在右邊方格裡 □

你的體重指數大於 35? (**B**MI) 是 □ 否□

你的年齡大過 50 歲?(**A**ge) 是 □ 否□

你的頸圍超過 40 厘米? (**N**eck size) 是 □ 否□

你的性別? (**G**ender) 男 □ 女□

如果身高是	厘米	147	152	157	163	168	173	178	183	188	193
並且體重大於	公斤	76	81	86	93	99	105	111	117	124	130

如果身高是	英尺 英寸	4’10”	5’0”	5’2”	5’4”	5’6”	5’8”	5’10”	6’0”	6’2”	6’4”
並且體重大於	磅	167	178	189	205	218	231	244	257	273	286

則體重指數大於 35

姓名________ 年龄________ 电话________ 填表日期________

推荐医生姓名________ 推荐医生电话________

STOP BANG 量表

你睡觉打呼吗？[**S**nore] 是 □ 否 □

你感觉白天疲劳或困倦吗？[**T**ired] 是 □ 否 □

有人发现你睡觉时有呼吸暂停吗？[**O**bserved stop breathing] 是 □ 否 □

你患高血压吗？[high blood **P**ressure] 是 □ 否 □

请数一下你的回答中有几个“是”

并把这个数字填在后面的方框里 □

你的体重指数大于35？[**B**MI] 是 □ 否 □

你的年龄大于50岁？[**A**ge] 是 □ 否 □

你的颈围超过40 厘米？[**N**eck size] 是 □ 否 □

你的性别？[**G**ender] 男 □ 女 □

如果身高是	厘米	147	152	157	163	168	173	178	183	188	193
且体重大于	公斤	76	81	86	93	99	105	111	117	124	130
如果身高是	英尺英寸	4'10"	5'0"	5'2"	5'4"	5'6"	5'8"	5'10"	6'0"	6'2"	6'4"
且体重大于	磅	167	178	189	205	218	231	244	257	273	286

则体重指数大于35

(PARE PANCADA)

Você ressona? Sim __ Não __

Você sente-se fatigado, cansado ou com sono durante o dia? Sim __ Não __

Alguém observou que você deixa de respirar enquanto você está a dormir? Sim __ Não __

Você tem hipertensão? Sim __ Não __

Por favor conte o número de respostas assinaladas "Sim" e escreva o número nesta caixa

I	I	P	G
IMC > 35	Idade > 50 a	Tamanho de pescoço > 40 cms> 15.7"	Gênero Macho

Se a altura em pés é :	4 '10"	5' 0"	5 '2"	5' 4"	5 '6"	5' 8"	5 '10"	6' 0"	6 '2"	6' 4"
E peso em lb:	167	179	191	204	216	230	250	258	272	287
Se a altura é cm:	147	152	158	163	168	173	178	183	188	193
E peso é kg:	75	81	86	92	97	104	113	116	122	129

Então IMC é> 35

STOP BANG

Do you **S**nore? **YES** __ **NO** __
Ikaw ba ay naghihilik? Oo ___ Hindi ___

Do you feel **T**ired, fatigued or sleepy during the day? **YES** __ **NO** __
Nararamdaman mo bang mapagod at antukin pag-araw? Oo ___ Hindi ___

Has anyone **O**bserved you stop breathing in your sleep? **YES** __ **NO** __
Mayroon bang nagsabi sa iyo na humihinto and iyong pag-hinga kapag ikaw ay tulog? Oo ___ Hindi ___

Do you have high blood **P**ressure? **YES** __ **NO** __
Mataas ba ang presyon ng iyong dugo? Oo ___ Hindi ___

If height is: Kung an taas ay:	ft. in.	4'10"	5'0"	5'2"	5'4"	5'6"	5'8"	5'10"	6'0"	6'2"	6'4"
& weight is > Kung ang bigat ay:	lbs.	167	179	191	204	216	230	250	258	272	287
If height is Kung an taas ay:	cm	147	152	158	163	168	173	178	183	188	193
& weight is > Kung ang bigat ay:	kg	75	81	86	92	97	104	113	116	122	129

Then your BMI is > 35

B - based on the above table, is your BMI >35? **YES** __ **NO** __
Binase sa table sa taas, ito ba ang iyong BMI > 35? Oo ___ Hindi ___

Is your **A**ge over 50 years? Ang edad mo ba ay 50? **YES** __ **NO** __

How old are you? ___________yrs Oo ___ Hindi __
Ilang taon ka na? ___________ taon

Is your **N**eck Size over 40 cm (15.7")? **YES** __ **NO** __
Ang sukat ba ng leeg mo ay lampas ng 40? Oo ___ Hindi ___

Gender – are you a male? **YES** __ **NO** __
- ikaw ba ay lalaki? Oo ___ Hindi ___

*Could you please count the number of "**Yes**" responses from the above 8 questions*
Puwede bang bilangin kung ilan ang sagot mo na "Oo" sa 8 tanong na tinanong, pagkatapos, ilagay sa loob ng
and put the number in this box: [ ]
kahon na ito.

Other: ______________________________

Thank you!!!
Salamat !!!

هل تعاني من الشخير؟	نعم	لا
هل تشعر بالتعب أو الارهاق أو النعاس أثناء النهار ؟	نعم	لا
هل لاحظ أحد توقف تنفسك أثناء نومك؟	نعم	لا
هل تعاني من ارتفاع ضغط الدم؟	نعم	لا

الرجاء حساب عدد إجاباتك بنعم ووضع الرقم في هذا المربع ☐

G	N	A	B
الجنس	قياس الرقبة	العمر	دليل كتلة الجسم
ذكر	>40cm >15.7”	> 50 سنة	>35

إذا كان الطول بالقدم و البوصة		6’4”	6’2”	6’0”	5’10”	5’8”	5’6”	5’4”	5’2”	5’0”	4’10”
و الوزن بالباوند	<	287	272	258	250	230	216	204	191	179	167
إذا كان الطول بالسنتميتر		193	188	183	178	173	168	163	158	152	147
و الوزن بالكيلوغرام	<	129	122	116	113	104	97	92	86	81	75

فإن دليل كتلة الجسم لديك يكون > 35

STOP BANG

S Вы храпите?	ДА__ НЕТ
T Вы чувствуете себя усталым или сонливым в течение дня?	ДА__ НЕТ
O Кто-либо засвидетельствовал что вы перестаёте дышать во сне?	ДА__НЕТ
P Вы страдаете от высокого кровянного давления?	ДА__ НЕТ

Пожалуйста подсчитайте количество ДА и запишите в этом прямоугольнике

B Индекс массы тела	>35 кг/м^2	ДА__ НЕТ
A Ваш возраст	> 50 лет	ДА__ НЕТ
N Окружность вашей шеи	>44 см	ДА__ НЕТ
G Пол	мужской	ДА__ НЕТ

если ваш рост	см	147	152	158	163	168	173	178	183	188	193
если ваш вес >	кг	75	81	86	92	97	104	113	116	122	129

Следовательно ваш Индекс массы тела **> 35** кг/м^2

STOP BANG

Da li **Hrčete**? Da __ Ne __

Da li se osjećate **Umorni** ili pospani u toku dana? Da __ Ne __

Da li je iko **Vidio** da prestanete disati dok spavate? Da __ Ne __

Da li imate povišen krvni **Pritisak**? Da __ Ne __

Molimo da saberete sve odgovore na koje ste odgovorili sa “Da” i stavite broj u kućicu.

B	A	N	G
BMI (Tjelesna masa)	**A**ge (Dob)	**N**eck size (Obim vrata)	**G**ender (Pol)
>35	>50 y	> 40cm > 15.7”	-Male (Muški)

Ako je visina	ft. in.	4’10”	5’0”	5’2”	5’4”	5’6”	5’8”	5’10”	6’0”	6’2”	6’4”
& težina >	lbs.	167	179	191	204	216	230	250	258	272	287

Ako je visina	cm	147	152	158	163	168	173	178	183	188	193
& težina >	kg	75	81	86	92	97	104	113	116	122	129

Tada je BMI > 35

STOP BANG

ΡοχαλίζειΣ ? **ΝΑΙ __ ΟΧΙ __**

Αισθάνεσαι κουρασμένος η νυσΤαλέος κατά την ημέρα? **ΝΑΙ __ ΟΧΙ __**

Έχει κανείς παρατηρήσει Οτι σταματάς να αναπνέεις στον ύπνο σου? **ΝΑΙ __ ΟΧΙ__**

Έχεις υψηλή Πίεση (υπέρταση)? **ΝΑΙ __ ΟΧΙ__**

Εάν έχεις ύψος:	ft. in.	4'10"	5'0"	5'2"	5'4"	5'6"	5'8"	5'10"	6'0"	6'2"	6'4"
& ζυγίζεις >	lbs.	167	179	191	204	216	230	250	258	272	287
Εάν έχεις ύψος	cm	147	152	158	163	168	173	178	183	188	193
& ζυγίζεις >	kg	75	81	86	92	97	104	113	116	122	129

Τότε το BMI σου είναι > 35

Με βάση τον άνω πίνακα, έχεις BMI >35? **ΝΑΙ __ ΟΧΙ __**

Είσαι πάνω από 50 ετών ? **ΝΑΙ __ ΟΧΙ __**

Πόσο χρονών είσαι ? _____ χρονών

Το μέγεθος τού λαιμού σου είναι πάνω από 40 εκ. (15.7")? **ΝΑΙ __ ΟΧΙ __**

Γένος – είσαι άντρας? **ΝΑΙ __ ΟΧΙ __**

Παρακαλώ πρόσθεσε τον αριθμό των ΝΑΙ απαντήσεων από τις 8 ερωτήσεις καί γράψε τον αριθμό στο κουτί αυτό : ☐

STOP BANG

ঘুমে কি নাক ডাকেন? হ্যাঁ __ না

দিনে কি ক্লান্ত, অবসন্ন অথবা ঘুম বোধ করেন হ্যাঁ __ না

কেউ কি আপনাকে ঘুমে আপনার শ্বাস রুদ্ধ হতে দেখেছয়ু? হ্যাঁ __ না

আপনি কি high blood **P**ressure এ ভুগছেন? হ্যাঁ __ না

আপনার উত্তর হ্যাঁ গননা করে বাকশতে লিখুন

B	**A**	**N**	**G**
BMI >35	বয়স >50 y	গলার মাপ > 40cm > 15.7"	Gender - Male

If height is	ft. in.	4'10"	5'0"	5'2"	5'4"	5'6"	5'8"	5'10"	6'0"	6'2"	6'4"
& weight is >	lbs.	167	179	191	204	216	230	250	258	272	287
If height is	cm	147	152	158	163	168	173	178	183	188	193
& weight is >	kg	75	81	86	92	97	104	113	116	122	129

Then BMI is > 35

STOP Скринінг Інструмент Синдрому Апное Уві Сні

Дайте відповідь на кожен з наступних питань Так чи Ні:

1. Ви голосно хропите під час сну (голосніше, ніж говорити або достатньо голосно, щоб бути почутим крізь зачинені двері)?	Так ☐	Ні ☐
2. Чи часто ви відчуваєте втому або сонливість протягом дня?	Так ☐	Ні ☐
3. Чи хто-небудь спостерігав зупинку вашого дихання під час сну?	Так ☐	Ні ☐
4. Чи є у вас високий кров'яний тиск або чи ви лікуєтесь від нього?	Так ☐	Ні ☐
5. Індекс маси тіла* (ІМТ) більше 35 кг/м^2?	Так ☐	Ні ☐
6. Вік старше 50 років?	Так ☐	Ні ☐
7. Окружність шиї більше 40 сантиметрів?	Так ☐	Ні ☐
8. Чоловіча стать?	Так ☐	Ні ☐

*Індекс маси тіла обраховується за формулою:

$$I = \frac{m}{h^2},$$

де:

- m — маса тіла в кілограмах
- h — зріст в метрах,

і вимірюється в кг/м^2.

S - האם את/ה נוחר/ת?
T - האם את/ה עייף/ה או ישנוני/ת במשך היום?
O - האם מישהו ראה אותך מפסיק/ה לנשום בלילה?
P - האם יש לך לחץ דם גבוה?

B - BMI>35
A - גיל מעל 50
N - היקף צואר מעל 40 ס"מ
G - גבר

References

1. Chung, F., Yegneswaran, B., Liao, P., Vairavanathan, S., Islam, S., Khajehdehi, A., & Shapiro, C. M. (2008). STOP questionnaire – a tool to screen patients for obstructive sleep apnea. *Anesthesiology, 108*(5), 812–821.

Representative Studies Using Scale

Farney, R. J., Walker, B. S., Rarney, R. M., Snow, G. L., & Walker, J. M. (2011). The STOP-Bang equivalent model and prediction of severity of obstructive sleep apnea: relation to polysomnographic measurements of the apnea/hypopnea index. Journal of clinical Sleep Medicine, 7(5), 459–465.

Gay, P. C. (2010). Sleep and sleep-disordered breathing in the hospitalized patient. Respiratory Care, 55(9), 1240–1254.

Senthilvel, E., Auckley, D., & Dasarathy, J. (2011). Evaluation of sleep disorders in the primary care setting: history taking compared to questionnaries. Journal of Clinicinal Sleep Medicine, 7(1), 41–48.

Note: It should be noted that this is one of two scales that are used in the title of this book (see Chap. 96 for THAT).

Tayside Children's Sleep Questionnaire (TCSQ) 93

Purpose Designed to assess disorders of initiating and maintaining sleep (DIMS) in children, the TCSQ consists of ten parent-reported items relating to sleep onset, night-waking, preferred sleep setting, and other sleep behaviors.

Population for Testing Developers recommend the scale for use with children between the ages of 1 and 5 years.

Administration The scale is a pencil-and-paper, parental report measure requiring approximately 5 min for completion.

Reliability and Validity In analyzing the scale's psychometric properties, developers McGreavey and colleagues [1] found an internal consistency of .85.

Obtaining a Copy A copy of the scale can be found in the original article published by developers [1].

Direct correspondence to:
Jacqui McGreavey
Health Centre, Victoria Street
Monifieth, Dundee
DD5 4LX, UK
Email: jacqui.mcgreavey@tpct.scot.nhs.uk

Scoring Though the scale contains 10 items, only the first nine are used in scoring. Parents are asked about their children's sleep habits over the previous 3 months – answers are collected using a five-point, Likert-type scale that ranges from 0 (indicating that the behavior never occurs) to 4 (meaning it happens every night). Initially, developers have suggested a cutoff score of 8 – a relatively value meant to identify mild sleep problems as well.

A. Shahid et al. (eds.), *STOP, THAT and One Hundred Other Sleep Scales*,
DOI 10.1007/978-1-4419-9893-4_93, © Springer Science+Business Media, LLC 2012

Tayside Children's Sleep Questionnaire

Questions

1. How long after going to bed does your child usually fall asleep.
2. The child goes to bed reluctantly
3. The child has difficulty getting to sleep at night (and may require a parent to be present)
4. The child does not fall asleep in his or her own bed
5. The child wakes up two or more times in the night
6. After waking up in the night the child has difficulty falling asleep again by himself or herself
7. The child sleeps in the parent's bed at some time during the night
8. If the child wakes, he or she uses a comforter (e.g. Dummy) and requires a parent to replace it
9. The child wants a drink during the night (including breast or bottle-feed)
10. Do you think your child has sleeping difficulties

Reference

1. McGreavey, J. A., Donnan, P. T., Pagliari, H. C., & Sullivan, F. M. (2005). The Tayside children's sleep questionnaire: a simple tool to evaluate sleep problems in young children. *Child: Care, Health, and Development, 31*(5), 539–544.

Representative Studies Using Scale

Johnson, N. and McMahon, C. (2008). Preschoolers' sleep behaviour: associations with parental hardiness, sleep-related cognitions and bedtime interactions. *Journal of Child Psychology and Psychiatry, 49*(7), 765–773.

94 Teacher's Daytime Sleepiness Questionnaire (TDSQ)

Purpose A short scale consisting of only ten items, the TDSQ was developed to assess evidence of sleep disturbances in children from the perspective of the child's elementary school teacher. The instrument queries several behavioral issues that may manifest as a result of disturbed sleep, including difficulty maintaining alertness, napping during the day, yawning, clumsiness, aggressiveness, and hyperactivity.

Population for Testing The scale was created for use with children aged 4–11 years.

Administration The TDSQ is a self-report, paper-and-pencil measure completed by the elementary school teacher of the child being assessed. It requires 3–5 min for completion.

Reliability and Validity The scale has been employed primarily in clinical settings, and thus, its psychometric properties have not been evaluated extensively. In an early study performed by developers, [1], the scale was found to possess seven factors with an overall internal consistency of .80. Additionally, scores on the TDSQ correlated significantly with the daytime sleepiness subscale of the Children's Sleep Habits Questionnaire (Chap. 21).

Obtaining a Copy A copy of the scale is available in the original article published by developers [1].

Direct correspondence to:
Judith A. Owens
Rhode Island Hospital, Division of Pediatric Ambulatory Medicine
Potter Building, Suite 200
Providence, RI 02903, USA

Scoring Respondents are provided with a three-point, Likert-type scale ranging from "never or rarely (less than once per week)" to "usually (every day)" and are asked to indicate how frequently the child in question demonstrates certain behaviors over the course of a typical week. A total score is calculated, with higher scores indicating greater daytime sleepiness. Scores can then be compared to additional measures of sleepiness and sleep disturbance in order to better understand the child's behavior across a wide range of settings.

A. Shahid et al. (eds.), *STOP, THAT and One Hundred Other Sleep Scales*,
DOI 10.1007/978-1-4419-9893-4_94,

Teacher's Daytime Sleepiness Questionnaire (TDSQ)

The following statements are about signs of daytime sleepiness in children. Think about a typical week for this child when answering the questions.

HOW OFTEN DOES THIS CHILD...
(Circle one answer for each question)

	1 Never or rarely (Less than once a week)	2 Sometimes (At least once a week)	3 Usually (Every day)
Have trouble staying awake in the morning	1	2	3
Have trouble staying awake in the afternoon	1	2	3
Take daytime naps?	1	2	3
Yawn during the day?	1	2	3
Seem clumsy or uncoordinated?	1	2	3
Disrupt school activities because of sleepiness?	1	2	3
Disrupt school activities because of irritability or aggressive behaviour?	1	2	3
Have a major discipline problem?	1	2	3
Appear hyperactive?	1	2	3
Complain about his/her sleep?	1	2	3

Reference

1. Owens, J.A., Spirito, A., McGuinn, M., & Mobile, C. (2000). Sleep habits and sleep disturbance in elementary school-aged children. Journal of *Developmental and Behavioral Pediatrics, 21*(1), 27–36.

Representative Studies Using Scale

Owens, J.A., Maxim, R., McGuinn, M., Nobile, C., Msall, M., & Alario, A. (1999). Television-viewing habits and sleep disturbance in school children. *Pediatrics, 104*(3), e27.

Time of Day Sleepiness Scale (TODSS)

95

Purpose Constructed using items taken from the Epworth Sleepiness Scale (ESS; Chap. 29), the ToDSS was designed to collect subjective assessments of sleepiness for three different times of day: morning, afternoon, and evening. The scale allows clinicians and researchers to assess daytime sleepiness across a variety of situations at several different points in time. While still a new instrument, the ToDSS may prove useful for those who need an efficient measure of changes in daytime sleepiness throughout the day.

Population for Testing The scale has been evaluated in a population of patients presenting for a sleep consultation at a clinic. Participants had a mean age of 47.5 ± 13.5 years.

Administration The scale is a self-report, paper-and-pencil measure requiring approximately 5 min for administration.

Reliability and Validity In an initial validation study conducted by Dolan and colleagues [1], developers found an internal consistency ranging from .87 to .9, and results on the ToDSS were highly correlated with scores obtained on the ESS. ToDSS scores decreased significantly following treatment for those patients with obstructive sleep apnea.

Obtaining a Copy A copy of the scale can be found in the original article published by developers [1].

Direct correspondence to:
Leon D. Rosenthal
Sleep Medicine Associates of Texas
5477 Glen Lakes Dr. Suite 100
Dallas, TX 75231, USA
Email: ldr@sleepmed.com

Scoring The scale is divided into three columns: morning (before noon), afternoon (from noon to 6:00 p.m.), and evening (after 6:00 p.m.). For each time-of-day column, respondents use a scale from 0 ("would never doze") to 3 ("high chance of dozing") to indicate the likelihood that they would fall asleep in certain situations. Scores are tallied for each column to provide a total score for the three different times of day. Total scores can then be compared.

A. Shahid et al. (eds.), *STOP, THAT and One Hundred Other Sleep Scales*,
DOI 10.1007/978-1-4419-9893-4_95, © Springer Science+Business Media, LLC 2012

TIME OF DAY SLEEPINESS SCALE

Modified—Morning-Afternoon-Evening

NAME____________________ **DATE**____________

In contrast to just feeling tired, how likely are you to doze off or fall asleep at each specified time of the day (in the morning, afternoon, and evening) in each of the following situations? Even if you have not done some of these things recently, try to work out how they would have affected you. For each time of the day, use the following scale to choose the most appropriate rating for each situation:

0= Would never doze
1= Slight chance of dozing
2= Moderate chance of dozing
3= High chance of dozing

	Chance of Dozing		
Situation	***Morning*** *Before noon*	***Afternoon*** *Noon-6pm*	***Evening*** *After 6 pm*
Sitting & reading....................................			
Watching TV....................................			
Sitting inactive in a public place(i.e.theater)....................			
As a car passenger for an hour without a break..................			
Lying down to rest....................................			
Sitting & talking to someone....................................			
Sitting quietly after a meal without alcohol......................			
In a car, while stopping for a few minutes in traffic..........			
Total			

Reference

1. Dolan, D. C., Taylor, D. J., Okonkwo, R., Becker, P. M., Jamieson, A. O., Schmidt-Nowara, W., & Rosenthal, L. D. (2009). The time of day sleepiness scale to assess differential levels of sleepiness across the day. *Journal of Psychosomatic Research, 67*, 127–133.

Representative Studies Using Scale

None.

Toronto Hospital Alertness Test (THAT)

96

Purpose Developers designed the THAT as a brief, self-report alternative to instruments like the Maintenance of Wakefulness Test and the Alpha Attenuation Test – time-consuming measures that require specialized laboratory equipment and advanced training to conduct. Consisting of ten items, the THAT presents several psychological states relating to alertness (the ability to think creatively, to concentrate, and to see details clearly, for example) and asks respondents to rate how often in the past week they have experienced those states. Just as the Epworth Sleepiness Scale (Chap. 29) acts as a complementary measure to the Multiple Sleep Latency Test rather than a pure facsimile, the THAT functions well in conjunction with the ZOGIM-A (Chap. 102), which measures a different facet of alertness.

Population for Testing The scale has been validated with a sample of patients referred to a sleep clinic for evaluation whose mean age was 42 ± 14.

Administration The scale is a self-report, pencil-and-paper measure requiring approximately 5 min for completion.

Reliability and Validity An initial psychometric evaluation of the scale [1] demonstrated an internal consistency of .96, and a test-retest reliability of .82. Results on the THAT also differed significantly for patients found to have narcolepsy.

Obtaining a Copy A copy of the scale can be found in the original article published by developers [1].

Direct correspondence to:
Colin M. Shapiro
MP7 # 421
Toronto Western Hospital
399 Bathurst Street, Toronto, ON
M5T 2S8

Scoring Respondents use a six-point, Likert-type scale to indicate how frequently they experience certain feelings relating to alertness. The scale ranges from 0 (meaning "not at all") to 5 ("all the time"), though it is reversed for the questionnaire's final two items to ensure respondent compliance. The scale provides a total score ranging from 0 to 50, with higher scores denoting greater levels of alertness.

A. Shahid et al. (eds.), *STOP, THAT and One Hundred Other Sleep Scales*,
DOI 10.1007/978-1-4419-9893-4_96, © Springer Science+Business Media, LLC 2012

Toronto Hospital Alertness Test (THAT)

This questionnaire tries to establish how alert you feel. In reporting your feeling, we would like you to consider your last week. Use the following scale to check one response for each question.

	Not at all	Less than ¼ of the time	¼ to ½ of the time	½ to ¾ of the time	More than ¾ of the time	All the time I was awake
During the last week, I felt	0	1	2	3	4	5
Able to concentrate						
Alert						
Fresh						
Energetic						
Able to think of new ideas						
Vision was clear, noting all details (e.g., driving)						
Able to focus on the task at hand						
Mental facilities were operating at peak level						
Extra effort was needed to maintain alertness						
In a boring situation, I would find my mind wandering						

Note: This scale contributed the second word in the title of this book (see Chap. 91 for STOP).

Reference

1. Shapiro, C.M., Auch, C., Reimer, M., Kayumov, L., Heslegrave, R., Huterer, N., Driver, H., & Devins, G. (2006). A new approach to the construct of alertness. *Journal of Psychosomatic Research, 60*, 595–603.

Representative Studies Using Scale

Moller, H.J., Devins, G.M., Shen, J., & Shapiro, C.M. (2006). Sleepiness is not the inverse of alertness: evidence from four sleep disorder patient groups. *Experimental Brain Research, 173*(2), 258–266.

Hossain, N.K., Irvine, J., Ritvo, P., Driver, H.S., & Shapiro, C.M. (2007). Evaluation and treatment of sleep complaints: patients' subjective responses. *Psychotherapy and Psychosomatics, 76*, 395–399.

Twenty-Item Toronto Alexithymia Scale (TAS-20) 97

Purpose Finding the psychometric properties of the original Toronto Alexithymia Scale to be flawed, developers created the TAS-20 – a revised measure consisting of 20 items divided into three separate factors, or domains of alexithymia. These factors are: the ability to identify feelings and to distinguish them from physiological sensations, the capacity to communicate those feelings to others, and the tendency to exhibit externally oriented thinking. Recent studies suggest that alexithymia may be particularly relevant to experiences of sleep: TAS-20 scores correlate highly with self-report measures of sleep quality [1], while polysomnographic evaluations have demonstrated decreased deep sleep in individuals with alexithymia [2]. Thus, sleep specialists may find the TAS-20 useful in identifying underlying causes of sleep complaints, in developing treatment plans, and in understanding patient motivations (for example, the ways in which cognitive factors may relate to CPAP compliance).

Population for Testing In a validation study conducted by developers [3], ages of student and patient participants ranged from 20 to 66 years.

Administration The self-report, pencil-and-paper scale requires between 5 and 10 min for administration.

Reliability and Validity According to developers' extensive evaluations of the scale's psychometric properties [3, 4], the TAS-20 possesses an internal consistency of .81 and a test-retest reliability of .77. Results on the TAS-20 were negatively correlated with measures of openness to experience and assertiveness.

Obtaining a Copy An example of the scale's questions can be found in the original article published by developers [3].

Direct correspondence to:
Graeme J. Taylor
Mount Sinai Hospital, Room 936
600 University Ave., Toronto, Ontario
M5G 1X5 Canada

Scoring Respondents use a five-point, Likert-type scale to indicate how well each item describes them. The scale ranges from 1 ("strongly disagree") to 5 ("strongly agree"), though five items are reversed to control for acquiescent responding. Higher scores denote more severe alexithymia.

References

1. De Gennaro, L., Martina, M., Curcio, G., & Ferrara, M. (2004). The relationship between alexithymia, depression, and sleep complaints. *Psychiatry Research, 128*(3), 253–258.
2. Bazydlo, R., Lumley, M. A., & Roehrs, T. (2001). Alexithymia and polysomnographic measures of sleep in healthy adults. *Psychosomatic Medicine, 63*, 56–61.
3. Bagby, R. M., Parker, J. D. A., & Taylor, G. J. (1994a). The twenty-item Toronto alexithymia scale—I. Item selection and cross-validation of the factor structure. *Journal of Psychosomatic Research, 38*(1), 23–32.

A. Shahid et al. (eds.), *STOP, THAT and One Hundred Other Sleep Scales*,
DOI 10.1007/978-1-4419-9893-4_97, © Springer Science+Business Media, LLC 2012

4. Bagby, R. M., Taylor, G. J., & Parker, J. D. A. (1994b). The twenty-item Toronto alexithymia scale—II. Convergent, discriminant, and concurrent validity. *Journal of Psychosomatic Research, 38*(1), 33–40.

Representative Studies Using Scale

Bazydlo, R., Lumley, M. A., & Roehrs, T. (2001). Alexithymia and polysomnographic measures of sleep in healthy adults. *Psychosomatic Medicine, 63*, 56–61.

Tani, P., Lindberg, N., Joukamaa, M., Nieminen-von Wendt, T., von Wendt, L., Appelberg, B., Rimón, R., & Porkka-Heiskanen, T. (2004). Asperger syndrome, alexithymia and perception of sleep. *Neuropsychobiology, 49*(2), 64–70.

98 Ullanlinna Narcolepsy Scale (UNS)

Purpose The UNS is an 11-item scale designed to evaluate a variety of symptoms relating to narcolepsy, including frequency of daytime narcoleptic episodes, muscle weakness associated with powerful emotions, and nighttime sleep latency.

Population for Testing The scale has been validated with both patient and control populations. Comparison groups were included to ensure that the scale could accurately distinguish between symptoms of narcolepsy and those of other sleep or fatigue-related issues (e.g., apnea, depression, sleep deprivation). The scale was administered to individuals aged 17–72.

Administration Requiring between 5 and 10 min for completion, the UNS is a self-report, paper-and-pencil measure.

Reliability and Validity A preliminary psychometric evaluation of the UNS [1] demonstrated a specificity of 98.8% and a sensitivity of 100% when a cutoff score of 14 is used. Additionally, a Chinese translation of the scale has been found to possess an internal consistency of .75 [2].

Obtaining a Copy An example of the scale's items can be found in the original article published by developers [1].

Direct correspondence to:
Christer Hublin
Department of Neurology
University of Helsinki, Haartmanink
4, SF-00290 Helsinki, Finland

Scoring Each item queries a symptom relating to narcolepsy – respondents use a scale ranging from 0 to 4 to indicate how frequently they experience those symptoms. Total scores can range from 0 to 44 with higher scores denoting greater narcoleptic tendencies. Developers suggest a cutoff score of 14 to achieve the greatest levels of sensitivity and specificity.

A. Shahid et al. (eds.), *STOP, THAT and One Hundred Other Sleep Scales*,
DOI 10.1007/978-1-4419-9893-4_98, © Springer Science+Business Media, LLC 2012

Ullanlinna Narcolepsy Scale

1. When laughing, becoming glad or angry or in an exciting situation, have the following symptoms suddenly occurred?

	Never	1-5 times during Lifetime	Monthly	Weekly	Daily or Almost Daily
Knees Unlocking	☐	☐	☐	☐	☐
Mouth Opening	☐	☐	☐	☐	☐
Head Nodding	☐	☐	☐	☐	☐
Falling Down	☐	☐	☐	☐	☐

2. How fast do you usually fall asleep in the evening?

>40 min 31-40 min 21-30 min 10-20 min <10 min

3. Do you sleep during the day (take naps)?

☐ No need ☐ I wanted but cannot sleep ☐ Twice weekly or less
☐ On 3-5 days weekly ☐ Daily or almost daily

4. Do you fall asleep unintentionally during the day?

	Never	Monthly or less	Weekly	Daily	Several times Daily
Situation					
Reading	☐	☐	☐	☐	☐
Travelling	☐	☐	☐	☐	☐
Standing	☐	☐	☐	☐	☐
Eating	☐	☐	☐	☐	☐
Other Unusual	☐	☐	☐	☐	☐

References

1. Hublin, C., Kaprio, J., Partinen, M., Koskenvuo, M., & Heikkila, K. (1994). The Ullanlinna narcolepsy scale: validation of a measure of symptoms in the narcoleptic syndrome. *Journal of Sleep Research, 3*, 52–59.
2. Wing, Y. K., Li, R. H. Y., Ho, C. K. W., Fong, S. Y. Y., Chow, L. Y., & Leung, T. (2000). A validity study of Ullanlinna narcolepsy scale in Hong Kong Chinese. *Journal of Psychosomatic Research, 49*(5), 355–361.

Representative Studies Using Scale

Hublin, C., Kaprio, J., Partinen, M., Koskenvuo, M., Heikkila, K., Koskimies, S., & Guilleminault, C. (1994). The prevalence of narcolepsy: an epidemiological study of the Finnish twin cohort. *Annals of Neurology, 35*(6), 709–716.

Ervik, S., Abdelnoor, M., Heier, M. S., Ramberg, M., & Strand, G. (2006). Health-related quality of life in narcolepsy. *Acta Neurologica Scandinavica, 114*(3), 198–204.

Verran and Snyder-Halpern Sleep Scale (VSH)

99

Purpose The scale was developed in order to assess the subjective sleep quality of hospitalized individuals – those without preexisting sleep difficulties. The VSH evaluates two domains of sleep experience: disturbance (including sleep latency, mid-sleep awakenings, soundness of sleep, and movement during sleep) and effectiveness (items relating to rest upon awakening, subjective quality of sleep, and total sleep period). Though the VSH was initially an eight-item scale, six additional items were added following psychometric evaluation in order to improve the range of difficulties queried by the scale. The newest version has yet to be validated.

Population for Testing The scale has been validated with a population of individuals with no history of sleep difficulties. Participant ages ranged from 20 to 78 years.

Administration Requiring between 10 and 15 min for completion, the scale is a self-report measure of subjective sleep.

Reliability and Validity A validation study conducted by developers Snyder-Halpern and Verran [1] demonstrated an internal consistency of .82. However, these psychometric properties apply only to the 8-item version of the questionnaire. The 14-item revised version has yet to be evaluated.

Obtaining a Copy An example of the scale's original eight items can be found in an article published by developers [1].

For the full scale, direct correspondence to:
R. Snyder-Halpern
St. Joseph's Hospital Centers
15855 Nineteen Mile Road
Mt. Clemens, MI 48043

Scoring The VSH uses a visual analogue scale examining sleep over the previous three nights. Responses are recorded along a 100 mm line, with 0 indicating that the sleep behavior or quality is not present, and 100 indicating that it is consistently experienced. The locations of the respondent's choices are measured in millimeters, and a global score is obtained by summing these each item score (items pertaining to mid-sleep awakenings, movement during sleep, and sleep latency are reversed before adding). Higher scores indicate better quality of sleep.

A. Shahid et al. (eds.), *STOP, THAT and One Hundred Other Sleep Scales*,
DOI 10.1007/978-1-4419-9893-4_99, © Springer Science+Business Media, LLC 2012

Verran and Snyder-Halpern Sleep Scale (VSH)

Did not awaken——Was awake 10 hours
Had no sleep——Had 10 hours' sleep
No sleep during the day yesterday——Slept 10 hours during the day
Did not sleep yesterday morning——Slept off and on yesterday morning
Did not sleep yesterday evening——Slept off and on yesterday evening
Fell asleep immediately——Did not fall asleep
Slept lightly——Slept deeply
Had no trouble with disrupted sleep——Had a lot of trouble with disrupted sleep
Didn't wake at all——Was awake off and on all night
Had no trouble falling asleep——Had a lot of trouble falling asleep
Didn't move——Tossed all night
Awoke exhausted——Awoke refreshed
After morning awakening, stayed awake——After morning awakening, dozed off and on
Had a bad night's sleep—Had a good night's sleep
Had enough sleep—Did not have enough sleep

Reference

1. Snyder-Halpern, R., & Verran, J. A. (1987). Instrumentation to describe sleep characteristics in health subjects. *Research in Nursing and Health, 10*(3), 155–163.

Representative Studies Using Scale

Higgins, P. A. (1998). Patient perception of fatigue while undergoing long-term mechanical ventilation: incidence and associated factors. *Heart and Lung, 27*(3), 177–183.

Reishtein, J. (2005). Sleep in mechanically ventilated patients. *Critical Care Nursing Clinics of North America, 17*(3), 251–255.

Call-Schmidt, T.A., Richardson, S. J. (2003). Prevalence of sleep disturbance and its relationship to pain in adults with chronic pain. *Pain Management Nursing*, 4(3), 124–33.

Visual Analogue Scale to Evaluate Fatigue Severity (VAS-F)

100

Purpose The scale consists of 18 items relating to the subjective experience of fatigue. Each item asks respondents to place an "X," representing how they currently feel, along a visual analogue line that extends between two extremes (e.g., from "not at all tired" to "extremely tired"). In contrast to discrete, Likert-type scales, the VAS-F places fewer restrictions on the range of responses available to individuals. However, the benefits of a visual analogue scale may be offset by the frequent reluctance of individuals to use the highest and lowest extremes.

Population for Testing The scale has been validated with adults aged 18–55 years.

Administration A self-report, paper-and-pencil measure, the scale requires between 5 and 10 min for completion.

Reliability and Validity Initial psychometric evaluations conducted by Lee and colleagues [1] have demonstrated a high internal reliability ranging from .94 to .96. Concurrent validity has been established with the Stanford Sleepiness Scale and the Profile of Mood States scale. Still, some have criticized the scale as ambiguous, suggesting that it is not sensitive to the distinction between fatigue and sleepiness [2].

Obtaining a Copy A copy can be found in the original article published by developers [1].

Direct correspondence to:
Dr. K.A. Lee
N411Y, Box 0606
Dept. of Family Health Care Nursing,
University of California
San Francisco, CA 94143-0606

Scoring Each line is 100 mm in length – thus, scores fall between 0 and 100. The instrument also possesses two subscales: fatigue (items 1–5 and 11–18) and energy (items 6–10). Though individuals do not require training in order to score the scale, developers are quick to point out that high levels of inter-rater reliability are vital if results are to be correctly interpreted.

A. Shahid et al. (eds.), *STOP, THAT and One Hundred Other Sleep Scales,*
DOI 10.1007/978-1-4419-9893-4_100,

Visual Analogue Scale to Evaluate Fatigue Severity (VAS-F)

ID #_________ Date___________

Time _________a.m. __________p.m.

We are trying to find out about your level of energy before and after your night of sleep. There are 18 items we would like you to respond to. This should take less than 1 minute of your time. Thank you.

DIRECTIONS: You are asked to circle a number on each of the following lines to indicate how you are feeling RIGHT NOW.

For example, suppose you have not eaten since yesterday.
What number would you circle below?

not at all hungry 0 1 2 3 4 5 6 7 8 9 10 extremely hungry

You would probably circle a number closer to the "extremely hungry" end of the line.
This is where I put it:

not at all hungry 0 1 2 3 4 5 6 (8) 9 10 extremely hungry

NOW PLEASE COMPLETE THE FOLLOWING ITEMS:

1. not at all **tired** 0 1 2 3 4 5 6 7 8 9 10 extremely **tired**

2. not at all **sleepy** 0 1 2 3 4 5 6 7 8 9 10 extremely **sleepy**

3. not at all **drowsy** 0 1 2 3 4 5 6 7 8 9 10 extremely **drowsy**

4. not at all **fatigued** 0 1 2 3 4 5 6 7 8 9 10 extremely **fatigued**

5. not at all **worn out** 0 1 2 3 4 5 6 7 8 9 10 extremely **worn out**

6. not at all **energetic** 0 1 2 3 4 5 6 7 8 9 10 extremely **energetic**

7. not at all **active** 0 1 2 3 4 5 6 7 8 9 10 extremely **active**

8. not at all **vigorous** 0 1 2 3 4 5 6 7 8 9 10 extremely **vigorous**

9.	not at all **efficient**	0	1	2	3	4	5	6	7	8	9	10	extremely **efficient**
10.	not at all **lively**	0	1	2	3	4	5	6	7	8	9	10	extremely **lively**
11.	not at all **bushed**	0	1	2	3	4	5	6	7	8	9	10	totally **bushed**
12.	not at all **exhausted**	0	1	2	3	4	5	6	7	8	9	10	totally **exhausted**
13.	**keeping my eyes open** is no effort at all	0	1	2	3	4	5	6	7	8	9	10	**keeping my eyes open** is a tremendous chore
14.	**moving my body** is no effort at all	0	1	2	3	4	5	6	7	8	9	10	**moving my body** is a tremendous chore
15.	**concentrating** is no effort at all	0	1	2	3	4	5	6	7	8	9	10	**concentrating** is a tremendous chore
16.	**carrying on a conversation** is no effort at all	0	1	2	3	4	5	6	7	8	9	10	**carrying on a conversation** is a tremendous chore
17.	I have absolutely **no desire to close my eyes**	0	1	2	3	4	5	6	7	8	9	10	I have a tremendous **desire to close my eyes**
18.	I have absolutely **no desire to lie down**	0	1	2	3	4	5	6	7	8	9	10	I have a tremendous **desire to lie down**

References

1. Lee, K. A., Hicks, G., & Nino-Murcia, G. (1991). Validity and reliability of a scale to assess fatigue. *Psychiatry Research, 36*, 291–298.
2. LaChappelle, D. L. & Finlayson, M. A. J. (1998). An evaluation of subjective and objective measures of fatigue in patients with brain injury and healthy controls. *Brain Injury, 12*(8), 649–659.

Representative Studies Using Scale

None.

Women's Health Initiative Insomnia Rating Scale (WHIIRS) 101

Purpose A brief, five-item scale evaluating insomnia symptoms, the WHIIRS was developed as part of a larger study investigating a range of health issues affecting postmenopausal women. The scale requires individuals to rate the quality of their sleep and the frequency with which they experience certain sleep problems, providing a total score that may be useful for both research and clinical purposes.

Population for Testing The scale has been validated with a large sample of women aged 50–70 years.

Administration Requiring between 3 and 5 min for completion, the scale is a self-report measure completed in a pencil-and-paper format.

Reliability and Validity An initial evaluation of the scale's psychometric properties [1,2] found an internal consistency ranging from .70 to .85 and a same-day test-retest reliability of .96.

Obtaining a Copy A copy is included in a study published by Levine and colleagues [1,2].

Direct correspondence to:
Douglas W. Levine
Section on Social Sciences and Health Policy
Department of Public Health and Sciences
Wake Forest University School of Medicine
Winston-Salem, North Carolina 27157
Email: dlevine@wfubmc.edu

Scoring Questions one through four are answered using a five-point, Likert-type scale (0 means that the problem has not been experienced in the past 4 weeks, while four denotes a problem that occurs at least five times a week). Respondents indicate how often they have experienced certain sleep difficulties over the past month, with higher scores denoting higher frequencies. Question five asks individuals to rate the quality of their sleep on a typical night. Total scores will fall between 0 and 20. Though no specific cutoff has been recommended, Levine and colleagues suggest that a .5 a standard deviation difference in mean scores on the WHIIRS between two treatment groups may indicate a significant difference.

A. Shahid et al. (eds.), *STOP, THAT and One Hundred Other Sleep Scales*,
DOI 10.1007/978-1-4419-9893-4_101, © Springer Science+Business Media, LLC 2012

Women's Health Initiative Insomnia Rating Scale

These questions ask about your sleep habits. Please mark one of the answers for each of the following questions. Pick the answer that best describes how often you experienced the situation in the past 4 weeks.

	No, not in past 4 weeks	Yes, less than once a week	Yes, 1 or 2 times a week	Yes, 3 or 4 times a week	Yes, 5 or more times a week
1. Did you have trouble falling asleep?	1	1	2	3	4
2. Did you wake up several times at night?	0	1	2	3	4
3. Did you wake up earlier than you planned to?	0	1	2	3	4
4. Did you have trouble getting back to sleep after you woke up too early?	0	1	2	3	4

5. Overall, was your typical night's sleep during the past 4 weeks:

Very sound or restful	Sound or restless	Average quality	Restless	Very restless
0	1	2	3	4

References

1. Levine, D. W., Kripke, D. F., Kaplan, R. M., & Lewis, M. A. (2003). Reliability and validity of the women's health initiative insomnia scale. *Psychological Assessment, 15*(2), 137–148.
2. Levine, D. W., Kripke, D. F., Kaplan, R. M., & Lewis, M. A. (2003). Reliability and validity of the women's health initiative insomnia scale. *Psychological Assessment, 15*(2), 123–136.

Representative Studies Using Scale

Brunner, R. L., Gass, M., Aragaki, A., Hays, J., Granek, I., Woods, N., Mason, E., Brzyski, R. G., Ockene, J. K., Assaf, A. R., LaCroix, A. Z., Matthews, K., & Wallace, R. B. (2005). Effects of conjugated equine estrogen on health-related quality of life in postmenopausal women with hysterectomy. *Archives of Internal Medicine, 165*(17), 1976–1986.

102 ZOGIM-A (Alertness Questionnaire)

Purpose Consisting of ten items, the ZOGIM-A was created as an efficient and inexpensive alternative to laboratory measures such as the Maintenance of Wakefulness Test (MWT). The scale evaluates a respondent's experiences with alertness over the course of the day, querying the subjective impact of environmental factors (e.g., caffeine, exercise), the anticipated benefits of increased energy levels, and the perceived proportion of the day spent at high levels of alertness. Just as the Epworth Sleepiness Scale (Chap. 29) acts as a complementary measure to the Multiple Sleep Latency Test rather than a pure facsimile, the ZOGIM-A functions well in conjunction with the THAT (Chap. 96), which measures a different facet of alertness.

Population for Testing The scale has been validated with a sample of patients referred to a sleep clinic for evaluation whose mean age was 42 ± 14.

Administration The scale is self-administered using paper and pencil requiring approximately 5 min for completion.

Reliability and Validity Shapiro and colleagues [1] evaluated the scale's psychometric properties and found an internal consistency ranging from .93 to .95 and a test-retest reliability of .68. Additionally, scores on the ZOGIM-A differed significantly for patients found to possess narcolepsy.

Obtaining a Copy A copy is included in a study published by Shapiro and colleagues (2006).

Direct correspondence to:
Colin M. Shapiro
MP7 # 421, Toronto Western Hospital
399 Bathurst Street
Toronto, ON, Canada M5T 2S8

Scoring ZOGIM-A items are scored using a five-point, Likert-type scale ranging from 1 ("extremely") to 5 ("not at all"). Summing the scores obtained on each item provides a global index – lower scores denote impaired alertness while higher scores indicate high alertness.

A. Shahid et al. (eds.), *STOP, THAT and One Hundred Other Sleep Scales*,
DOI 10.1007/978-1-4419-9893-4_102, © Springer Science+Business Media, LLC 2012

ZOGIM-A

This brief questionnaire deals with your level of alertness. Use the following scale to check one response for each question.

Alertness can be affected by different experiences. How might your alertness be affected by each of the following?	Not at all 5	Slightly 4	Moderately 3	Largely 2	Extremely 1
a. Losing about 30 min of nighttime sleep.					
b. Doing about 30 min of exercise.					
c. Not drinking coffee or other foods that contain caffeine.					
d. Taking a 1-week vacation.					
e. Forgetting about your worries.					
If you were more alert	Not at all 5	Slightly 4	Moderately 3	Largely 2	Extremely 1
a. Would you be able to organize your day-to-day activities more effectively?					
b. Would you be able to complete your tasks more methodically?					
c. Would your new ideas occur to you more readily?					
d. Would you make fewer careless mistakes?					
e. What proportion of the day do you feel a high level of alertness?	5 90-100%	4 50-90%	3 10-15%	2 0-15%	1 0%

Reference

1. Shapiro, C. M., Auch, C., Reimer, M., Kayumov, L., Heslegrave, R., Huterer, N., Driver, H., & Devins, G. M. (2006). A new approach to the construct of alertness. *Journal of Psychosomatic Research, 60*(6), 595–603.

Representative Studies Using Scale

Hossain, N., Irvine, J., Ritvo, P., Driver, H. S., & Shapiro, C. M. (2007). Evaluation and treatment of sleep complaints: patients' subjective responses. *Psychotherapy and Psychosomatics, 76*(6), 395–399.

Kayumov, L., Brown, G., Jindal, R., Buttoo, K., & Shapiro, C. M. (2001). A randomized, double-blind, placebo-controlled crossover study of the effect of exogenous melatonin on delayed sleep phase syndrome. *Psychosomatic Medicine, 63*, 40–48.

Appendix

The enclosed set of 12 short questionnaires will give most clinics a quick overview of the sleep issues of most patients. If you would like to have the scoring sheets for these scales, please contact us and we will be pleased to send them to you.

1. The Epworth Sleepiness Scale (ESS), a widely used measure of sleepiness
2. The Fatigue Severity Scale, a widely used measure of fatigue
3. The Toronto Hospital Alertness scale (THAT), an easy-to-use measure of alertness
4. Owl Lark Self-Test, helps assess body clock rhythm
5. Athens Insomnia Scale, to quickly assess features of insomnia
6. STOP BANG, easy-to-use inquiry regarding sleep apnea
7. The Restless legs questionnaire helps to detect Restless Legs syndrome and the
8. CAGE – a quick screening measure for alcohol dependence
9. CES-D, screen for mood-related problems which is common in patients with sleep disorders
10. Zung Anxiety scale
11. Illness intrusiveness scale
12. FACES adjective checklist

A. Shahid et al. (eds.), *STOP, THAT and One Hundred Other Sleep Scales*,
DOI 10.1007/978-1-4419-9893-4, © Springer Science+Business Media, LLC 2012

Epworth Sleepiness Scale

Name: ______________________________ Today's date: ____________

Your age (Yrs): __________ Your sex (Male = M, Female = F): ______

How likely are you to doze off or fall asleep in the following situations, in contrast to feeling just tired?

This refers to your usual way of life in recent times.

Even if you haven't done some of these things recently try to work out how they would have affected you.

Use the following scale to choose the **most appropriate number** for each situation:

0 = would **never** doze
1 = **slight chance** of dozing
2 = **moderate chance** of dozing
3 = **high chance** of dozing

It is important that you answer each question as best you can.

Situation	Chance of Dozing (0-3)
Sitting and reading ____________	___
Watching TV ____________	___
Sitting, inactive in a public place (e.g. a theatre or a meeting) ____	___
As a passenger in a car for an hour without a break ______	___
Lying down to rest in the afternoon when circumstances permit ____	___
Sitting and talking to someone __________	___
Sitting quietly after a lunch without alcohol ______	___
In a car, while stopped for a few minutes in the traffic ______	

THANK YOU FOR YOUR COOPERATION

© M.W. Johns 1990-97

FATIGUE SEVERITY SCALE

During the past week, I have found that:	Strongly Disagree			Neither Agree Nor Disagree			Strongly Agree
1. My motivation is lower when I am fatigued.	1	2	3	4	5	6	7
2. Exercise brings on my fatigue.	1	2	3	4	5	6	7
3. I am easily fatigued.	1	2	3	4	5	6	7
4. Fatigue interferes with my physical functioning.	1	2	3	4	5	6	7
5. Fatigue causes frequent problems for me.	1	2	3	4	5	6	7
6. My fatigue prevents sustained physical functioning.	1	2	3	4	5	6	7
7. Fatigue interferes with carrying out certain duties and responsibilities.	1	2	3	4	5	6	7
8. Fatigue is among my three most disabling symptoms.	1	2	3	4	5	6	7
8. Fatigue interferes with my work, family, or social life.	1	2	3	4	5	6	7

TORONTO HOSPITAL ALERTNESS TEST (THAT)

This questionnaire tries to establish how alert you feel. In reporting your feeling, we would like you to consider your last week. Use the following scale to check one response for each question.

During the last week I felt:	Not at all	Less than ¼ of the time	¼ to ½ of the time	½ to ¾ of the time	More than ¾ of the time	All the time I was awake
	0	1	2	3	4	5
1. Able to concentrate						
2. Alert						
3. Fresh						
4. Energetic						
5. Able to think of new ideas						
6. Vision was clear noting all details (e.g. driving)						
7. Able to focus on the task at hand						
8. Mental facilities were operating at peak level						
9. Extra effort was needed to maintain alertness						
10. In a boring situation, I would find my mind wandering						

THE OWL LARK SELF-TEST

With these last 19 questions do your best. Select one answer that makes the most sense to you.

1. Considering only you own "feeling best" rhythm, at what time would you get up if you were entirely free to plan your day? (Choose time period by circling 5, 4, 3, 2 or 1)

5	4	3	2	1
5 am noon – 6.30 am	6.30 am – 7.45 am	7.45 am – 9.45 am	9.45 am – 11.00 am	11.00 am – 12 noon

2. Considering only you own "feeling best" rhythm, at what time would you go to bed if you were entirely free to plan your evening(Choose time period by circling 5, 4, 3, 2 or 1)

5	4	3	2	1
6 pm – 9 pm	9 pm – 10.15 pm	10.15 pm – 12.30 am	12.30 am – 1.45 am	1.45 am – 3 pm

3. If there is a specific time at which you have to get up in the morning, to what extent are you dependent on being woken up by an alarm clock?
   - Not at all dependent ☐4
   - Slightly dependent ☐3
   - Fairly dependent ☐2
   - Very dependent ☐1

4. Assuming adequate environmental conditions, how easy do you find getting up in the morning?
   - Not at all easy ☐1
   - Not very easy ☐2
   - Fairly easy ☐3
   - Very easy ☐4

5. How alert do you feel during the first half hour after having woken in the mornings?
   - Not at all alert ☐1
   - Slightly alert ☐2
   - Fairly alert ☐3
   - Very alert ☐4

6. How is your appetite during the first half hour after having woken in the mornings?
   - Very poor ☐1
   - Fairly poor ☐2
   - Fairly good ☐3
   - Very good ☐4

7. During the first half hour after having woken in the morning, how tired do you feel?
   - Very tired ☐1
   - Fairly tired ☐2
   - Fairly refreshed ☐3
   - Very refreshed ☐4

8. When you have no commitments the next day, at what time do you go to bed compared to your usual bedtime?
   - Seldom or never later ☐4
   - Less than one hour later ☐3
   - 1-2 hours later ☐2
   - More than tow hours later ☐1

9. You have decided to engage in some physical exercise. A friend suggests that you do this one hour twice a week and the best time for him is between 7:00 – 8:00 am. Bearing in mind nothing else but you own "feeling best" rhythm, how do you think you would perform?
   - Would you be in good form ☐4
   - Would be in reasonable form ☐3
   - Would find it difficult ☐2
   - Would find it very difficult ☐1

10. At what time in the evening do you feel tired and as a result in need of sleep?

5	4	3	2	1
8 pm – 9 pm	9 pm – 10.15 pm	10.15 pm – 12.45 am	12.45 am – 2 am	2 am – 3 am

11. You wish to be at your peak performance for a test which you know is going to be mentally exhausting and lasting for two hours. You are entirely free to plan your day and considering only your own "feeling best" rhythm, which ONE of the four testing times would you choose?
    - 8:00 – 10:00 am ☐6
    - 11:00 am –1:00 pm ☐4
    - 3:00 pm – 5:00 pm ☐2
    - 7:00 – 9:00 pm ☐0

12. If you went to bed at 11:00 pm, at what level of tiredness would you be?
    - Not at all tired ☐0
    - A little tired ☐2
    - Fairly tired ☐3
    - Very tired

14. One night you have to remain awake between 4– 6:00 am in order to carry out a night watch. You have no commitments the next day. Which ONE of the following alternatives will suit you best?
    - Would NOT go to bed until watch was over ☐1
    - Would take a nap before and sleep after ☐2
    - Would take a good sleep before and nap after ☐3
    - Would take ALL sleep before watch ☐4

15. You have to do two hours of hard physical work. You are entirely free to plan your day and consider only your own "feeling best" rhythm, which ONE of the following times would you choose?
    - 8:00 am – 10:00 am ☐4
    - 11:00 am – 1:00 pm ☐3
    - 3:00 pm – 5:00 pm ☐2
    - 7:00 pm – 9:00 pm ☐1

13. For some reason you have gone to bed several hours later than usual, but there is no need to get up at any particular time the next morning. Which ONE of the following events are you most likely to experience?

☐4 Will wake up at usual time and will NOT fall asleep again
☐3 Will wake up at usual time and will dose thereafter
☐2 Will wake up at usual time but will fall sleep again
☐1 Will NOT wake up until later than usual

16. You have decided to engage in hard physical exercise. A friend suggests that you do this for one hour twice a week and the best time for him is between 10:00 – 11:00 pm. Bearing in mind nothing else but your own "feeling best" rhythm, how well do you think you would perform?

Would you be in good form	☐1
Would be in reasonable form	☐2
Would find it difficult	☐3
Would find it very difficult	☐4

17. Suppose that you can choose your own work hours. Assume that you worked a FIVE-hour day (with breaks) and that you job was interesting and paid by results. Which five consecutive hours would you select?

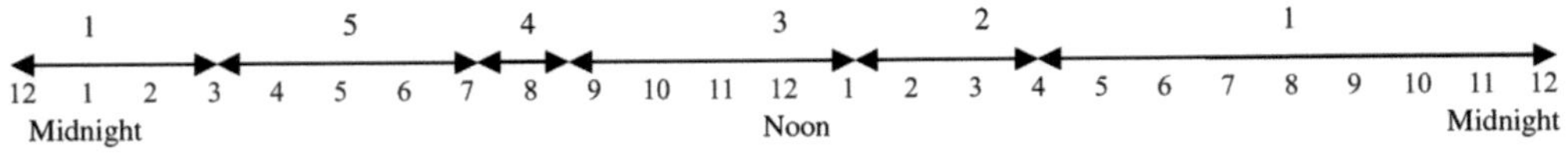

18. At what time of the day do you think that you reach your "feeling best" peak?

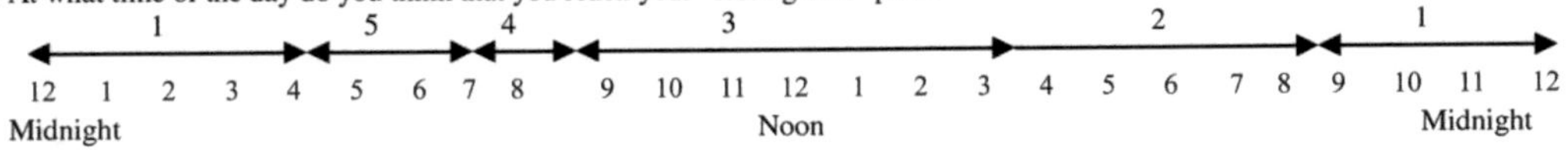

19. One hears about "morning" and "evening" types of people. Which ONE of these types do you consider your self to be?

Definitely a "morning" type?	☐6
Rather than a "morning" than an "evening" type	☐4
Rather more an "evening" than a "morning" type	☐2
Definitely an "evening" type	☐0

ATHENS INSOMNIA SCALE

This scale is intended to record your own assessment of any sleep difficulty you might have experienced. Please, check (by circling the appropriate number) the items below to indicate your estimate of any difficulty, provided that it occurred at least three times per week during the last month.

3. Sleep induction (time it takes you to fall asleep after turning-off the lights)

0: No problem	1: Slightly delayed	2: Markedly delayed	3: Very delayed or did not sleep at all

4. Awakenings during the night

0: No problem	1: Minor problem	2:Considerable problem	3: Serious problem or did not sleep at all

5. Final awakening earlier than desired

0: Not earlier	1: A little earlier	2: Markedly earlier	3: Much earlier or did not sleep at all

6. Total sleep duration

0: Sufficient	1:Slightly insufficient	2:Markedly insufficient	3: Very insufficient or did not sleep at all

7. Overall quality of sleep (no matter how long you slept)

0: Satisfactory	1:Slightly unsatisfactory	2: Markedly unsatisfactory	3: Very unsatisfactory or did not sleep at all

8. Sense of well-being during the day

0: Normal	1:Slightly decreased	2: Markedly decreased	3: Very decreased

9. Functioning (physical and mental) during the day

0: Normal	1:Slightly decreased	2: Markedly decreased	3: Very decreased

10. Sleepiness during the day

0: None	1: Mild	2: Considerable	3: Intense

STOP-BANG

STOP

Do you **S**nore?	Yes ❑	No ❑
Do you feel **T**ired, fatigued or sleepy during the day?	Yes ❑	No ❑
Has anyone **O**bserved you stop breathing in your sleep?	Yes ❑	No ❑
Do you have high blood **P**ressure ?	Yes ❑	No ❑

Please count the number of "Yes" responses and put the number in this box ❑

	B	**A**	**N**	**G**
	BMI	Age	Neck Size	Gender
	>35	>50 y	> 40cm > 15.7"	- Male
See pg. B		F	B	F

If height is	4'10"	5'0"	5'2"	5'4"	5'6"	5'8"	5'10"	6'0"	6'2"	6'4"
& weight is >	167	179	191	204	216	230	250	258	272	287

Then BMI is > 35

RLS QUESTIONNAIRE

Please, answer the following questions according to your best knowledge! Where you can choose between **Yes** or **No,** circle the appropriate.

1. Does it happen or did it happen earlier that you experienced recurrent unpleasant sensation or tingling in your legs, while sitting or laying down? .... **Yes / No**

   If **Yes,** how would you describe this sensation? (circle one):

   a. painful **b. unpleasant** **c. both painful and unpleasant**

2. Does it happen or did it happen earlier that you repeatedly felt an urge to move your legs while sitting or laying down?... **Yes /No**

   If yes, do you need move your whole body not only your legs?..**Yes / No**

   THIS FEELING, THAT YOU HAVE TO MOVE, IS SOMETIMES SO PRESSING THAT YOU CAN NOT RESIST IT… YES / NO

   OR YOU JUT SIMPLY HAVE TO MOVE YOUR ARMS OR LEGS?... YES / NO

3. Do your legs jump or move a lot involuntarily while sitting or laying down?...**Yes / No**

   If **yes**, do you think that the sensations in your legs and the movements are connected?.....**Yes/ No**

   If **yes**, how often do these involuntary movements occur (circle only one answer):

   seldom **occasionally** **frequently** **almost always**

   Do these involuntary movements occur only before you fall asleep?...................................**Yes/ No**

4. Do you feel, or did you feel earlier that there are recurrent periods when you are so *itchy, you can not stay in one place* or you have to move your arms or legs?... **Yes /No**

Continue to answer the following questions **only** if you answered **yes** to at least one of the previous questions. If you answered **no** to all of the above questions, please go to the next page.

5. When these sensations or movements occur, are they worse while you have a rest (while sitting or laying down) than during physical activities?.. **Yes / No**

6. If these sensations or movements are present and you get up walking, are they improving or do they disappear while you are walking? Please, try to remember, that you may have observed that these sensations or movements are getting worse again when you stop walking, but they are less cumbersome while you are walking?..**Yes/ No / Don't Know**

Continue to answer the following questions only if you answered **yes** to both of the last two questions. If you answered no to question 5 or 6, please go to the next page.

7. If these sensations or movements are present are they gettng worse in the evening or during the night?.**Yes / No**

8. Not NOW, but when these sensations or movements have started, and perhaps they were not as bad as they are now, were these sensations or movements getting worse in the evening or during the night?...............**Yes/ No**

CAGE

It is an instrument used to screen for alcoholism.

Two 'yes' response indicates that the client should be investigated further.

1 Have you ever felt you needed to **Cut** down on your drinking?

2 Have people **Annoyed** you by criticizing your drinking ?

3 Have you ever felt **Guilty** about drinking ?

4 Have you ever felt you needed a drink first thing in the morning (**E**ye –opener) to steady your nerves or to get rid of a hangover?

CENTER FOR EPIDEMIOLOGIC STUDIES DEPRESSION (20)

Below is a list of the ways you might have felt or behaved. Please indicate how often you have felt this way DURING THE PAST WEEK.

0 = Rarely or None of the Time (Less than 1 Day)
1 = Some or a Little of the Time (1 - 2 Days)
2 = Occasionally or a Moderate Amount of Time (3 - 4 Days)
3 = Most or All of the Time (5 - 7 Days)

	DURING THE PAST WEEK:	Rarely/ None	Some/ A Little	Occasionally/ Moderately	Most/ All
1.	I was bothered by things that usually don't bother me .	0	1	2	3
2.	I did not feel like eating; my appetite was poor.	0	1	2	3
3.	I felt that I could not shake off the blues even with help from my family or friends.	0	1	2	3
4.	I felt that I was just as good as other people	0	1	2	3
5.	I had trouble keeping my mind on what I was doing.	0	1	2	3
6.	I felt depressed.	0	1	2	3
1.	I felt that everything I did was an effort.	0	1	2	3
2.	I felt hopeful about the future.	0	1	2	3
3.	I thought my life had been a failure.	0	1	2	3
4.	I felt fearful.	0	1	2	3
5.	My sleep was restless.	0	1	2	3
6.	I was happy.	0	1	2	3
13.	I talked less than usual.	0	1	2	3
14.	I felt lonely.	0	1	2	3
15.	People were unfriendly.	0	1	2	3
16.	I enjoyed life	0	1	2	3
17.	I had crying spells.	0	1	2	3
18.	I felt sad.	0	1	2	3
19.	I felt that people disliked me.	0	1	2	3
20.	I could not get "going".	0	1	2	3

ZUNG ANXIETY

HOW OFTEN HAS EACH OF THE FOLLOWING STATEMENTS APPLIED TO YOU DURING THE PAST 2 WEEKS.

1 = NONE OR A LITTLE OF THE TIME 3 = GOOD PART OF THE TIME
2 = SOME OF THE TIME 4 = MOST, OR ALL, OF THE TIME

	NONE			MOST
1. I feel more nervous and anxious than usual	1	2	3	4
2. I feel afraid for no reason at all	1	2	3	4
3. I get upset easily or feel panicky	1	2	3	4
4. I feel like I'm falling apart and going to pieces	1	2	3	4
5. I feel that everything is all right and nothing bad will happen	1	2	3	4
6. My arms and legs shake and tremble	1	2	3	4
7. I am bothered by headaches, neck and back pains	1	2	3	4
8. I feel weak and get tired easily	1	2	3	4
9. I feel calm and can sit still easily	1	2	3	4
10. I can feel my heart beating fast	1	2	3	4
11. I am bothered by dizzy spells	1	2	3	4
12. I have fainting spells or feel like fainting	1	2	3	4
13. I can breathe in and out easily	1	2	3	4
14. I get feelings of numbness and tingling in my fingers and toes	1	2	3	4
15. I am bothered by stomach aches or indigestion	1	2	3	4
16. I have to empty my bladder often	1	2	3	4
17. My hands are usually dry and warm	1	2	3	4
18. My face gets hot and blushes	1	2	3	4
19. I fall asleep easily and get a good night's rest	1	2	3	4
20. I have nightmares	1	2	3	4

ILLNESS INTRUSIVENESS RATING SCALE

Please circle the one number that best describes your current life situation. If an item is not applicable, please circle the number (1) to indicate that this aspect of your life is not affected very much. Please do not leave any items unanswered.

HOW MUCH DOES YOUR SLEEP PROBLEM AND/OR ITS TREATMENT INTERFERE WITH YOUR:

	Not very much						Very much
1. Health	1	2	3	4	5	6	7
2. Diet	1	2	3	4	5	6	7
3. Work	1	2	3	4	5	6	7
4. Active Recreation (e.g., sports)	1	2	3	4	5	6	7
5. Passive Recreation (e.g., reading, listening to music)	1	2	3	4	5	6	7
6. Financial Situation	1	2	3	4	5	6	7
7. Relationship With Your Partner	1	2	3	4	5	6	7
8. Sex Life	1	2	3	4	5	6	7
9. Family Relations	1	2	3	4	5	6	7
10. Other Social Relations	1	2	3	4	5	6	7
11. Self-Expression/Self-Improvement	1	2	3	4	5	6	7
12. Religious Expression	1	2	3	4	5	6	7
13. Community and Civic Involvement	1	2	3	4	5	6	7

FACES ADJECTIVE CHECKLIST

Below is a list of words that describe feelings people have. Please read each one carefully. Then circle the ONE number corresponding to the adjective phrase that best describes **HOW YOU HAVE BEEN FEELING DURING THE PAST WEEK INCLUDING TODAY**. If you are unfamiliar with any of the words, please circle the question mark (?) to the right of the rating scale. The numbers refer to the following descriptive phrases:

1.	Fatigued	0	1	2	3	4	?	26.	Comatose	0	1	2	3	4	?
2.	Worn-out	0	1	2	3	4	?	27.	Unconscious	0	1	2	3	4	?
3.	Exhausted	0	1	2	3	4	?	28.	Dormant	0	1	2	3	4	?
4.	Wacked-out	0	1	2	3	4	?	29.	Bombed	0	1	2	3	4	?
5.	Drained	0	1	2	3	4	?	30.	Blurry-eyed	0	1	2	3	4	?
6.	Pooped	0	1	2	3	4	?	31.	Vigorous	0	1	2	3	4	?
7.	Overtired	0	1	2	3	4	?	32.	Full of pep	0	1	2	3	4	?
8.	Weary	0	1	2	3	4	?	33.	Lively	0	1	2	3	4	?
9.	Tired	0	1	2	3	4	?	34.	Charged-up	0	1	2	3	4	?
10.	Spent	0	1	2	3	4	?	35.	Wide-eyed	0	1	2	3	4	?
11.	Bushed	0	1	2	3	4	?	36.	Energetic	0	1	2	3	4	?
12.	Out of Steam	0	1	2	3	4	?	37.	Carefree	0	1	2	3	4	?
13.	Frazzled	0	1	2	3	4	?	38.	Active	0	1	2	3	4	?
14.	Limited Endurance	0	1	2	3	4	?	39.	Cheerful	0	1	2	3	4	?
15.	Achy Muscles	0	1	2	3	4	?	40.	Alert	0	1	2	3	4	?
16.	Indolent	0	1	2	3	4	?	41.	Snoozy	0	1	2	3	4	?
17.	Languid	0	1	2	3	4	?	42.	Sleepy	0	1	2	3	4	?
18.	Soporific	0	1	2	3	4	?	43.	Drowsy	0	1	2	3	4	?
19.	Lassitude	0	1	2	3	4	?	44.	Slumber	0	1	2	3	4	?
20.	Supine	0	1	2	3	4	?	45.	Heavy-eyed	0	1	2	3	4	?
21.	Accidie	0	1	2	3	4	?	46.	Half-Awake	0	1	2	3	4	?
22.	Phlegmatic	0	1	2	3	4	?	47.	Sluggish	0	1	2	3	4	?
23.	Line of Least Resistance	0	1	2	3	4	?	48.	Yawning	0	1	2	3	4	?
24.	Jaded	0	1	2	3	4	?	49.	Dozy	0	1	2	3	4	?
25.	Apathetic	0	1	2	3	4	?	50.	Somnambulant	0	1	2	3	4	?

Index

A. Shahid et al. (eds.), *STOP, THAT and One Hundred Other Sleep Scales*,
DOI 10.1007/978-1-4419-9893-4, © Springer Science+Business Media, LLC 2012

S

T

U

V

W

Z

MIX
Papier aus verantwortungsvollen Quellen
Paper from responsible sources
FSC® C105338

If you have any concerns about our products, you can contact us on
ProductSafety@springernature.com

In case Publisher is established outside the EU, the EU authorized representative is:
Springer Nature Customer Service Center GmbH
Europaplatz 3, 69115 Heidelberg, Germany

Printed by Libri Plureos GmbH
in Hamburg, Germany